Family Secrets

Family Secrets

Risking Reproduction

in Central Mozambique

Rachel R. Chapman

Vanderbilt University Press ■ Nashville

© 2010 by Vanderbilt University Press
Nashville, Tennessee 37235
All rights reserved
First printing 2010

This book is printed on acid-free paper made from fiber that
meets the requirements of the independent Sustainable Forestry
Initiative program, ensuring that it comes from a responsibly
managed North American forest. *www.sfiprogram.org*
Manufactured in the United States of America

Library of Congress Cataloging-in-Publication Data

Chapman, Rachel Rebekah, 1961–
Family secrets : risking reproduction in central
Mozambique / Rachel R. Chapman.
p. ; cm.
Includes bibliographical references and index.
ISBN 978-0-8265-1717-3 (cloth ed. : alk. paper)
ISBN 978-0-8265-1718-0 (pbk. ed. : alk. paper)
1. Maternal health services—Utilization—Mozambique.
2. Health behavior—Mozambique. 3. Pregnant women—
Mozambique. I. Title.
[DNLM: 1. Maternal Health Services—utilization—
Mozambique. 2. Anthropology, Cultural—Mozambique.
3. Social Conditions—Mozambique. 4. Women's Rights—
Mozambique. WA 310 HM7 C466f 2010]
RG966.M85C53 2010
362.19'82009679—dc22
2010020350

For my mothers and fathers
brothers and sisters
Solea and James

In memory of George Povey

Contents

Acknowledgments

Graça Machel opened my eyes to the human costs of the right-wing insurgency that our government supported in Mozambique and moved me to commit to practical and socially conscious work there. Prexy Nesbitt, Steve Gloyd, Kathy Sheldon, and Steve Tarcynski connected me to the Mozambique Support Network and helped build the bridge I crossed to the country. James Pfeiffer's true partnership gave me the courage to make it happen. Without these people this book would not exist. Thank you all.

Javelina Aguiar, my wise teacher and research partner, opened the path to Mucessua, made me part of her family, and mothered my first pregnancy. I am forever indebted to her. I am also indebted to the Mucessua party structure, especially the Mozambican Women's Organization (OMM) and the late Sr. Jaime Taunga, first bairro secretary. I thank the people of Mucessua, especially the women who shared their homes and stories. The preventable loss of so many lives and the continued hardships for all those left behind keep me focused.

I thank the Manica Province and Gondola District Health Directorates, especially my counterpart, Sr. Davissone, who introduced me to the people and land of Manica; Florencia Floriano, the provincial director of maternal and child health; the late Sr. Machobo, provincial director of the Manica Community Health Department; provincial epidemiologist Dr. Jim Black; Gondola District directors Sr. Manuel and Sr. Carmagira; Nurse Mentira and Sister Shika at the Gondola maternity ward; and the Gondola Community Health director, Sr. Maguaze.

The administrative, logistical, and program teams of Mozambique Health Committee were invaluable in their support. I thank Nancy Ibrahimo, Moises Metuque, Isaias Sitoe, and Susana Knip in the Chimoio office; my Mozambique Health Committee colleagues Lucy Ramirez, Yves Lafort, Claire Metraud, Jorine Muiser, and Kathy Hubenet; and Diana McCleod, Peggy Reihle, the late George Povey, Tatiana, and Lisa in Seattle headquarters. Srs. Traquino, Mario, Fernando, Machado, and Madeira provided transport and keen commentary on whatever was the subject of the day. In Maputo, thanks to Dr. Julie Cliff, Kery Sylvester, Isabel Casamira, and Ana Laforte at the University of Eduardo Mondlane and Anamarie Jurg and Tomas Taju at the

Ministry of Health. I thank my mentor and National Institutes of Health MIRT field advisor Dra. Rosa Marlene Manjate Liquela, previously national director of the Mozambique National STD/HIV/AIDS Control Program.

I thank Claudia Mitchell-Kernan, Karen Brodkin Sacks, Susan Scrimshaw, Carole Browner, Robert Edgerton, Osman Galal, Edward Alpers, Gail Harrison, and Gery Ryan at UCLA for their expertise and feedback on early iterations of this work. I thank Ann Walters, Joe, Zue, Fredito, Gloria Wekker, Alycee, Ran, Iris and Atalya Boytner, Jane, Keiko, Jill, and Fatimata for support of every kind. Many thanks to Mel Goldstein, Janet McGrath, Atwood Gaines, Sue Hinze, and Rhonda Williams for strong mentorship at Case Western Reserve University; and to Monica, Elysee, Susan, Sue, Gillian, Cynthia, and Stephanie, my Cleveland sister circle.

In Seattle I thank Nancy, Amy, Gitana, Vito, and the five-star staff at Hedgebrook Writing Retreat, as well as Loreen, Nassim, and all my Hedgebrook sisters who are out there "authoring change," for the opportunity to finish the manuscript in a room of my own and with inspiration. At the University of Washington, I thank Simon Ottenberg, Lorna Rhodes, Mimi Kahn, and Stevan Harrell for thoughtful feedback on the prospectus, and Janelle Taylor and Celia Lowe for sharing their manuscripts and experience. Thank you, UW writing women Angela Ginorio, Shirley Yee, Michelle Habell-Pallan, Susan Glenn, Kathy Friedman, and Sonnet Retman. Special thanks to Devon and Elaine Peña for such careful reading and superb guidance, and to Marlaine Figueroa-Grey, my superlative graduate research assistant.

Robbie Davis-Floyd was midwife to this book, and Leith Mullings and Caroline Bledsoe were doulas who said, "Push," at just the right time. Amy Kaler gave expert advice on all things Shona. *Tatenda.* Thank you to two anonymous reviewers for thoughtful critique and great direction. I am so grateful to the timely perfectionism of Christine Duell, my personal editor, and Sally Brown, my generous indexer.

I could not have wished for a better editor than Michael Ames, who believed in this project and made me a better writer. Thank you. Having the gift of Malangatana's artwork grace the cover of the book is the greatest honor I could hope for. *Obrigada.* I dedicate this work to the Mozambique he envisions.

Lastly, I thank my families—my parents—Lois and Paul for finding me, and Marie, rest in peace, and R. for being found. Thank you, Jean Pfeiffer, for giving me a second home and space to do my work. Thank you to my soul kin—Gloria Wekker, Alycee Lane, Ahoua Kone, Barbara Wallace, Ann Evans, Julia Vest, Tammy Elser, Molly Galusha, and, especially, Medria, my spirit guide. Finally, I thank James and Solea for their love and patience. James read this book ten thousand times, and each time gave me courage to keep going and make it better.

Research for this book was also made possible by generous grants from the UCLA Department of Anthropology, the Fogarty Foundation Minority International Research and Training Program (MIRT), and the National Institute of Child Health and Development (NICHD), and by two generous grants from Hedgebrook Writing Retreat.

To Mozambique, thank you, *masvita, ndinotenda, obrigada. A luta continua.*

All births have multiple meanings. The world we are born into determines the range of choices we have, the costs of our decisions, and the fate of our creativity. When we need a specific outcome, we tell and use stories to change the odds, so that whatever we have decided in that moment must survive might have a sliver of a chance to do so.

Family Secrets

CHAPTER 1

Reproduction on the Margins

It is early morning, and patches of mist linger by the roadside. I yawn as I stand in line at the little bakery in the town of Gondola, where I frequently buy loaves of warm bread to eat with Dona Javelina Aguiar, my research assistant, before heading out for a day of work. On these mornings, Javelina's two sons and a flock of cousins and neighbors' children dart in and out of the doorway, mixing play and chores. Neighbor women and female relatives stop by to chat with us and politely nibble slices of bread, the sharp teeth of gossip and restrained daintiness masking grumbling hunger. Slowly, I am becoming a familiar sight. With my car and gifts of food, diapers, and medicine, my connections to the government health care system and foreign doctors, and my pay to research assistants in U.S. dollars, I am a significant resource. Because connection to me is seen as potentially valuable, I am also a cause of dangerous envy among some community members being directed at those closest to me, like Javelina.

As we blow the chill off the mornings with heavily sugared tea, I imagine I fit in, sitting and chewing over the troubles of the day before, and the costs and cures for the ills of the *nova vida*, as many Mozambicans have dubbed the volatile times we are living in at the end of the war of destabilization.[1] *Nova vida* means "new life" in Portuguese, but the phrase is usually brandished in conversations like a winning hand of cards to trump other explanations for bad news, to bemoan rising crime, to complain about not being able to make ends meet, or to describe new imports—technology, fashion, media. However, the phrase is especially useful to expound on the impertinence of youth, especially girls, and the new ways of life associated with the rapacious cities, experienced or imagined, that seduce young people and steal their respect for their elders and elders' ways.

Rushing to get an early start at Javelina's, I scoop up four hand-sized oval loaves, still warm from the brick oven and powdery with flour, and hold them in one arm as I carefully lay my payment of four tattered thousand-*metical* notes on the counter. That is the equivalent of about one day's wages for Javelina's husband, Casimiro, who works as a guard at the Avibela poultry-processing factory up the road.

Suddenly, I hear, "*Faz favor*, please, Mrs.! Mrs.! My sister!" A man's voice is frantically calling, and then someone tugs my sleeve from behind. "Please help me," the man implores. "My wife is giving birth, and we have no transport to the hospital. Please! All my children have been born at the hospital. Could you please come with me?" His face contorts as he tries to catch his breath, and he trembles.

In the few steps between the bakery door and the familiar white four-wheel-drive vehicle that belongs to the nongovernmental health organization I work for, I think I understand that the man's wife has gone into labor at home. "She is quite near, just here below the bakery." He gestures toward Bairro Mucessua, the neighborhood where I am conducting research on prenatal care.[2] "You can get there no problems, my sister. There is no danger," the man promises. The maternity clinic is across the road in the opposite direction, just minutes away by vehicle.

Arranjar (arrange), *desviar* (divert), *colocar* (connect), *confusão* (confusion), and *jeito* (knack) are the handful of Portuguese words that I learned quickly in Mozambique and that eventually helped explain anything going on around me that I could not quite figure out. The man seems earnest enough, but the situation still feels like a *confusão*, a confusing, unclear, and potentially ill-advised *desvia* (diversion) from my morning plan. A bit unsure, I ask the hired driver, "Senhor Mario, can we try?" Used to my frequent detours, Senhor Mario nods and starts the engine. Soon we are turning off the paved Beira Corridor, the main thoroughfare snaking through the town of Vila Gondola on its way from the Zimbabwe border to the west, to the port city of Beira on the Indian Ocean to the east. The truck bumps down a dirt road carved and curved by the wet-season rush of rainwater toward River Mucessua, for which the bairro was named, a polluted brown stream in that early dry-season month of April.

At the foot of a towering breadfruit tree, its exposed gray roots tangling in all directions and digging into the red dust like hundreds of arms and bony fingers, what existed of the road ends. I turn to tell the man that we cannot risk driving any farther, but he has vanished with a slam of the door. He hurtles through backyards, under lines of drying laundry, and finally ducks into a house to the right and below where the truck has stopped on the embankment of bony roots and fine red earth. Senhor Mario kills the engine, and I leap out.

People preparing for their day pause to stare, water dripping from their faces or balls of corn meal hovering halfway to their mouths, as I charge through their backyards after the man, apologizing on the run. At the house where the man stopped, the front courtyard is empty. Many footprints have disturbed the broom designs left in the red earth by the morning sweeping, intended to neaten the yard and to scatter malingering night-traveling spirits. I approach the earth-and-pole construction with clothes drying on its thatched roof of dried reeds alongside scraps of rusted metal, a soda can, and a few chipped, white-enamel-covered tin plates and cups. From behind the house, a woman's voice instructs harshly, "*Faz força! Faz força!*" (Use force! Use force!).

The door opens abruptly, releasing a faint whiff of cooking smoke, and the man steps out with a barefoot girl of twelve or thirteen in a bright green minidress, her eyes cast down, rural-girl demure. "Please, follow this girl behind the house. Could you go? Please!" He pushes me slightly with one shaky hand, sweating now in his gray suit, yellowing white shirt, and shabby but well-shined brown leather shoes. Reluctantly, I allow myself to be led by the girl down a narrow path beside the house and peer around the corner. I have never seen a live birth, except what little I saw of myself giving birth to my daughter seven months earlier in a clinic in Harare, Zimbabwe.

To the side of a small garden of tall corn, a naked woman lies back, propped on her elbows atop an empty relief-aid corn sack. Two older women kneel beside her, one at her hip, the other at her bottom, each holding one of her knees. From the purple skin folds between her legs bulges the crowning head of her baby—swirls of black hair covered in blood and white paste. The girl in peacock green stands a minute in the midst of the rustling green corn, biting her knuckles and looking respectfully off into the distance. Then, with the slightest nod in my direction, she bends forward and retreats into the darkness through the low rear door of the house.

"*Bom dia,*" I call out, and then, "Is she all right? Is everything all right? Hello?" I call louder, stuck to my spot by the corner of the house. The women's serious faces register attentiveness, but not alarm, as if everything might be going normally so far.

"Come and help us, sister," the older of the two birth assistants implores me without looking up.

"It looks as though you are doing fine," I say. "You don't need me. I'll . . . I'll be right here with the car when you need to go to the hospital. That is all I know how to do." I stand limply, almost wringing my hands, never coming out from behind the wall. I do not know how to help, and I feel the naked woman on the ground does not deserve to have a useless stranger staring at her. But considering the pain and concentration twisting her face, I see she is not even aware of our conversation or my presence. I back away, stumbling in my haste back up the little pathway between the mud wall and stalks of corn.

In front of the house, the suited man is dripping sweat as he sits on a tree stump, his head resting in his hands, his cigarette smoking at his forehead.

"Everything seems to be going fine," I report.

"Jesus," he says, more imploring than swearing, and not hearing or not responding to my news. "This is my seventh child. All the others were born in the hospital." Now I hear something like shame pinching his voice at the thought of his wife giving birth on the ground under the sky. He seems proudly *assimilado* (the Portuguese term for Europeanized Mozambicans allowed certain privileges and opportunities within the colonial government structure), a man with city contacts and city ways. I suspect he thinks I am a nun from a local mission maternity clinic, known during the colonial period for being the first facility in the area to offer clinical birth conditions to rural communities for the price of a newborn Catholic. He also seems afraid.

The girl slips quietly out of the house and comes to sit down on a pile of dirt in the front yard, poking at the ground with a stick and stealing sideways looks at me. I leave the father and his trembling cigarette to sit with her.

"Is it your mother back there giving birth?" I ask.

"No. My mother is one of the other ladies, the prophet who cures women who are without a child."

"So, you've seen lots of babies being born before, then?"

"No. But I have heard it happening before—terrible!"

I do not know what else to say, or how much time has gone by. We fall silent.

The man begins to pace, finishes his cigarette, and strides, agitated, over to us. "I have only been away in the city at my second house. The time for the birth had passed, and I was called away from my wife by business in Chimoio [the Provincial capital]"—and perhaps his "around the corner" woman, I am thinking, jaded.[3] "While I was gone, my wife and her sister arranged to come to this prophet to ask for help bringing on the labor. I know what they feared." My assumption was that they feared late birth was the result of sorcery sent by another woman. "Now you see? While the three were praying here, the pains began suddenly, and my wife has been forced to give birth right there where she is. I arrived here looking for her, only to find her already too far. I ran back to town for help and saw your truck there outside the bakery. What could I do? Can't you help her?"

The only health care I personally gave women in the prenatal care study I was conducting was in the form of iron and folic acid supplements supplied by a Peruvian doctor I worked with and, whenever I could purchase them, tubes of tetracycline ointment for rampant pinkeye infections. Nevertheless, it was widely believed in Mucessua that I was helping pregnant women. Many people thought I was a nun from some foreign mission.

As my unease intensifies, it is also becoming clear to me that this birth at the prophet's house may have been planned. It was most likely the man's absence at precisely the expected time of birth that made the woman and her sister choose to go to the prophet and not to the maternity clinic. If they feared that the man had another lover on the scene, the vulnerable pregnant woman would not risk seeing this other woman while on the way to the hospital or in labor, and thus exposing herself to the potentially fatal ceremonial "heat" the other woman might be carrying from sexual relations with this man. This heat from a spouse's lover is considered strong enough to harm and even kill a birthing woman, her newborn, or both. The prophet could provide spiritual protection during the birth from complications like prolonged or obstructed labor that are believed to be the result of sexual infidelity on the part of either partner. Embedded in the man's nervous tirade, I imagine I hear what sounds like a confession.

Before I can respond, from behind the house, the quivering wail of a newborn squeezes tears into my eyes, and the man exhales, it seems for the first time. Being male, he is not welcome behind the low, square house where his wife lies beside a vegetable garden, so I jump up to see how everyone is doing. As I get to my feet, the prophet-healer pushes out her front door, winding a long piece of red thread around one hand. Turning directly outside the doorway, she reaches up into the roof and pulls something from the thatching. As she comes closer I see that the small brown patch in her palm is a rusted razor blade she had stored alongside the dishes, empty can, and drying clothes. "Please wait a minute," I beg her and fly back to the car to get a new razor blade from the medicine kit behind the front seat. I pour out the entire contents of the kit while Senhor Mario leans silent against the truck. Not a single razor blade is left.

I dash once more through the backyards, my speed piquing the neighbors' interest. Skidding down into the prophet's yard and shaking my head, I extend my empty palms to her. Miserable, I follow her wide backside, wrapped in a dark blue traditional cloth over a worn dress, around to the garden behind the house. The mother is now squatting on her heels on the burlap sack where she had been lying. To the side of her right foot lies a pale, purplish baby, eerily quiet on a square of smudged sheet over the red dust. The baby girl is breathing, and vernix covers her skin and hair. All around, the tall corn shivers and whispers in the breeze.

"The other one won't come," says the woman who must be the birthing woman's sister, referring, I soon realize, to the placenta. The crouching mother whimpers, as her sister pushes a dented tin cup to her lips, spilling dark liquid into her mouth and down her chin. Grabbing the cup, the mother downs the contents, grimacing, and slumps heavily onto her hands and knees with a groan.

When my daughter, Solea, was born seven months earlier in a clinic in Harare, Zimbabwe, the two Shona midwives assisting my birth had gently tried to dissuade me from putting her immediately to my breast to nurse. They advised me to have a shower first because I was "dirty" from the birth. By "dirty" they meant unclean not so much from the bodily fluids of my exertion as from the liminal, potentially dangerous journey to motherhood I had just come through. I was "hot" from this sacred and highly charged rite of childbirth and might pass that heat through my milk to my infant, making her sick. Moments later, the Polish obstetrician, who had been attending other patients and missed the entire birth, burst into the delivery room and ordered me to suckle my daughter to help birth the placenta while she kneaded my uterus through my abdomen. The placenta had indeed pushed out promptly, accompanied by breathtaking stabs of pain.

"Sometimes putting the baby to suck at the breast can cause the contractions to come again and push 'the other' out," says a voice that sounds far away, but comes out of my own mouth. All three women stare at me, momentarily frozen, and then return to their coaxing and pushing with renewed vigor, ignoring my unacceptable suggestion. The mother flails, her head lolling.

"Maybe you could try massaging," I dare, remembering the pictures in my worn copy of David Werner's *Where There Is No Doctor* of a woman cupping handfuls of a pregnant woman's belly between her hands like a huge mound of bread dough to stem postpartum hemorrhaging.[4]

"You do it, sister," says the older of the two assisting women. I shake my head, my uselessness making me nauseous. Why, why was I an anthropologist? "I can take you to the maternity clinic," I offer again, wretched. This suggestion sparks the first real panic from the three women, who all move at once. The mother says something and thumps down backward on the corn sack, panting irregularly. As the sister pushes hard into the mother's belly, which seems to recede endlessly, the prophet asks me, "Could you bring the nurse from Koro?" Koro was the local name for a farm run by an English missionary couple fifteen kilometers down the Beira Corridor. They offered primary health services and medicines to anyone who came for them whether or not they could pay the low fees, but asked for work on the mission grounds or fields in return. They were especially known for treating people in what were still, in 1995, called RENAMO zones—areas controlled or largely inhabited by peasants believed to be loyal to antigovernment, RENAMO forces during the war. Even with the ceasefire in 1992, the government was still not delivering health services to these areas. "The maternity clinic is so much closer. I can get you there quickly." "Please, please bring the nurse from the Koro," the prophet said, begging this time.

I sprinted to the truck. They must know some reason why we should not move the woman with the placenta still inside her, I tell myself. I can imagine the women's fears of confronting the nurses at the government clinic with this disaster in progress. Women gossiped that nurses at the district maternity clinic refused to assist a delivery unless a woman brought her filled-out prenatal care card and paid a large cash bribe. I had heard claims that without the payment, the nurses might send you home, leave you to deliver alone, or even kill your infant at birth. The high local rates of neonatal deaths and stillbirths did nothing to quell these suspicions. Three such accusations of infant murder by a nurse at the maternity clinic were brought to the local district-level tribunal between 1995 and 1998, but dismissed.[5] Though an estimated 60 percent or more of all births in the area were home births, all three of these women would certainly be berated for bringing a failed home birth to the hospital. If the woman or newborn died, perhaps the prophet would be blamed and charged with a crime. Yet, in the cover of the small corn patch, word of any deaths would stay hidden in the bairro, a haunting rumor of misfortune, sorcery, and malevolent spirits.

I sympathized with the women's plight, but it would take half an hour to go to the mission and back, with no guarantee of finding anyone there to help. Perhaps the mother was already hemorrhaging. At the truck, I cry, "Senhor Mario, let's go to the maternity ward!" The five-minute careen back up the bumpy path and over the Corridor and five more minutes down another dusty road to the government maternity clinic lands us a world away from the woman and her baby in the corn.

We arrive at the Gondola District maternity clinic, a low, whitewashed structure built during the colonial period as a clinic for African employees of the Mozambique Railway Company that now serves a population of 500,000 people without the benefit of running water. As I enter, a wave of air fetid with urine, sour breast milk, menstrual blood, Dettol antiseptic cleanser, and human waste assaults my nose. The waiting room is packed with waiting pregnant women, women waiting with babies, and children waiting to be weighed and vaccinated. Doubtless some of the infants in that room are making their first appearance at the maternity ward after a home delivery. I knock and, without waiting, push open the door to the examination room, where the two nurses on duty are conducting a prenatal exam. A young woman lies passively on the worn metal examination table with her yellow dress pulled up to her ribs and her underpants at her ankles while the two nurses discuss something unrelated to her.

"*Desculpe* [Forgive me]," I mumble. I was a familiar and welcome colleague who often brought supplies and offered transport when possible. Both nurses smile at me. "Dona Raquel! *Como esta* [How are you?]?" Their faces slam shut, however, as I tell my story. "Could one of you come back with me?"

"*Com çerteza, não* [Certainly not]," Enfermeira Julia snaps. "There are too many other women to attend to here. We cannot simply leave our post because someone is too lazy to come here, and prefers to give birth in the street."[6]

"Besides, what would happen if the woman dies out there where we have no materials to work with? We might be held responsible!" adds Enfermeira Monica.

"But can I move her with her placenta still inside her?

"*Não tem problema*. No problem. There is no danger."

I shiver, hearing those words for the second time that day. I accept the huge wad of sterile cotton thrust at me to put between the new mother's legs to catch the blood en route, and run out.

This time dashing through the backyards I do not greet or apologize. Rushing past the man, I charge behind the house with the cotton. The mother is on her knees again, mouth open, drooling. I pray that the massage suggestion has done less harm than good. The baby is still on the ground, now loosely wrapped in the gray smudged piece of sheet. "The nurses wanted to come, really," I lie, "but they are busy with other women. We have to get her to the maternity, now! We must go!" I pantomime how to use the cotton, and then hustle up to the front yard to explain to the man what is happening.

Almost immediately the new mother stumbles out the front doorway of the house, steered by her sister and the prophet-healer. Ashen and drenched with sweat, she has been clothed hurriedly in what I can tell is her good dress, straining violet sateen bunched around her waist, and a *capulana*—a bright yellow swath of printed cotton cloth—wrapped from her waist down. Another cloth wrap is anchored somehow between her legs to help hold the cotton wads from the maternity clinic. The whole ensemble is not working. Blood drips down her legs into the dust around her bare feet. With her placenta still attached inside her, she holds her ghostly infant in the sheet. One at each arm, the prophet-healer and the sister maneuver her along like a flimsy puppet. I follow behind them with the father, our shiny shoes connecting the dots of blood. Standing atop her dirt pile, the girl in tropical green watches stone-faced and silent as our tiny, horrid parade winds through the neighbors' backyards.

When we arrive at the truck, everyone but the shaking mother and I fuss about soiling the truck's meticulously clean interior. The sister heaps the mother into the backseat tangled up with the baby, the capulana cloths, the blood-soaked cotton, and the now crimson-stained purple dress, shoves her own hip up and slides in after her. The husband rides outside in the back of the pickup. I ride in the front passenger seat beside Senhor Mario, his face coiled in disgust, as if he smells something rotten. The prophet-healer stays behind waving with exaggerated cheeriness.

Turning back once in my seat I catch a glimpse of the mother, who is trembling as if she is very cold, a look of awe and joy on her face as she stares intently into the tiny face of her daughter clutched in her arms.

Ten minutes later, at the maternity hospital, the sea of pregnant women and mothers with babies parts to let our bad luck through. I see the mother, her small, silent bundle, and her sister only as far as the door of the *sala do parto* (birthing room). There, the two nurses, with smiles on their mouths but not in their eyes, thank me rigidly for bringing them this emergency and shut the peeling door in my face. I drift back to the truck, unaware of anyone in the waiting room. Outside, Senhor Mario is scrubbing the backseat of the truck with a rank, moldy rag. A pair of bloody footprints waits on the floor of the back seat to be erased.

This is my clearest memory from Mucessua, Mozambique, captured in my field journal on that day, April 14, 1995. It is an arrival story, but not mine alone. When the events of this day took place, I had lived and worked in Mozambique for more than two years. Yet, it took the convergence of these people, in this setting, enacting the unfolding drama that shaped the precarious circumstances of this baby's birth for me to grasp why pregnancy in Mozambique was a well-kept *segredo da casa*, a family secret. This tiny girl entered the world dragging behind her the dawning of my insight into her complex world like a twin placenta—slippery, iridescent, and vibrant. In Mozambique, as in many parts of the world, to give birth is called *dar luz*—to give light, to enlighten—and witnessing birth without taking the special precautions known to seasoned midwives can be powerful enough to render you blind.

The incident also captures my uneasy role as a participant-observer of Mozambican women's lives in limbo, caught between hope and fear, death and life, at the end of two wars and the beginning of a new struggle with deepening poverty and HIV/AIDS. Conjuring it up still floods me with residual panic brought on by my feelings of helplessness. It did not matter that I worked for a maternal and child survival project that was assisting the Ministry of Health to implement a Safe Motherhood Initiative (SMI). SMI is an international maternal health strategy developed by the World Health Organization (WHO 1985b, 1994) to provide high-quality maternal health services to reduce the number of women injured, incapacitated, or killed by preventable and treatable complications during pregnancy or childbirth (Bolton et al. 1989: 80). Only by chance had I crossed the path of that man on that morning. It did not matter that the Mozambique Ministry of Health had been implementing a Safe Motherhood Initiative for more than a decade through public education programs utilizing posters, radio announcements, public assemblies, and vaccine campaigns. The Mozambique SMI also involved a nationwide effort to identify high-risk obstetric cases and to transfer obstetric emergencies to appropriate care facilities. Health care workers, local leaders, and village elders all joined community health mobilizations to promote early initiation of prenatal care and trained attendants at births. None of it mattered. A woman was lying just minutes away from a maternity clinic where life-saving care was available with her life seeping out of her into the earth. Why?

Was it lack of information, of motive, transport, education, social support, or her husband's permission? Was it her religious beliefs or cultural practices, or inadequate micronutrients in her diet? Was it her unceasing triple burden of backbreaking work on her agricultural plot, at her home, and at the market selling produce that delayed her? Or was it her inability to pay a cash incentive to clinic nurses and her resulting fear of ill treatment at the maternity hospital whose walls, services, and staff morale were crumbling under severe budget cuts in the public sector? Current public health discourse puts forward many competing hypotheses about why so-called high-risk women underutilize reproductive health services all over the world. The results are the same. Women die from largely preventable pregnancy- and birth-related causes in huge numbers—more than half a million women each year, 99 percent of these in so-called developing countries (WHO/UNICEF/UNFPA 2004). In sub-Saharan Africa, 1 in 16 women dies in childbirth. The meaning of this statistic in terms of actual lives lived and lost can be fully appreciated only when compared, for example, to the lifetime risk of dying from a maternity-related cause in the U.K., which is 1 in 8,200 (UN Mozambique 2008). Maternal mortality has recently been called "the most dramatic health inequality on the planet" (Bunting 2008).

When I first visited Mozambique in 1990, the country was still at war, and, not surprisingly, maternal death rates, a "most immediate and visible index of scarcity and unmet needs," were at elevated levels (Scheper-Hughes 1992: 25). At an estimated 1,500 per 100,000 live births, the maternal mortality rate in Mozambique was among the highest in the world, alongside Bangladesh, Nigeria, Chad, Pakistan, and Afghanistan (Povey 1990; WHO 1991). In 1995, the national maternal mortality rate was estimated to be around 980 per 100,000 live births, ranging from 320 to 2,000, depending on the region (UNDP Mozambique 1998). At that time, it was projected that one in nine women would die of pregnancy- and birth-related causes (WHO/UNICEF 1997), and back-street abortions were estimated to be responsible for 16 to 18 percent of all maternal deaths (Granja 1996).[7] A decade later, the lifetime risk of maternal death in Mozambique was reported to have improved slightly, to 1 in 14 women (WHO/UNICEF/UNFPA 2004). Today, however, escalating HIV/AIDS infection rates as high as 28 percent of the adult population and 40 percent of pregnant women in the central provinces of the country make pregnancy and birth ever more risky processes for Mozambican women and their infants. We know that without treatment, an estimated 30–40 percent of HIV-positive women will pass HIV to their infants (ANECCA 2004).

Low attendance of clinical prenatal care and maternity services is not unique to Mozambique. For decades, governments across the developing world and international donors have sponsored the Safe Motherhood Initiative (SMI). Yet, despite this initiative and the growing availability of routine malaria prophylaxis as well as screening for HIV/AIDS and other sexually transmitted infections in prenatal clinics, women in impoverished settings routinely delay prenatal care visits to clinics until late in their pregnancy or avoid them altogether. Health care providers are frequently frustrated by what they see as a recurrent pattern of confounding reproductive health behaviors: the most vulnerable women are often those who elude medical surveillance, monitoring, and intervention, falling through the cracks in troubling and persistent ways. Health care specialists ask why high-risk women in communities that experience excessive maternal and infant morbidity and mortality do not use prenatal care services, especially when they are accessible—located within a short walking distance and free of charge.

Over the past decade, global awareness about maternal mortality in the developing world and the importance of improving prenatal care interventions has increased dramatically (Bunting 2008). Until recently, however, few studies of maternal mortality have paid attention to local experiences of reproductive vulnerability or specifically addressed the prenatal care strategies of women in developing countries from an ethnographic perspective (Adetunji 1996). The processes by which impoverished women make reproductive health care choices during pregnancy and birth remain largely unexamined (Chapman 2004). Despite the lack of information about the pregnancy management strategies of impoverished women, below the surface of standard discourse on maternal mortality in developing countries linger deeply embedded assumptions that poor women are incompetent and somehow undeserving health consumers (Marshall 1988). Such assumptions barely mask "blame the victim" attitudes among many biomedical health workers and health policy makers in government ministries, international development organizations, and donor agencies. Remarks by a UNICEF spokesperson presenting a keynote address at an international conference on maternal mortality and the Safe Motherhood Initiative in Bangladesh capture this perspective: "Who is it that dies most from maternal mortality most often? People who do not listen to the doctors, are neither educated nor motivated, without time or money, and so forth. In other words, those less likely to have sought prenatal care" (Rohde 1995: S5).

It is on the "and so forth" and "in other words" of this quotation that I aim to shed some light—*dar luz*. Not enough is known about the circumstances in communities that have been targeted by the Safe Motherhood Initiative in Mozambique, elsewhere in the developing world, and in pockets of the industrialized and postindustrial global North where global-South conditions of poverty prevail. When these communities have been examined, there has been scarce consideration of the social and health costs of economic inequality and "abjection," the term James Ferguson uses to describe "the combination of an acute awareness of a privileged 'first class' world, together with an increasing social and economic disconnection from it" (Ferguson 2006: 166). What are women's perceptions of their own reproductive vulnerabilities? How do women imagine, understand, and act upon these threats in their daily lives? What is the relationship between women's perceptions of reproductive vulnerability and their health strategies, decisions, and practices?

Many of the standard public health hypotheses seem inadequate to account for the gap between first- and third-world maternal mortality rates or the distance between the Gondola maternity clinic and the woman birthing in the garden. An ever-growing list of "risk factors" associated with adverse maternal outcomes casts a net so wide as to be ineffective, catching most of the population of Mozambican women of reproductive age. The focus on risk factors, in turn, gives rise to an equally long list of behavior change models that simply ignore cultural and structural constraints and the complex interface between the two. As Paul Farmer has pointed out: "This sort of analysis . . . gives short shrift to history and political economy and admits no consideration to the adverse impact of colonial and neocolonial policies, to say nothing of racism or gender inequality" (Maternowska 2006: x). It was clear that to understand why a woman lay dying minutes away from the maternity clinic, I needed to consider the broader political, economic, and social forces at work. Why was the maternity hospital so overburdened and understaffed, with long lines, rare electricity, and no running water? Why was there only one doctor for every 100,000 Mozambicans? Why was there just one ambulance serving 500,000 people in Gondola District? What social forces had prompted the women to seek the spiritual protection and expertise of a prophet-healer during birth? I knew that some of the answers to my questions lay buried in Bairro Mucessua.

Into the Bairro

Bairro Mucessua is a neighborhood of about five thousand on the outskirts of the town of Vila Gondola in Manica Province, a province of about one million people at the center of the nation of Mozambique. I worked there as the assistant to the director of health education for Manica Province from 1993 to 1995, following the ceasefire of Mozambique's seventeen-year war of destabilization between the ruling party, Frente de Libertação de Moçambique (FRELIMO), and the insurgent army, Resistência Nacional Moçambicana (RENAMO) backed by the apartheid governments of Rhodesia and South Africa. This period also marked the eve of the emergence of the country's HIV/AIDS epidemic, a circumstance postponed by the violence of war, which stopped foot and vehicle movement across Mozambique's borders with Malawi, Zimbabwe, and South Africa, —countries that by the 1990s were already hard-hit by HIV/AIDS. I conducted fieldwork on pregnancy and prenatal care in Bairro Mucessua during this time, and returned for a year in 1998 to complete my work. Most importantly, I lived, worked, became pregnant and gave birth, and shared life with my husband and daughter in this part of Central Mozambique for nearly four years between 1992 and 1999, and continue to return periodically. What I learned most about Mucessua came from the moments between the interviews and questionnaires.

To see Bairro Mucessua as I have come to see it between 1991 and 2010 is to encounter a wider Mozambican society marked by historical upheavals and deep contradictions—a "combination of extreme disruptions and continuities in older patterns of domination and inequality" (Alexander 1994: 1). Unpacking these contradictions means placing my account of women's reproductive stress and resilience in Mucessua on the larger stage of post-Independence Mozambique during the years of a growing debt crisis and economic restructuring. In 1992, war had recently ended with a ceasefire in October; multiparty elections were held in 1994. The fragile peace and democracy, however, had brought no prospect of meeting even basic needs, let alone prosperity, to the majority of Mozambicans. On the contrary, the government Poverty Alleviation Unit estimated that for most of the population, poverty in Mozambique increased after the end of the war (Hanlon 1996: 17). The country remains one of the world's poorest, ranked 168 out of 177 in the 2005 Human Development Report (UNDP 2005). These high rates of poverty and the scarcity of health services are the legacy not only of warfare, but also of colonial exploitation, natural disaster, and state planning failures. Living day to day in this world, I learned that I would find only some of the answers to my questions in Mucessua.

The current obstacles and opportunities in women's lives in Central Mozambique have a long history. During the colonial period, opportunities created by women's roles in cash cropping and crop expansion were limited by the inequitable terms of colonial exchange of goods (Alpers 1975). Further embedding these gender-linked relations to production, the exportation of male laborers from the region to South Africa, Rhodesia, and Portugal's other colonies heightened community dependence on unpaid female subsistence cultivation. This pattern of labor migration has created a labor reserve in which women are primarily responsible for the social costs of reproduction—bearing and raising the next generation of laborers, as well as nurturing laborers when they are incapacitated by sickness or accident or simply age. Forced male and female labor, called *chibalo* under the Portuguese, and the extraction of male labor for export were also associated with a particular cluster of health consequences, including seasonal starvation and high infant and maternal mortality (Raikes 1989). The unequal terms of trade that evolved in the region before colonial contact and intensified throughout colonial occupation set in motion the process of exploitation and impoverishment that Mozambique struggles with today (Isaacman 1996; Isaacman and Isaacman 1983; Hanlon 1996; Pfeiffer 2005).

Mozambique's more recent history of colonial resistance and independence, the externally promoted internal war of destabilization, widespread dislocation of rural populations, and continued male labor migration have had a profound and immediate influence on the society. These forces have continuously ruptured and reorganized patterns of social organization, with important implications for women's health. With the cessation of war-related violence, millions of refugees returned to Mozambique from neighboring countries. Many *deslocados*—people displaced from their homes within the country—began to return to and resettle their ancestral farmlands. Yet, in many cases, deslocados chose to remain in the crowded peri-urban areas they fled to for safety during the war, aspiring to access new opportunities in the postwar economy and hoping their children would benefit from the infrastructure of towns like Gondola—the water, sanitation, schools, and health care that only slowly were being extended to rural, war-torn areas. In Bairro Mucessua the daily lives and destinies of longtime residents and deslocados have become entangled in the overcrowded quarters of the busy neighborhood.

Some claim, however, that the most obvious cause for the continued level of suffering in Mozambique since the end of the war has been the World Bank and the International Monetary Fund's Structural Adjustment Programs (SAPs) (Hanlon 1996: 15).

SAPping Mozambique's Health

After Independence in 1975, the new government in Mozambique embraced the comprehensive primary health care model elaborated at a historic 1978 conference in Alma Ata. The new public-sector system provided basic services through a tiered network of linked hospitals, health centers, and health posts. The national Ministry of Health coordinated its programs through ten Provincial Health Directorates, each of which provided support to ten to twenty-five district directorates responsible for the management of health facilities. The system centers on the horizontal integration of basic services delivered at facility level; diagnosis and basic care for common illnesses are broadly offered at all levels of the health care system. Referral systems link the levels of care within districts and provinces. At the hospital level, services are differentiated and specialized, while at lower levels, services are more integrated, as fewer staff combine multiple functions to deliver them. Some specific programs, such as TB, antenatal care, and health education services, remain comparatively more vertical in orientation, from the national level down through provinces and districts to facilities, with varying degrees of integration with other services at each level.

In the early years of Independence, Mozambique's overall primary health care system expanded to an impressive number of facilities, allowing broad geographical coverage, and an essential-drug system provided critical medicines to most facilities. However, the system was underresourced, with major workforce shortages at all levels, training deficits, and frequent stockouts of materials and medicines. Management inadequacies were particularly problematic, given the small pool of higher-level health workers. Finally, primary health care was further undermined by the decades-long war supported by the apartheid governments of Rhodesia and South Africa, followed by severe government spending cutbacks imposed by structural adjustment programs under the direction of the International Monetary Fund (IMF) (Pfeiffer et al. 2008).

Mozambique joined the IMF and World Bank at the height of the war of destabilization in 1984, and then implemented a modified form of World Bank–mandated SAPs in 1987. In Mozambique as elsewhere around the globe, SAPs involved the World Bank's neoliberal "universal recipe for economic recovery" (Federici 2004: 9)—liberalization of currency controls, elimination of subsidies and barriers to imports, refocusing of the economy toward exports, and most critically, disinvestment of the state from the provision of public services (with the exception of the military) and privatization of land and means of production in order to help service Mozambique's significant foreign debt. Devastating cuts have been made in the state's welfare programs in favor of a more privatized economy. Aimed at shrinking government spending, these austerity policies jeopardize the nation's ability to provide food security, health care, education, and other social services (Demble 2002; Gunewardena 2002). The two most important IMF controls were cuts in government spending and cuts in credit to the economy (Hanlon 1996: 19). "In short, the cost of social service is transferred from the public sphere back to the domestic sphere" (Bolles 2002: 10; Bujra 1986; Brown 2005).

So far, the balance sheet of structural adjustment in Mozambique, as elsewhere in Africa, is bleak: "capital flight, collapse of manufactures, marginal or negative increase in export incomes, drastic cutbacks in urban public services, soaring prices and a steep decline in real wages" (Rakodi 1997, qtd. in Davis 2004: 20). Overwhelmingly, these policies have also led to the rapid demise of core public infrastructure, such as provision of water and sanitation, public education, and public health, with a resulting increase in mortality rates (Cooper 2008: 92). Rigorous research and analysis confirm the deleterious effects of such neoliberal policies, with some critiques coming from Bretton Woods and other institutions that were among the fundamental architects of structural adjustment and liberalization. Patrick Bond cites the "devastating conclusions" of a mid-2005 study by London research and advocacy charity Christian AID (Bond 2007: 173):

> Trade liberalisation has cost sub-Saharan Africa $272 billion over the past 20 years. Had they not been forced to liberalise as the price of aid, loans, and debt relief, sub-Saharan African countries would have enough extra income

to wipe out their debts and have sufficient left over to pay for every child to be vaccinated and go to school. Two decades of liberalisation has cost sub-Saharan Africa roughly what it has received in aid. Effectively, this aid did no more than compensate African countries for the losses they sustained by meeting the conditions that were attached to the aid they received.

In Mozambique's health sector, the reductions in government expenditure led to several changes that resulted in the spiraling deterioration of the health system. National health spending was gouged 80 percent, representing a reduction in the percentage of the national budget spent on health from 10.7 percent in 1981 to 4.4 percent in 1988 (Cliff 1991: 28) and 2.7 percent in 2004 (UNDP 2008). With the effects of inflation and devaluation added, the real value of health expenditure was estimated to have fallen from U.S. $4 per person in 1981 to less than $0.05 per person in 1988. Another aspect of the reform included an increase in outpatient fees and the introduction of new inpatient fees that created access barriers to the poorest. Drug prices also rose, resulting in a significant drop in the number of patients able to afford medication. As the government sector worked to make ends meet in the face of a growing deficit, international donors and loan agencies, especially the large multilateral organizations such as the World Bank and UNICEF, gained increasing influence in health policy making. These agencies literally call the shots in the development and implementation of national- and provincial-level health programming in ways that seriously fragmented FRELIMO's innovative primary health care approach (Cliff 1991: 29; Hanlon 1996: 19).

FRELIMO's turn to the West epitomized by the implementation of SAPs was not enough for the United States, and in 1990, Mozambique was forced to accept a much harsher IMF-controlled "economic stabilization package" locally known as Programma de Reforma Economica (PRE) (Hanlon 1997: 19). The new measures focused primarily on further cutting government spending and cutting credit to the economy, which led to a decrease in GDP per capita, industrial production, and exports. Inflation rose from 33 percent in 1990 to 70 percent in 1994. At the same time, government salaries were slashed to below living wages. According to Hanlon (1997: 19), the socioeconomic effects of PRE spread in ways that affected health care and education:"A doctor earned $350 a month in 1991, $175 in 1993 and now takes in less than $100 dollars a month. For a nurse or teacher, monthly salaries fell from $110 to $60 to $40—not enough to support a family. Corruption rose rapidly as people sought extra money to survive; teachers demanded that pupils pay for extra lessons, while women arriving at maternity hospitals to give birth needed to bring a dollar or two to pay the midwife."

Women health workers were especially hard-hit by the rise in prices compared to wages, especially female heads of households and single women (Cliff 1991: 30). Growing despondency among inadequately paid health workers led both male and female health workers to reduce their hours in search of supplemental income, to abandon their regular posts, or to charge unauthorized fees to see patients either in the clinic or at their homes. Health posts were often empty for days or even weeks at a time as health workers attended seminars hosted by nongovernmental organizations that often provided per diems equivalent to monthly government salaries. Medicines in government pharmacies became increasingly expensive and less available except to those able to pay the inflated prices of stock diverted from formal channels into personal stashes and the informal market—a practice locally called some version of the Changana term *dumba nenge*, or "run for your life." Corruption and privatization were increasingly attractive temptations to workers laboring under such conditions (Cliff 1991: 30; Sheldon 1994). It is not surprising that the quality of health care fell precipitously.

Endangering Safe Motherhood

Weakened by years of war, and bending to pressure from international financial institutions and their political sponsors, by the mid-1980s, the Mozambican government moved away from its primary health ideals toward a selective health strategy promoted by international aid donor agencies. A selective health approach emphasizes vertical programming, for example, concentrating resources to address the problem of "maternal mortality" rather than creating a broader focus on women's health. This orientation contrasts with the state's previous horizontal emphasis on comprehensive primary health care as a central component of its agenda for social transformation. To address maternal mortality, Mozambique joined the international effort and implemented its own Safe Motherhood Initiative (SMI). In Mozambique, the SMI was cosponsored by the World Bank and the U.S. Agency for International Development (USAID), both well known for their protracted institutional commitment to population control in the third world (Alexander 1990; Hartmann 1987; Mass 1976), and their enthusiastic policy support for vertical medical programming like SMI. This support, however, also represented a powerful means of pushing a population control agenda on third-world governments by tying much-needed aid for maternal-child health services to successful implementation of family-planning programs.

The proposed strategy of the SMI in Mozambique included upgrading all levels of care within the maternal health services (Povey 1990).[8] Many aspects of Mozambique's SMI plan to upgrade the availability, accessibility, and quality of essential obstetric care remain unrealized due to resource limitations. Since the late 1970s, however, state maternity clinics have provided several prenatal services demonstrated to reduce maternal and infant mortality and morbidity. These interventions include folic acid and iron supplementation; screening for and treatment of anemia, tuberculosis, and malaria; tetanus immunization; detection and care of pre-eclampsia; and beginning in the late 1980s, screening for and treatment of syphilis and other sexually transmitted infections.[9] Nutritional counseling is provided for pregnant mothers and for caretakers of weaning infants. All maternal and infant health services were, and continue to be, officially free of charge. Since 1980, prenatal care services also include screening women at high risk for problems in pregnancy, obstetric complications, or both in order to refer them to the appropriate level of care for treatment.[10]

In spite of public health messages and Ministry of Health guidelines, most pregnant women in Manica Province, where I lived and worked, delayed prenatal care until after the first trimester. In 1994, a study of 1,016 women utilizing state prenatal care services reported that an estimated 69 percent of all pregnant women in the district of Gondola initiated prenatal care in a state clinic at some point during pregnancy (Lafort 1994). The mean time for initiating prenatal care, however, was during the sixth month of gestation. An estimated 44 percent of women in the district who initiated prenatal care did not return to give birth in a health facility. An estimated 57 percent of births in the province were home births (INE 1999). These patterns of late initiation of prenatal care and home birth were the same for women throughout the area regardless of distance from a health facility. Lafort (1994) concluded that no parallel prenatal care system existed in the region. Health care providers in the formal sector were frequently exasperated by this "noncompliance." Why weren't women coming into the clinics when they were told to come in?

While expansion of the health system has been vital to improving reproductive health care delivery in Mozambique, the changes have fallen short of intended goals. Underlying the proposed strategy is a mainstream demographic view of fertility as an isolated, biological event that ignores the wider array of factors contributing to the current situation of women's health, including reproductive health. Reproduction is not only a biological process, but also "an ongoing social and political construction that may begin long before and continue long after the biological fact of parturition" (Greenhalgh 1994; see also Bledsoe 1990; Browner and Sargent 1996). As a sociocultural construction, reproduction involves accessing a wide range of cultural resources and social institutions, including "factors articulated in social values, legal systems and production structures that govern society's view of the duties and rights of women, foremost among them being the reproductive function of women" (El-Mouelhy et al. 1989: 9).

As a political construction, reproduction entails the negotiation of power relations at many and often conflicting levels (Greenhalgh 1994: 4). Solving the problem of maternal morbidity and mortality, then, is not merely an epidemiological project, as Mozambique's plan for addressing it implies. As Soheir Morsy (1995a: 172) observes: "The project that poses a greater challenge as an object of intellectual discourse, not to mention as a framework for political activism, transcends the disentanglement of primary determinants of maternal mortality from webs of epidemiological variables. It is the investigation of the historical and social factors that produce risk factors that are then constructed as medicalized risk categories."

Indeed, there is no mystery about what causes maternal mortality in Mozambique or anywhere else. It is widely agreed that the six most prevalent causes of maternal mortality worldwide—hemorrhage, hypertensive disorders, sepsis, unsafe abortion and its sequelae, and anemia (Goodburn and Campbell 2001)—can be seen as mere endpoints on the maternal road to death. This road to death involves a combination of three core factors, including not only high-risk pregnancies but also socioeconomic disadvantage and lack of access to health care (Senanayake 1995: S11). Many contributors at the 1995 Fifth International Conference on Maternal and Neonatal Health in Dhaka, Bangladesh, stressed this point. As one speaker summarized: "The most striking aspect of maternal and child deaths is the sheer scale of the problem: 1,400 young women and 39,000 children die every day worldwide, and almost all these deaths are preventable. A closer look reveals something equally striking: the underlying causes of maternal and child death are essentially the same" (ibid.).

Currently, the Safe Motherhood Initiative in Mozambique addresses only the high-risk pregnancy aspect of the three-lane road to maternal death. The core element of the national program is based on WHO's risk approach (WHO 1978a; WHO/UNICEF 1980): beginning in 1980, a pregnancy control form for health personnel to fill out during initial prenatal examinations was introduced in antenatal clinics throughout the country "to monitor pregnancies and to help direct specialist care to mothers at greatest risk" (Jelley and Madeley 1983a: 111). Ideally, this system identifies women at high risk for pregnancy or obstetric complications in order to refer them to the appropriate level of care for treatment. In practice, because of its low sensitivity and high rate of false positives, the risk approach has come under growing criticism as being a poor predictor of complications (Rohde 1995). It is now widely agreed that many emergency pregnancy and birth complications cannot be predicted or prevented. Therefore, consistent prenatal visits, timely detection of problems, and availability of competent emergency obstetric care are critical aspects of reproductive health strategies aimed at decreasing maternal deaths (Coria-Soto et al. 1997).

It might be expected, then, that early detection of pregnancy or obstetric complication would depend on early prenatal exams and on women going to adequately equipped health facilities to give birth. Yet, research conducted three years following the implementation of the risk strategy in health facilities in Mozambique's capital, Maputo, found that the women most at risk for pregnancy and obstetric complications were not the highest users of government prenatal care services. Data also showed that women at high risk for complication underused prenatal services in comparison to those identified as being at lower risk (Jelley and Madeley 1983a: 111).

Given the limited definition of risk underlying the Safe Motherhood Initiative in Mozambique, such findings would seem to confound the proposed medicalized solution to the problem of maternal mortality. What is being left out of the equation? The assessment of reproductive risk factors must include confronting socioeconomic disadvantage and lack of access to health care. However, instead of addressing these issues, proponents of the risk approach resort to explanations that obscure these forces and even blame the most vulnerable communities for the crisis conditions under which they labor to bear and raise children (Mullings 1995). This is the approach still promoted by international agencies and imposed by international aid donors in Mozambique and other developing countries.

Ignoring the historically specific context of maternal mortality, development discourses frequently justify the implementation of deadly economic restructuring policies throughout "developing countries" while simultaneously encouraging women's and community involvement in "sustainable" development programs (World Bank 1993). This conflicting development framework belatedly acknowledges women's entrenched contribution to the production of household health at the same time it charges women with the responsibility for health, not to mention blaming them for "maldevelopment." This policy shift toward community empowerment diverts attention from the inability of national governments to bring about long-awaited state services and infrastructure and to live up to their obligation to provide good health care for all (Morsy 1995a: 172). It also serves to mask the role of international intervention in undermining state stability and stymieing the provision of public social services.

When applied to Mozambique, these dynamics are particularly insidious. Paradoxically, current economic restructuring policies in Mozambique are implemented by the primary sponsors of Safe Motherhood—the IMF, World Bank, and USAID. These policies have forced such great reductions in popular-sector spending that it is virtually impossible for the Ministry of Health, even with major donor inputs (Hanlon 1997: 19; Cliff 1991), to offer the services or facilities that could adequately address the need for emergency treatment of maternal complications that result in maternal and neonatal deaths. Even the provision of basic services that might assist in the detection or prevention of or appropriate attention to such emergencies is a strain on the system.

There are other reasons why the SMI risk approach is likely to fail those women who are most at risk of negative infant or maternal outcomes. Embedded in it is an anticipatory notion of risk in which the concepts of "predisposition" to illness or health complications and "inherent" risks are central (Nelkin 2003: vii). This model defines risk as the statistical probability of an event's occurring within a population, a possible future occurrence of biological harm. The programmatic corollary to an inherent risk orientation, in this case predisposition to pregnancy or obstetric complications, is systematic detection of future risks. Such an approach to risk keeps the focus of both sickness and its prevention or treatment in the domain of an individual whose health is of concern (Tesh 1988).

This concept of risk also carries with it implicit notions about agency, or lack thereof. "Risk," as a health term, suggests that sources of sickness or various kinds of threats to health are simply out there and that the key lies in determining the nature of the barrier those at risk might put up. This agencyless model of illness causality may be in keeping with public health models that assume pathogens do not have a mind of their own. However, as I learned in Mozambique, inherent biological risks are not the only or the most salient threats to women at whom SMI is directed (Chapman 2003; Jelley 1983a,b; Ndyomugyenyi, Neema, and Magnussen 1998; Sargent and Rawlins 1991).

Recent literature on health risks indicates growing awareness that risk is socially constructed and that "risk perceptions depend less on the nature of a hazard than on political, social, and cultural contexts" (Nelkins 2003: viii). There has even been a call for "ethnographies of risk management within households and communities that pay attention to social risk" (Nichter 2003: 29). However, the possible mechanisms through which social threats influence health seeking have been understudied and misinterpreted. As Nichter has suggested, understanding when social threats outweigh the biologized risk categories prioritized in clinical settings can help us identify why preventive health measures are taken up in some cases and rejected in others (ibid.). We need "finer grained assessments of how individuals actually cope with states of vulnerability" (Lupton 1999: 102–3, qtd. in Nichter 2003: 28). Such assessments are crucial not only to better understand the role of lay risk perceptions in health decision making and to help direct services, resources, education, and outreach where most needed, but also to accurately expose the costs of social inequalities in terms of restricted life chances and increased social suffering. In the chapters that follow, I sift just such a more finely grained assessment from the women's stories.

SAPs and the Social Environment

Less obvious and less well documented than SAPs' effects on health and health care in Mozambique is the disturbing effect on the social environment of the poisoned chalice of economic stabilization policies (Cooper 2008). The removal of price protections for basic commodities, of subsidies for rural agricultural producers, and of free education and health services has been especially hard on women (Hanlon 1996; Cliff 1991). Rising costs of living and the introduction of fees for school and medical care have made access to money more important to survival than it has ever been. Yet women are frequently without adequate education and skills to compete for waged labor and unable to make ends meet through subsistence farming alone. At the same time, increased privatization, the monetization of formerly communal work-exchange practices, and increasing competition for land and jobs have intensified women's workloads as subsistence cultivators (MOPF 1998: 312). In the face of all these forces, cash-poor women experience multiple levels of vulnerability—biological, social, and economic. They balance uneasily on the boundaries of wage and subsistence economies, as they navigate life in underresourced peri-urban enclaves that are the borderlands between urban and rural cultures and spaces. These hybrid spaces are increasingly familiar features that cling to the hems of "urban spatial explosion" in much of the developing world (Guldin 1997: 44). In these borderlands, crime and crowd retribution are constants. Violent occurrences, heightened tension, and interpersonal conflicts are everyday experiences as people compete for limited resources in crowded quarters.

The growth of slums and the movement of surplus population from rural areas to urban and peri-urban slums have been described as the most tangible consequences of neoliberalism. This trend reflects a shift in patterns of global economic policies, writes Mike Davis, who describes "systemic underdevelopment in which the compact of unequal exchange (that is the root of African nations debt crisis) is replaced by pure neglect: in the slums of the post-colonial era, survival has become a game of intense *self*-exploitation, running the gamut from informal service work to biomedical labor (the sale of organs or the participation in clinical trials)" (Davis 2004: 7).

These politics of abandonment have also engendered change at the microlevel as individuals are forced to reorganize around limited household resources, especially the coping strategies and inventiveness of women on one hand and mounting crime and violent gangs on the other (Davis 2004: 20). Another feature of these new slum countergeographies of survival in Mozambique has been the explosion of sex work in urban and rural settings. Here, as elsewhere around the globe, this upsurge in microexploitation signals how market forces and the importance of monetary payments have seeped into the most intimate of social relationships with striking consequences—the commodification of reproduction.

The Commodification of Reproduction

Because the way monetary exchanges have permeated Mozambican social relationships is my central concern in this book, I explore the concept of commodification of reproduction in some depth. Anthropologists use the term "commodification" to refer to a wide range of circumstances, consequences, and processes by which something or someone is turned into or comes to be looked upon or sold as a commodity (Taylor 2004: 12). Definitions and applications of the concept diverge widely. Some scholars recognize commodities as such by virtue of their being situated in a context that includes the presence of a "cash nexus" in which people, goods, and services are exchanged for money. Others apply the concept of commodification more generally to any social process by which people, objects, or acts become exchangeable in a marketplace. One such process might be through loss or erasure of identity or place (ibid.: 12–13).

Marx distinguished persons from things, but defined commodities as both product and process. Commodities, he wrote, were "in the first place, an object outside us, a thing that by its properties satisfies human wants of some sort or another" (1978: 199). Yet commodities were also process: "The wealth of those societies in which the capitalist mode of production prevails, presents itself as 'an immense accumulation of commodities,' its unit being a single commodity" (Marx 1976: 125). Marx placed this process of commodification at the heart of capitalist social relations, the route whereby an economic system becomes one in which "exchange value dominates production to its whole depth and extent" (Marx 1973: 188). He also stressed the negative transformative *qualities* of commodification (Davis Floyd 2004: 219) as both process and relationship, the means by which a commodity must be divorced from the social conditions of its production and rendered "exchangeable" with other commodities. This is fetishism, the means by which a commodity becomes infused with the magical "life" of its "value" while its "necessarily social" labor time remains invisible, obscured, and mystified (Taylor 2004: 189). The concept of commodification communicates this relationship or dynamic of separation and mystery manifested by this process of fetishism.

There are, however, dangers in uncritically applying categories derived from European realities to African contexts like postwar Mozambique (Crehan 1997: 16). For example, anthropologist Igor Kopytoff has explored the process of commodification and the uneasy and culturally specific distance between categories of "persons" and categories of "things" in both Western and African contexts. He proposes that the "Western" moral discourse eschewing the commodification of children and, by extension, of human reproduction might have rather recent roots—in nineteenth-century (public at least) growing discomfort regarding "any social arrangement reminiscent of slavery." Yet, using African social institutions as his point of reference, Kopytoff points out that kinship at its core is intertwined with "the production and acquisition of human capital" and with rights in human reproductive labor power, such as rights over bodies, feelings, services, sexuality, and reproductive capacities. Given this intimate link between kinship and rights in and power over others, there may be a certain ubiquitous, even "natural" tendency toward "economism" in human relationships, Kopytoff suggests: "Many, indeed most, human societies have found the invasion of kinship by economics rather congenial. . . Innumerable societies have framed various social arrangements—such as inheritance, co-residence, marriage, reproduction, rights over children, and adoption—in terms of concrete rights-in-persons, rights transacted through payments in things, animals, commodities, and money" (2004: 272).

Regarding social life in African cultural settings, Crehan suggests we harness the concepts of use-value and exchange-value to capture the dual dynamic of commodification as process and relationship/dynamic.[11] *Use-value* identifies the qualities or properties of an object or the specific nature of a service in terms of satisfying any kind of human need. *Exchange-value* is solely a quantitative measure referring to the value of one object or service in relation to that of other goods. Crehan also carefully distinguishes between "commoditization" (the term she prefers) and "monetization": "Commoditization refers to production geared around exchange; goods and services are produced in order to be exchanged. Monetization refers to the process whereby exchange comes to use a universal equivalent (some form of money) in which the relative values [exchange value] of different goods can be expressed" (21).

Drawing on these concepts to describe changing social life in two settings in 1980s rural Zambia, Crehan identifies two often incompatible mechanisms of distribution and access to resources. One set of transactions relied on money and exchange value of goods, and the other depended directly on mobilizing use-value through relationships between people created by kinship. Crehan calls these respectively a "culture of contract" and a "culture of reciprocity" (184). These two economies mapped two distinct terrains of social interactions and social relationships underlying the processes by which the social product was distributed and individuals obtained access to resources. Residents in these two towns agreed that the increasing monetization of social life in rural Zambia led to a lament for the "breakdown of old morality and the new overwhelming dominance of money" (146). Despite increased monetization and the potential to buy certain kinds of labor, men's access to female social reproductive labor depended very much on marriage. While certain kinds of labor were seen as "located within a moral domain, some relationships were appropriate to organize through market mechanisms; others [especially cultivation of the daily staple sorghum for home consumption] were more properly organized through marriage" (160).

Crehan finds that in the Zambian context, because of the increasing fragility of rural subsistence and in the absence of a state-provided safety net, tensions accrued around ruptures of kinship-based rights and responsibilities to distribute surplus production and especially the use-value of women's labor. In an environment of growing resentments and suspicions, witchcraft practices and accusations emerged as a discourse that named these tensions. Dealing with witchcraft allowed the articulation of and analysis of unmet needs and expectations within an increasingly discordant set of kin relations strained by new intrusions of monetization in the context of palpable and growing material inequalities. These tensions were not so much over the treatment of persons as things or the social as economic. Rather, it was the overlapping of moral and material anxieties about the ways money was shifting distribution of and access to labor and goods and creating new vulnerabilities. These are the shifts and the attendant "new" vulnerabilities that I seek to track down in Central Mozambique, particularly the processes by which new vulnerabilities productively create new geographies of violence (Bogues 2005: 3) and also countergeographies of survival.

The vulnerability, conflict, and violence against women that increasingly accumulate around the distribution of the social product in the form of women's reproductive and social reproductive labor are not new phenomena at all (Merchant 1980; Fortunati 1995; Mies 1986; Silverblatt 1987; Beckles 1995; Bush 1990). As Sylvia Federici argues, the expropriation of the reproductive labor power of peasant households has been accomplished over time not only by the privatization of land and enclosure of the commons. Also key have been increased taxation, the commutation of labor services for wage labor from which women were systematically driven, the extension of state control of every aspect of reproduction through the medicalization of birth, and the violence and terror of the European witch hunts of the sixteenth and seventeenth centuries. These forces and processes served to effectively alienate women from their own power in and control over their bodies and labor power.

Combined with colonization, slavery, and the extraction of material and labor resources from the colonies, these processes that captured women's reproductive labor power while rendering it invisible enabled the first primitive accumulation of capital—the historical process on which Marx premised the development of capitalist relations (Federici 2004: 12). Also called "primitive appropriation" the extraction of labor value by means of conquest and plun-

der (97) has been a universal process in every phase of capitalist development that recurs in response to crises in capitalist accumulation and serves to
lower the cost of labor and obscure the exploitation of women and colonial
subjects (16–17).

> Not surprising, then, if large-scale violence and enslavement have been on
> the agenda, as they were in the period of "transition," with the difference
> that today the conquistadores are the officers of the World Bank and the
> International Monetary Fund, who are still preaching the worth of a penny
> to the same populations which the dominant world powers for centuries
> robbed and pauperized. Once again, much of the violence unleashed is
> directed against women, for in the age of the computer, the conquest of the
> female body is still a precondition for the accumulation of labor and wealth,
> as demonstrated by the institutional investment in the development of new
> reproductive technologies that, more than ever, reduce women to wombs.
> (17)

Identifying these spasms of enclosure, violence, and enslavement as they
persist in the present helps us understand the general pressures that condition the crisis of reproduction in Mozambican households, and the specific
reproductive pressures many Mozambican women face today. In Mucessua,
these not so new inequalities and enclosures fuel competition among women
for scarce monetary and land resources from men in ways that rearrange the
gender relations of reproduction. Increasingly, monetary payments are expected for local gender socialization practices throughout the reproductive
cycle. This has been accompanied by a shift to payments of cash instead of
gifts, cattle, tools, and labor for seduction fees, bridewealth payments, and
the offerings of respect paid for birth assistance. For some time, *lobolo*—
bridewealth payments made by the groom's family to the bride's family to
formalize marriage bonds between lineages—have been made in cash.

More recently, the price demanded for bridewealth has skyrocketed, and
money is increasingly demanded in place of the ritual gifts of respect paid by
suitors for *masunggiro*, or the virgin seduction fee—a customary payment to
a girl's parent by her first sexual partner—and for payments from the families of birthing women to midwives for birth assistance. These deep-rooted
reproductive practices, which have traditionally been means of controlling
male and female sexuality and organizing reproductive labor, have been altered by monetization, but they remain resilient, even as they are being reinvented as cultural practices in the current socioeconomic context. Pregnancy
for Mozambican women is embedded in this socially and politically charged
reproductive cycle that is fraught with heightened potential for both material
profit and social discord.

The stakes are high, for, as Federici and others have insisted, it is the reproductive and social reproductive labor of women that "re/produces the commodity of labor power. It is transformed into the wages of the current or future worker and as such is *commodified*, produces an exchange value rather than simply the utility or use value of labor" (Lilley and Shantz 2004; emphasis mine). Yet this work is neither paid nor socially valued:

> The exchange value [of reproductive labor] is cashed not by the house-worker but by the bearer of the labor power that the houseworker has reproduced. There is an assumption that the wage, the price paid by the boss for labor power, includes a payment for the costs of reproduction. If the worker is to bring their labor power to work everyday then they must be able to renew that labor power, with food, clothing and shelter, at an acceptable level to allow them to keep working at an adequate capacity.
>
> The problem with this assumption of course is that the payment is made to the worker, the bearer of the labor power commodity, rather than to the people, usually women, who have done the bulk of the work necessary to re/produce the commodity labor power. (Lilley and Shantz 2004)

It is the unpaid productive and reproductive labor of women that generates the surplus value that often provisions peasant and proletariat men and the national elite. Foreign banks and corporations take this value away in profit and call it wealth and economic growth. Under neoliberism, with more pressure on the household to sustain and reproduce itself with fewer and fewer inputs, it should be no surprise that women's unwaged reproductive labor is pushed further and further into the market. Fayorsey has examined these dynamics in Ghana. She describes the agency of urban Ghanaian women to negotiate complex relationships with multiple male partners over sex, pregnancy, childbirth, and children as a means to leverage the best material and social condition for themselves and their kin. She describes the sum of processes involved in pregnancy and childbirth as "a process which can be likened to 'buying' and 'selling' in the market place," which she labels "commoditization of reproduction" (1993: 21).

I expand Fayorsey's term "commoditization of reproduction" to include the sum of social relations of reproduction across the life cycle—that is, all the social relationships of power involved in reproduction—that have become monetized. "Commoditization of reproduction" thus encompasses all processes and practices related to social and biological reproduction, including pregnancy and childbirth, in which the exchange of money has replaced exchanges of labor, trust, respect, and other forms of social indebtedness and interdependence. The body politics that emerge when reproduction is commoditized signal a new "regime of value" (Appadurai 1996). In Mozambique, this regime pushes bodies into new courses of action and changes the meaning and motives of the contacts that link bodies in embraces, relationships, and kinship-based obligations for mutual support. It also turns some contacts into contracts. This shift is characterized by the erosion of women's sources of material subsistence and social support networks, and by intensified intrahousehold inequality, distrust, and conflict.

Women's bodies often bear the brunt of clashes that erupt when sex, marriage, birthing, and babies have monetary value to social actors with competing interests (see Fayorsey 1992 for the trend in Ghana). As pregnancy is itself a sign of good fortune and impending social wealth in Mucessua, it has the potential to arouse jealousy and distrust between neighbors and competition between women already sharing the attention and material and social-sexual capital of men through formal and informal polygynous arrangements. In addition to being at risk for pregnancy and birth complications, women are responsible through childbearing for balancing the debt incurred when their families receive elevated monetary bridewealth payments. Changes ripple throughout the reproductive cycle in this environment, which has been "infused with powerful possibilities, both threatening and alluring. These possibilities include not only the emergence of commodities and market exchanges, but also . . . the possibility of making any object into a commodity by transacting it in the appropriate (or inappropriate) manner" (Weiss 1996: 8). These gendered politics of reproduction further stimulate the dangerous cycle of pressure women are already under to bear children.

In response to these conditions, women in Mucessua experienced mounting fear of exposure to attacks on their reproductive capacity through witchcraft and sorcery practices, known locally as *feitiço*. Women's interpretations of feitiço as threats to reproductive health are elements of a culturally cogent system of social checks and balances that resonates in this atmosphere. As infertility and child mortality endanger women's social status and their ability to maintain relationships that mediate key material and social resources, women are intensely fearful of reproductive risks stemming from conditions of inequality, jealousy, and competition. Despite their fear of feitiço and high risk for pregnancy and birth complications, many Mozambican women with access to clinical maternity services delayed or avoided clinical prenatal consultations and hospital births. This avoidance limits opportunity for early detection and treatment of preventable complications (Murata et al. 1992), including anemia, syphilis, malaria and, more recently, mother-to-child transmission of HIV/AIDS.

Frequent reproductive complications and loss led pregnant women in Mucessua to seek protection among a vibrant array of alternative health care options that existed outside the formal government-run biomedical facilities. Instead of attending the prenatal clinic, they self-treated with local plants they collected in the bush or bought in the open-air market stalls, and with pharmaceuticals purchased in the open market or the only pharmacy. They went to Pentecostal and African Independent churches that offered healing through prayer, fasting, and laying on of hands. They patronized faith-healing prophets who cast out harmful spirits and used holy water in baths, enemas, emetics, and purgatives. They sometimes sought *curandeiros*—indigenous healers who consulted spirits through possession and other divination practices and used plant and nonplant preparations—and visited herbalists who used only plant-based therapies. They were customers of traveling nurses and drug vendors from Zimbabwe and South Africa selling pills and injections. Some women patronized Koro, the British mission-run clinic 15 kilometers away. This variety of options, or pluralism of the health system, has its roots in Mozambique's history and rapidly transforming political economy.

Even with scant access to and little control over material reserves and despite tremendous time and work constraints, pregnant women in Mucessua often generated the substantial social and economic capital necessary to leverage some control over their own reproductive experiences and to influence the physiological and social outcomes of pregnancy. They attempted to reduce their chances of reproductive loss, both in terms of infant and child survival and in terms of reproductive threats to securing relationships, making alliances, forming valued social identities, and attaining senior female status and some social and economic autonomy.[12] Such status was attained in the local social economy only by becoming the mother of children who survived to carry on the lineage name of a man who would claim paternity.

Mozambican women's efforts to protect themselves from reproductive harm constitute a paradox. On one hand they reflect "the destructive signature of poverty and oppression written on individual and social bodies" (Scheper-Hughes 1992: 533). On the other, they reflect the creative if sometimes contradictory means by which women attempt to survive and insist on continuity in the face of destitution and possibility. Why were women avoiding prenatal care? Or were they?

In Central Mozambique, as elsewhere in the world, women's concerns about what most health practitioners define as biological and medical risks were often expressed in terms of, overlapped with, or were completely eclipsed by social threats (Nichter 2003: 29; Nichter 2002; Etuk, Itam, and Asuquo 1999; Asowa-Omorodion 1997; Adetunji 1992; Sesia 1997; Eggleston 2000). For women in this world, reproductive vulnerability stems from public knowledge of their pregnant condition. The Shona word for a woman whose pregnancy is apparent from the swelling of her body is *chikotsa*, meaning either the one who sees, or the one who hides in order to conceal, save, or keep. For women in Mucessua, prenatal care is a process of layering protection against the reproductive threats they perceive around them with more help from church pastors, prophets, and indigenous healers, who deal directly with their perceptions of pregnancy threats as primarily social—and less from the formal biomedical system, which does not. Silence and secrecy are the first forms of prenatal care.

The Politics of Reproduction

My goal in writing *Family Secrets* is to provide insight into this paradox of practical health service use and global health challenge. I present a close look at the conditions of vulnerability and marginality that mediate women's use of health services directed specifically at them, and at the nature of the state policies and practices behind these services. I examine how, in a time of sweeping economic restructuring, communities, relationships, and lives unravel in ways that need to appear on the cost-benefit analysis ledgers of governments and multilateral lending institutions, but do not. The responsibility for the policies that render some lives surplus while creating wealth and profit elsewhere can too easily be displaced onto those very communities whose relative surplus value is being extracted or whose surplus lives leave few options but self-exploitation.

The character of livelihoods pursued on the margins of formal economic relationships and investments is often represented as the reason for the devaluation of life in the shadows of globalization, rather than the result of underinvestment and overexploitation. I seek to reframe reproductive risks (WHO 1978a; World Bank 1993), as reproductive threats that are historically contingent, sociopolitical constructs, and the biopolitics of women's long-standing and emergent reproductive health practices as "sites of struggle where women's bodies clash with capitalism" (Lilley and Shantz 2004). As both the subject of intellectual inquiry and the basis for political action, there is a need for local accounts of the particular ways that women's productive and reproductive bodies bear the brunt of subsidizing the "new international economic order" (Navarro 1986: 217–19), and the particular ways that they seek to "mitigate, resist and undo" these forces (Geronimus 1994).

Anthropological studies have not traditionally linked reproductive behavior to broader social processes and structural principles (Browner and Sargent 1996). Rather, anthropological approaches to the study of reproduction and especially of reproductive health seeking have focused on beliefs and values as they relate to reproductive behaviors and on the construction of explanatory models (Maternowska 2006: 37). This approach was grounded in the assumption that the main cause of underutilization of health services or of failure to conform to health promotion and disease prevention recommendations are incorrect "beliefs" informed by a coherent local explanatory model (Atkinson and Farias 1994).

Increasingly, however, anthropologists have begun to examine the relationship between pregnancy risk perceptions, the efforts women make to influence pregnancy course and outcome, and structural constraints on both risk perceptions and reproductive health decision making (Jok 1998; Madhaven and Bledsoe 2001; Browner 2001; Bledsoe with Banja 2002; Allen 2002; Inhorn 2003b). Engagement by medical anthropologists with the political economic aspects of reproduction has contributed to new interpretations of fertility and population studies data (Maternowska 2006: 37). For example, Mamdani's important study of the failure of family-planning programs in Manipur, India, signaled a shift toward a more critical framework for the study of fertility and fertility control across cultures (Mamdani 1973). As Sargent and Cordell (2003: 1971) found among Malian women immigrants in Paris, and Feldman-Savelsberg (1994) found among women in Cameroon, women in the most impoverished communities must carefully strategize their reproductive choices as they confront disintegrating social cohesion and increasing economic competition.

A new framework emerges when analysis places reproduction at the center of social theory, and when it calls attention to the impact of global processes on everyday reproductive experiences—a politics of reproduction (Ginsburg and Rapp 1995). As a theoretical point of reference, the politics of reproduction places women's everyday desires, disappointments, and creativity at the center of analysis. It calls attention to how the organization of reproduction in any society is a cultural construction shaped by social and political power at work on several interacting levels, including the semiotic and biophysical. A feminist approach to the politics of reproduction examines links between reproduction and gender organization and questions the mechanisms by which gender inequalities are produced, revealed, and challenged (ibid.: 6).

Recent studies from this perspective have, to some degree, two common aims—to transform traditional anthropological analyses of reproduction and to clarify the importance of making reproduction central to social theory (Ginsburg and Rapp 1995). For example, Soheir Morsy's analysis (1995a) of maternal mortality in Egypt considers the impact of historical changes in Egypt's state policies on women's health in conjunction with women's role in production and social reproduction. She illuminates the mechanisms by which state policies regarding maternal and child health prioritize population control strategies imposed by international aid donors. In another important example that takes a feminist politics of reproduction approach, Susan Greenhalgh's study (1994) of fertility and China's one-child birth rule reveals the ways that women have been both victims and agents of state control over childbearing. Joining three fields of anthropological inquiry—feminist, demographic, and political economic—Greenhalgh describes how peasant resistance to the state birth control policy, while successfully subverting the one-child rule, put women's bodies at risk and reinforced women's social subordination by reproducing the patriarchal and state-defined gender preference for sons over daughters.

These studies demonstrate the valuable ways in which reproduction provides an important terrain for the study of individual and community survival. Traditional anthropology's preoccupation with local-level holistic analyses associated with the "natural history" of human reproduction over the life cycle has been greatly expanded by the feminist agenda to bring reproduction to the center of social theory. Paying attention to the impact of larger processes on everyday reproductive pedagogies and daily reproductive practices produces a useful framework for understanding health decision making and directing services, resources, education, and outreach where they are needed most. As I followed women in Bairro Mucessua who were seeking safe passage through pregnancy and childbirth, a portrait emerged of a world in rapid transition and reproduction on the margins.

Mapping the Course of the Book

Three aspects of the birth I described at the beginning of this chapter help map the course I take through this book. First, this moment revealed key elements of the gendered dynamics of inequality at the roots of Mozambique's medically plural society. The relationships among the participants, setting, and unfolding drama of this event not only help explain women's seeking of various health options but also map the landscape in which they may find different healing options more or less available and more or less acceptable. I approach medical pluralism in Gondola as an array of healing sites from which women sought health care—not as separate systems or sectors (Kleinman and Kleinman 1980, 1986), but as options in a total social system (Stoner 1986: 47) "written into the 'natural' symbols that the body affords" (Comaroff 1985: 7). I focus on identifying therapeutic alternatives, recording women's uses of those therapeutic alternatives, and interpreting the signifying practice entailed by those choices, that is, "the process through which persons, acting on an external environment, construct themselves as social beings" (ibid.).

Within this framework, I emphasize the metamedical nature of the experience of pregnancy, not as illness, but as a transformative bodily process through which social categories and political power relations are expressed and social life organized. I document the ways that Mozambican women are responding to social and economic pressures they believe constitute the greatest threats to their reproductive and social health and to their unborn children. This case study paves the way for a better understanding of the costs of expanding inequality and the increasing commodification of social relationships in this moment of intensified global integration (Hart 2002: 13).

Second, the birth scenario raises questions about the adequacy of anthropological understandings of witchcraft and sorcery in contemporary African contexts. Rather than disappearing, so-called occult practices flourish in response to the deepening inequalities associated with the marginalization and commodification of social life in this particular chapter of "modernity" (Geschiere 1997). These inequalities spring from a world society whose exclusive membership combined with its ever-greater exposure "leaves most Africans today excluded from the economic and institutional conditions that they themselves regard as modern." How do we confront an analytic modernity that must be defined, in part, by the ways it "impede[s] and frustrate[s] African claims on the political and economic conditions of life that are normally characterized as modern" (Ferguson 2006: 167)? In what ways might we usefully consider the flourishing of witchcraft and sorcery alongside growing Pentecostal and African Independent church participation not only as complex responses to a "shared historical present" of the unequal, if alternative, modernities (Appadurai 1996; Hannerz 1996)? Might these African institutions be a product of global inequalities, and the shifting social forms that both enact and entrench the deeply gendered nature of these inequalities (White 2007)?

In Mucessua, social and spiritual threats shaped women's risk perceptions and informed their pregnancy actions. Their struggles to control reproduction and manage pregnancy propelled them to seek protection for themselves, their unborn infants, and their future fertility. I argue that localized and interpersonal experiences of inequality are played out through the daily drama of spiritual and social reproductive threats. I seek to expand the definition of reproductive health risks to include not only biological and social risks, but also the structural constraints and conjectural possibilities (Jessop 1982) —the structural violence—that stem from the economic and social marginalization of women and men in globalization's shadows, lack of access to basic resources, and systematic deficiencies in the health system. Strategies for surviving in this tension-ridden and materially impoverished environment have led to new ways to manage pregnancy risks and new prenatal practices, and have supported the sinuous nature of Mozambican gender roles.

For many in Mozambique, the primary and most feared cause of sickness lies in people's ability to make others suffer through witchcraft or sorcery. The language of "maternal vulnerability" and "reproductive threats" is more appropriate and potentially more useful than the language of "at risk," "pregnancy and maternal risks," or "obstetric risks," as I will show. What is needed is a deeper understanding of how inequalities associated with structural adjustment policies percolate into people's lives and social worlds and haunt their intimate relationships and decisions.

To arrive at this deeper understanding, I situate women's perceptions of and responses to reproductive threats in Bairro Mucessua in relation to their vulnerability in the *nova vida*—from economic marginalization to eroding social support. Women's economic marginalization is linked to changes in household structures and expectations. In turn, expectations and obligations between living and nonliving kin in the spirit world are central to the Shona healing system. Mozambique Shona healing beliefs and practices are embedded in the institution of kinship and in the institutions of witchcraft and sorcery, exposing the "dark side of kinship, . . . aggression within the family, where there should be only trust and solidarity" (Geschiere 1997: 11).

The third aspect of the birth story that guides the course of this book is its insistence that we see that as reproductive practices change, so do expectations of and resistances to the daily social performance of gender. What Dorothy Hodgson calls "these 'local' responses and resistances" constitute a critical reworking of the notion of Mozambican modernity. As Hodgson observes:

> Gender relations, in Africa as elsewhere, have never been merely a self-contained matter of "local" ideas or "local" practices. Throughout history and across space, "local" gender relations and ideologies have been constituted in interaction with translocal material, social and cultural processes; both men and women take advantage of the opportunities and constraints provided by these translocal flows to either reinforce or renegotiate not only their relationships, but their dominant concepts of masculinity and femininity as well. These "local" responses and resistances have, in turn, produced what Watts calls "a working and reworking of modernity. . . . Globality and locality are inextricably linked, but through complex mediations and reconfigurations of 'traditional' society; the nonlocal processes driving capital mobility are always experienced, constituted and mediated locally." (Hodgson 1997: 111)

The commodification of core reproductive practices aggravates women's economic vulnerability, and gets played out in terms of social, spiritual, and reproductive risks related to witchcraft and sorcery. The long-standing reproductive practices of masunggiro (seduction fees) and lobolo (bridewealth payments) intended to control sexuality and reproductive labor have been altered by monetization but remain significant, if reinvented, in the current social economy. The commoditization of reproductive practices appears to have fractured critical sources of social support necessary for safe motherhood. The event of pregnancy presents a prism through which to view these daily effects of growing inequality in women's lives. As Leith Mullings notes: "In the global context of population policies, disease, and disasters of all kinds, local populations seek to envision continuity through children and to act to ensure that continuity" (1995: 123).

In the next chapter, I locate Bairro Mucessua and myself as researcher in time and space. Chapter 3 lays out the specific constellation of political and historical factors that localize women's reproductive vulnerability in Mozambique today. This chapter situates women's reproductive vulnerability in the broader historical context of social and economic restructuring at the household, community, and nation-state levels.

In Chapter 4, I place the meanings and experiences of pregnancy in Mucessua within a larger, culturally defined reproductive cycle, which includes the social reproductive structures by which communities envision, organize, and attempt to ensure and control their continuity through children. Chapter 5 examines the related influences of growing commodification of social life and increasing female economic marginalization on specific reproductive practices: virginity examinations, virgin seduction fees, bridewealth payments, and childbirth assistance.

Chapter 6 answers the question: Why do women in Mucessua routinely delay or avoid clinical prenatal care? I follow women through pregnancy and analyze the patterns of health care seeking that emerge.

Chapter 7 focuses on local concepts of reproduction and the underlying theories of illness and health through which Mucessuan women give meaning to their experiences of vulnerability during pregnancy.

In Chapter 8, I look at how attention to the dynamics of secrecy and hiding during pregnancy is more crucial than ever in providing effective HIV/AIDS treatment to women and in the prevention of mother-to-child transmission of HIV. Why do HIV-positive pregnant women and their HIV-exposed infants fall through the cracks of HIV/AIDS treatment opportunities, even as services have become more accessible?

If you are wondering what became of the birthing mother and her newborn girl, I confess I do not know. When I returned to the maternity clinic the next day to check on them, the nurses told me that the two had gone home earlier that morning. Where? They did not know. I returned to the prophet-healer, who said she was not certain where the woman lived and gave me vague directions that, after much searching in another bairro, led me to a house that might have been her home. No one was there, and the neighbors reported that they had not seen the inhabitants recently. I returned several times during my remaining months in Mozambique, but never found the woman. Not knowing the ending to that story, I am left with questions, secrets, silence, and a stream of hypotheses about why so-called high-risk women underutilize reproductive health services. Searching for answers has kept me on the road to Mucessua.

CHAPTER 2

The Road to Mucessua

Radical hope first drew me to Mozambique. In 1989, I was active in the anti-apartheid movement in Los Angeles, California, where I worked with a local branch of a national grassroots organization, the Mozambique Support Network. Its objectives were community outreach and education about Mozambique and the externally funded civil war there that began soon after Mozambican Independence in 1975. Our group's messages focused on U.S. involvement in that war of destabilization and exposed the effects of South Africa's apartheid policies on the frontline states—Mozambique, Angola, Swaziland, Lesotho, and Namibia—which share part or all of their borders with South Africa. We always brought the message back home by comparing South African apartheid with institutional and interpersonal racism and state violence against people of color in the United States, a message reinforced by the 1992 Rodney King police abuse case not-guilty verdicts and the ensuing mass uprisings. We publicized Mozambique's forward-looking constitution, a blueprint for a society free of race, class, and gender bias. For all these reasons, Mozambique's history and struggle resonated with me.

In his opening speech at the 1973 founding conference of the Organização das Mulheres Moçambicanas (OMM), the Organization of Mozambican Women, Samora Machel, the first president of Independent Mozambique, spoke of the commitment of the socialist government of the Frente de Liberação de Moçambique (FRELIMO) to women's participation in the new nation state:[1]

> The emancipation of women is not an act of charity, the result of a humanitarian or compassionate attitude. The liberation of women is a fundamental necessity for the revolution, the guarantee of its continuity and the precondition for its victory. The main objective of the revolution is to destroy the system of exploitation and build a new society which releases the potential of human beings, reconciling them with labour and with nature. This is the context within which the question of women's emancipation arises.

Indeed, FRELIMO had begun to put these words into action even prior to Independence. Many women had joined the party during the opposition movement as political mobilizers, some holding positions of leadership. Many more women took up arms and fought in the women's military detachment. In 1973, FRELIMO helped organize OMM, a democratic popular organization mobilized to address the issues of women's integration in the anticolonial movement; women worked side by side with men in seizing freedom for Mozambique from the Portuguese in 1975 (Isaacman and Isaacman 1983: 91; 1984). The long-term goals were to articulate and implement social changes necessary for women's emancipation as a critical aspect of the broader struggle for human liberation. This vision for improving women's lives eventually propelled me across the globe to Mozambique.

A View from *o Ceu* (the Sky)

Looking down from the airplane window between the national capital, Maputo, and Beira, the capital of Sofala Province, the landscape is parched and grayish with the exception of a few orange-red dirt roads. All the fields look drab and sparse, like hair on a malnourished child. I am surprised by all the neat rows of houses and neighborhoods so far away from any city or town. I wonder what the different patterns of cultivation of the land mean, orderly and measured in some places and crazy-quilt in others. I can see where a river once snaked, a ribbon of lush green growth curving and then ending.

We have gained altitude quickly, and the land below fades even further behind what looks like smoke. Through a layer of yellowish haze high above the land we climb up and up to a strip of blue sky, my ears popping and stomach unsettled. Below are fewer patches and more large shapes—former lakes? A town sparkles briefly through the cloud smog as we skim over, along a new horizon of the smoke against a light blue sky. Now rivers and careful, well-defined fields in different shades and shapes, scattered houses, then just stretches of grasslands.

Only recently can you arrive in the center of Mozambique by commercial plane and land in the Beira airport on the coast. The glare of the sun on the tarmac as you disembark momentarily blinds you and the dense heat blurs your senses. It is useful to locate yourself by map as you drive away from the aqua sea to Manica Province. Manica Province is located at the waist of Mozambique where it bends slightly toward the Indian Ocean. At the navel of Manica Province is the district of Gondola. Gondola is part of the central plateau area of the province, called the Manica-Chimoio-Sussundenga peneplain; its altitudes range from 400 to 700 meters. The boundary between the central plain and the low-lying plain to the south is marked by prominent escarpments formed by a series of major geological faults. On the central plain itself, however, the topography of Gondola is gently undulating to flat, with broad ridges and isolated, steep-sided inselbergs. Vegetation on the plain originally consisted of old-growth, semi-deciduous, high-rainfall Miombo woodland, the main species being *Brachystegia spiciformis, B. boehmii,* and *Julbernadia globiflora.* However, due to past cultivation cycles the vegetation is now largely secondary growth.[2]

The general climate of this region is warm and humid, with two distinct seasons—a rainy season from November to March and a dry winter season from May to August, with April torn in half by thunderstorms and brief tropical downpours. The average total annual rainfall on the peneplain is about 1,000mm, increasing to 1,500mm and more as elevation increases to the north and west, and decreasing to as little as 500mm to 600mm as elevation slopes down into the Save River valley. At this altitude, mean monthly and daily temperatures on the central plateau are more constant throughout the year than in the western mountains. Average temperatures ranging from 17°C to 20°C in the summer season (representing the main growing season) combine with a rainy season and growing season of 150 days or more to produce a climate very favorable for crop growing. This hospitable climate and the zone's characteristic well-drained, red, sandy, clay loam soil help explain the relatively high level of colonial and postcolonial commercial development and current heavy settlement by the family farming sector in the Gondola District area (MAARP 1995a: 6–30; Tique 2002).

First Steps

During my first trip to Mozambique, in 1991, the war of destabilization was still under way. Traveling by day and returning to the capital city, Maputo, before dark and a possible rebel attack, I spent several weeks making a short documentary film about a woman's agricultural collective, *Primeiro de Maio,* May First, located on the outskirts of Maputo in an area circling the city called the Green Zones.[3] What struck me most about this community was the near absence of men and the fierce, animated pride among the women of Primeiro de Maio. The twenty-eight-member cooperative included one man. Another man had been hired on a temporary basis to plow the fields with his tractor, and another to paint the chicken coops. But it was women who ran the collective, organized finances, worked in the fields, sold the produce, made plans for the use of profits, cooked meals, and took care of their own and each other's children in a busy and happy *crèche* (day care for young children and babies).

The children sang at the top of their lungs under the direction of their shy and gentle teacher and caretaker, twenty-year-old Augustina:

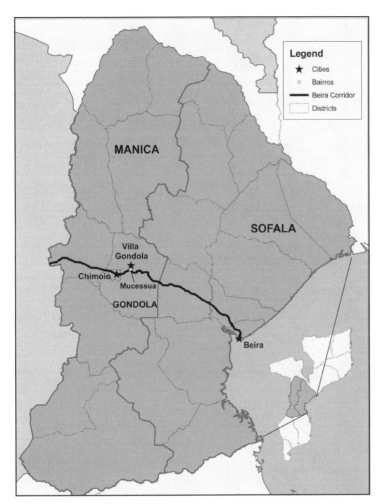

Manica and Sofala Provinces, Central Mozambique.
Inset: Mozambique.

The crèche is a garden.
The children are flowers.
The teacher is a gardener,
who waters us with love.

The women spoke openly about the ways their conventional domestic and productive roles had already changed as a result of the war. Many people were forced from rural, ancestral lands and separated from members of their families by flight from violence and by death. And yet, despite the constant presence of war, there was great eagerness and excitement among the women of the collective at the efficacy and achievement they felt in successfully running their large farm, which produced eggs and vegetables to sell in the city. They believed that the efforts of the independent Mozambican government to collectivize labor, to nationalize land, education, and health care, and to create communal villages, and its promise to bring women into the decision-making process at every level of the political system, still signaled real changes for women's control over their own lives and the lives of their children. This was just the kind of optimism for improving women's lot in life that I had idealistically anticipated in my sojourn to Mozambique.

Two years later, in 1993, I returned to Mozambique as a full-time employee of a small U.S. nongovernmental organization (NGO), the Mozambique Health Committee (now Health Alliance International). Based in Central Mozambique, this project was and continues to be run out of the International Health Program at the University of Washington School of Public Health. My position was assistant to Senhor Paulinho Davisson, provincial director of health education for Manica Province and its population of one million. In this capacity I was involved in many activities, including rural community health assessment research; the development of maternal and child health education materials; HIV/AIDS education in rural villages, factories, and secondary schools; latrine building and other sanitation projects; and vaccination campaigns.

It was, however, as an organizer of community health councils that I gained a local reputation, and this story unfolds out of my experiences in this specific relationship to a community. Participation in the community council program laid the groundwork for the questions I would later explore. Through my role in the project I gained familiarity and trust in Bairro Mucessua, where I would later conduct extensive field research. Working with the community councils, I met the woman who would become my primary research assistant, Dona Javelina Aguiar. Most critically, however, I experienced firsthand the struggle for control over health and healing as I watched health issues debated from different perspectives within the health hierarchy—foreign health development experts and administrators, biomedically trained Mozambican health professionals, popular healers, religious specialists, and laypeople.

A View from *a Rua* (the Road)

Coming to Bairro Mucessua by car from either direction, you must first arrive at the administrative center of Gondola District, Vila Gondola, at one time a key stopping point on the colonial Beira Railway Company line that ran from the border of then Southern Rhodesia to the once-bustling port of Beira. Over time, Vila Gondola became a truck and bus stop sandwiched between the railroad tracks and the Beira Corridor, a single-lane, pothole-filled tarmac road that links landlocked and resource-rich Zimbabwe to the

Indian Ocean. Today, Gondola is a dilapidated town, still organized around and spread outward from the Gondola Railway Station. Along its dirt roads are charred and rusting parts of abandoned civilian and military vehicles and houses and shops with deteriorating walls, crumbling stairs and porches, and missing doors and windows—ghostly shadows of colonial and state ambitions aborted by war and poverty.

The concentration of people in Gondola, as well as of private and state investment, reflects the concentration of colonial enterprise in the area, the degree to which postindependence state ventures reproduced colonial patterns, and the population movement and destruction that followed the most recent war. The Corridor's relative safety made it a haven where people from surrounding districts could escape the violence of the war and a site for continued investment (Alexander 1994: 4).

The Corridor brought to Gondola hordes of people fleeing the war. Many of these deslocados are the inhabitants of Bairro Mucessua. Forced or removed from their lands by war or famine, deslocados did not flee the country but remained, "dislocated," "out of articulation," with their way of living, which was tied to a specific piece of land where their ancestors lie buried (Galli 2003; Gengenbach 1998). Deslocados became squatters in Mucessua, with even less access to resources than the extremely poor majority of the community. People with resources and education tended to live closer to town or in the provincial capital, Chimoio. Most deslocados and recent returnees from refugee camps have been absorbed over time into the bairro or returned in the aftermath of the ceasefire to their rural, ancestral, and thus sacred lands (Hughes 1999). The Beira Corridor also meant business for the small, bustling Gondola open market, the dingy bars and shops, and the barefoot vendors hawking wares of doughy fried pastry balls, tangerines, and bananas to any stopping vehicle. It also meant transport for goods and people to bigger markets, to the city of Beira to the east and the town of Chimoio and the border with Zimbabwe to the west.

Leaving the Beaten Path

While working in the Provincial Health Directorate I frequently heard my clinical health care colleagues complain that women were not coming into prenatal clinics until late in their pregnancies, not coming in until they were already in labor and arriving to give birth, or not coming in at all. Many women came into the clinics only after giving birth at home in order to have their babies weighed, vaccinated, and registered in the maternity ward birth registry. Health workers in the formal sector also complained that too many of the women who came only to give birth had serious complications stemming from improper care during attempted home deliveries, especially orders to push before complete dilation and the use of potent indigenous herbal medicines to bring on or speed up labor. When home deliveries went awry, these complications ended up as hospital emergencies, often too late for intervention.

As the assistant to the director of health education in Manica Province, I was assigned to help create community health councils throughout the province (Alinsky 2001). The main objective of reviving the community health council project in the 1990s was to improve village health status by enlisting the participation and support of locally identified community leaders to help increase participation in preventive health activities like prenatal care. In development terms, our strategy was to "empower" communities to identify local health problems and then to discover their own "sustainable" solutions using local resources (World Bank 1993).

During the implementation of this project, however, tensions emerged around the competition between community leaders and health personnel for ownership of the councils. To whom did the councils belong? That is, whose bidding were they to do? My orientation led me to insist that the councils belonged to the voluntary members themselves and to the communities they had come together to serve. My Mozambican health professional colleagues, however, saw the councils' primary reason for existence to be educating and influencing local people to participate in existing preventive health programs in the formal health sector—vaccination campaigns; prenatal, family-planning, and child health clinics; and environmental sanitation mobilizations. All involved generally felt that the first year of the community council project met with both successes and failures (Alinsky 2001; Gurolla-Bonilla 1995). Despite doubt about the sustainability of the councils without the input of wealthy international NGOs, the project was held up as a model for national replication.

As part of the protocol for community needs assessment and group health discussions with community councils, I always asked the women participating in the councils about their primary health concerns and "felt health needs." Time after time, they responded that the greatest health problems women faced were their own sickness and death during pregnancy and childbirth and the illness and death of their infants and children. Infertility was also a frequent complaint. From women's jokes about adultery, I learned about the generations-old fears that extramarital sex causes prolonged or difficult labor and sudden illness in a breast-feeding child. Many conversations included comments about the constant difficulties of pregnant and birthing women and revealed a great general awareness of the importance of prenatal care.

Yet, despite their awareness of the high maternal and infant morbidity and mortality, community leaders and other laypeople did not articulate a link between women's late initiation of prenatal clinic visits in the formal health system and their risk of complications in pregnancy and childbirth. In fact, extreme distrust of the formal medical system prevailed, so widespread that many mothers of pregnant adolescents, for example, opted for their daughters to avoid formal prenatal care altogether. According to national maternal health norms, all adolescent pregnancies were identified as high-risk obstetrics (ARO or *alto risco obstetrico*, Pt.) because of the high potential among that age group for pregnancy complications such as anemia and obstetric emergencies like obstructed labor due to cephalo-pelvic disproportion.[4] At the level of the community, however, this medical statistic translated into awareness that adolescents were especially likely to be transferred to the provincial hospital to give birth. Because their *lugar do parto*, the birth canal and vaginal opening, might be too small, the baby must be removed by *uma operação* (cesarean section). To assure that their daughters avoided this fate—being sent to the city without relatives to bring food and bedding to the laboring mother, or even hot water for bathing—many mothers did not allow their adolescent daughters identified as ARO to return for follow-up visits at the maternity clinic, preferring to prepare them for birth at home with indigenous medicines and perineal massage to stretch the *lugar do parto*.

It soon became evident that the formal sector was only one option among many that women turned to for reproductive health care. My primary research assistant, Javelina, turned out to be an expert on the subject. She had experienced infertility in her first marriage and been divorced as a result. Twelve years and numerous treatments from many sources later, she gave birth to her first son. With Javelina's help, I sought out local healers, herbalists, prophets, and spirit diviners who treated reproductive health problems. The Pentecostal and African Independent churches seemed to be doing the most for pregnant women and mothers. From weekly meetings to teach women proper hygiene during pregnancy and outline appropriate lengths of time for postpartum sexual abstinence, to laying on of hands and group fasting, casting out spirits, and prescribing holy-water baths, enemas, emetics, and purgatives, churches were indeed offering a wide range of treatments for women's reproductive health ailments. While the maternity clinic failed to bring most women in before their sixth month of pregnancy, churches were seeing women before conception, and more frequently and more consistently throughout pregnancy. Women were getting prenatal care in their first two trimesters, but not from the maternity clinic.

That pregnant women went late to the formal health sector was well documented. A study of the prenatal syphilis-screening program that was part of the Safe Motherhood Initiative in Manica Province confirmed what the formal health sector knew anecdotally: counter to existing public health education messages, pregnant women in the general population were not following the "norm" of initiating prenatal consultations in the formal sector during the first trimester of their pregnancies; they generally came in during their second or third trimester, and inconsistently. According to Lafort's study of 1,016 pregnant women, an estimated 69 percent of all pregnant women in the district of Gondola, where Bairro Mucessua is located, initiated prenatal care in a government clinic at some time in their pregnancy. Of these, 82 percent came in after the fourth month of pregnancy. The median time for initiating prenatal care in the formal sector was 5.8 months gestation for the entire sample, and 6.0 months in Gondola. Of the women seen at a biomedical facility for prenatal care, 44 percent did not return to give birth in the formal sector. The remaining 31 percent of pregnant women were assumed to have avoided the formal maternal health clinics altogether (Lafort 1994).

These data from Lafort's study suggested a multilayered problem. The figures had serious implications for screening and treating sexually transmitted infections, as well as for identifying and monitoring high-risk births. However, as might be expected, individuals and groups with disparate points of view and agendas interpreted the data differently. From the perspective of the staff at biomedical maternity facilities, the data pointed to a case of "non-compliance" with national norms conveyed through health education messages and "underutilization" of antenatal services. Lafort, a Belgian physician with long medical experience in Mozambique, had concluded in his study that due to the estimated high number of women who came into the formal system, it was unlikely that there existed any other parallel "system" of prenatal care being used by pregnant women (Lafort 1994: 10).

I believed there was too little data available to accurately assess alternative reproductive health options available to pregnant women. No one had ever asked women themselves what else they were doing, just focused on what they were not doing. Systematic information was needed concerning both women's central motives and strategies for seeking prenatal care and the local context of political uncertainty and economic insecurity in which individual women and households were making reproductive health care decisions and giving meaning and organization to the process of reproduction. I set out to explore women's reproductive choices and behavior relating to pregnancy and childbirth in a complex, medically plural system.

Why did women routinely avoid prenatal care or initiate prenatal consultations in the formal biomedical health sector late (second or third trimester) in their pregnancies? My search for answers to this question drew me further and further into the fragile and often messy terrain of human lives. I uncovered layer upon layer of threats to women that informed each aspect of the unfolding drama of reproduction, as well as reproductive loss and death. I found I could understand each layer of women's vulnerability and their efforts to overcome it in Bairro Mucessua only by delving into the historical and political context of postwar Mozambique via what Marcus and Fischer (1999: 86) have called "an interpretive anthropology fully accountable to its historical and political-economy implications." This approach obliges me to be accountable in my analysis to the influence of the broader forces of gender-power relationships and socioeconomic destabilization. At the same time, I must stay grounded in the everyday textures and rhythms of the love and labor of making ends meet when they do not. Paul Farmer has called this "an interpretive anthropology of affliction" (1992: 256).

People do not often stand still in the face of hardship. Rather they perform all manner of what Leith Mullings has termed "transformative action"—the daily labor of surviving under great adversity—which involves two kinds of efforts: "efforts to sustain continuity under transformed circumstances and efforts to transform circumstances in order to maintain continuity" (Mullings 1995: 133). Some social analyses have criticized this attempt to document the tiniest slivers of human agency for leading to overly romanticized claims of class resistance and culture change. More frequently, this kind of social reproductive labor remains unseen, unacknowledged, its labor value taken for granted. And yet, awareness of this frequently invisible toil, usually unpaid and most often done by women, could lead to an accounting and valuation in which the rewards of such effort are not simply another week, another day, another hour of life, but an experience of a week, day, or hour of living that creates hope or meaning and thus purpose to continue. We should not underestimate the material, social, and political value of this work but rather examine and understand it.

In an important extension of James Scott's seminal work detailing everyday forms of peasant resistance, which he called "weapons of the weak"— "the ordinary weapons of normally powerless groups" (1985: 29)—Leith Mullings elucidates another set of such weapons. Wielded in the domain of social reproduction, transformative labor describes the positive force of the labor power of "prosaic but constant struggle" not between the peasantry and those who exploit them, but among peasants themselves for their daily survival. Mullings's notion of transformative work requires us to recognize that even the smallest activities reveal human agency and its limits (Ginsburg and Rapp 1995: 11; Scott 1990). However, in research on reproduction, until recently, two concepts of culture and human agency have dominated thinking in anthropology and demography. Carter (1995: 55) calls these the passive concept, which represents people as mindlessly following cultural norms, and the active concept, which portrays individuals as conscious decision makers who purposefully choose their fertility levels through abstract reason. He criticizes both models, maintaining that the passive notion of culture that denies human agency does not hold up in the face of ethnographic evidence, and that the notion that people act as rational utility maximizers is untenable because maximization is too complex and time consuming to account for daily, ongoing cognitive processes.

A reinterpretation of the core anthropological concepts of culture and agency offers a solution to the conundrum of attributing agency to de-mographic actors without endowing them with utility-maximizing ratio-nality. Drawing on the work of Anthony Giddens (1979) and Jean Lave (1988), anthropologists interested in the demographic aspects of fertility have made significant advances in reconceptualizing reproduction as a so-cially constructed process. Carter, for example, usefully redefines human agency,

> not as a sequence of discrete acts of choice and planning, the standard view, but as a reflexive monitoring and rationalization of a continuous "flow of conduct," in which practice is constituted in dialectical relation between persons acting and the setting of their activities. In this way, both cultural concepts—the values assigned to different behaviors—and political economy—the forces creating the setting—become ingredients to, rather than external to, action, and the human agent is placed center stage. (Carter 1995: 55)

Indeed, however constrained their options were by the local, national, or even international setting, women in Mucessua acted to mix the ingredients of their own reproductive lives. Neither passive rule followers nor equation-running maximizers, Mucessuan women undertook shifting and often para-doxical efforts to protect themselves from reproductive risk, sustain daily life, and create new life under changing conditions made difficult by new inequalities. Their efforts indicate an intricate and contested nature of local cultural logic. Pregnant women sought to protect their bodies in ways that had meaning on multiple levels: as individual, biological entities; as actors in various social relationships constantly redefined in terms of emergent mate-rial conditions; and as members of the larger, changing body politic. At each level, every day, women labored, played roles, assumed and lost value, experi-enced vulnerability, and sought to protect themselves.

A Path through the Thorns: Research Methods and Site

The original goal of my research was to establish a practical knowledge base about women's reproductive choices and health-seeking behavior dur-ing pregnancy in a complex medically plural system where the socialist gov-ernment had made access to comprehensive primary health care a central component of the independent state agenda for social transformation (Walt 1983). While there was a high coverage of women by the government-run prenatal clinics in Manica Province, a majority of women initiated consul-tations after their first trimester of pregnancy, and more than half did not return to give birth at the maternity ward (Lafort 1994).

I established a number of research objectives to answer the specific question: Why do women routinely initiate prenatal care consultations in the formal biomedical health sector late (second or third trimester) in their pregnancies? These were: to provide an ethnography of pregnancy focusing on community knowledge, attitudes, and beliefs about pregnancy and prenatal health care; to identify and analyze patterns of prenatal health care–seeking of a representative sample of pregnant women; to identify and describe the wide range of health care facilities and providers women used during pregnancy and childbirth; and to create a taxonomy of pregnancy conditions and treatments.

I gathered data from formal interviews and reproductive health questionnaires with eighty-three women of reproductive age, during pregnancy and after birth, from life histories and compound mapping with a subset of women from the pregnancy case study group and from focus group sessions with women, adolescent girls, and men across the bairro. My first objectives with the focus groups were to introduce myself across the community and check the feasibility of the project by gauging women's openness to participating, and to recruit pregnant women into the case study group. I then intended to explore the range of women's attitudes, practices, and options related to pregnancy, prenatal care, and reproductive health–seeking.

In addition, I collected data on health care alternatives in Mucessua through in-depth interviews of formal and informal-sector health care providers, including doctors, nurses, midwives, diviner-healers, church prophets and pastors, herbalists, pharmacists, and health administrators; and I conducted observations at their sites of practice. I participated in the daily activities of women in Mucessua and coincidentally was pregnant and gave birth during the research period. In many ways, being pregnant made possible the intimacy I eventually was able to establish with many of the women in the study. From their perspective, my being pregnant for the first time and far away from my mother made me the object of pity and maternal concern. I was quickly taken under their wings and taught what to do and not to do for a healthy pregnancy and birth.

The Side of the Road

Bairro Mucessua is located on the south side of the Beira Corridor, which is its northern border, as the road passes through the center of Vila Gondola. Mucessua is bounded on the east and west by trickling riverbeds, with River Mucessua to the east, from which the bairro gets its name. On foot, Bairro Mucessua is accessible from the Corridor by myriad dusty footpaths and four sandy dirt roads that are sometimes impassable by car. During the rainy season these roads are eroded into deep ruts of red mud. The footpaths descend gently between the single row of shops, including a bar, a pharmacy, a bank, and a bakery, past the stone Catholic Church and the secondary school, all next to the crumbling asphalt of the Beirra Corridor. The paths wind past clusters of cement houses built during the colonial period along-side and behind the shops of European and Indian merchants and function-aries, and past the fine dwellings of the rare Mozambican railway employee with resources to construct them.

According to the local oral history of Mucessua, a Portuguese settler opened up the first road in the bairro in the 1940s to access land granted by the Companhia de Moçambique to develop commercial tangerine or-chards for export. Africans then lived widely dispersed in rural, patrilineal kinship-based compounds. The first three cement houses in Mucessua, built in the 1950s, belonged to Indian and Portuguese merchants. A Mozambican, Senhor Quingue, built a fourth house from materials bought with money he earned shoveling coal on the railway. Quingue owned all the land sur-rounding his cement house and planted it with corn and millet. He lives in the same house today, but instead of crops, small, wooden pole-frame and mud-brick houses of squatters, refugees from the war of destabilization, clut-ter the slopes behind it. Now over sixty, Senhor Quingue remembers the encroachment beginning in the early days of the anticolonial struggle with the Portuguese for Mozambican Independence: "Even before the war with RENAMO, I saw people begin to move onto my land. They wanted to live close to the town. I didn't turn them away because it was also a time of war. In those days the distrust between Portuguese and African began."

Many of the older one- and two-story cement buildings of the colonial period in Gondola are faded and in disrepair. Their dirty milk-white, shell, or blue-green walls are stained from the rusty red cloud of the dust that settles on everything—on the occasional glass windows, and here and there on the decorative hand-painted tiles and the ornate, whitewashed, wrought iron gates and window bars brought by settlers from Portugal, on the undersides of goats and chickens, on the legs and mostly bare feet of people going to and from fields and market, and on the children, sometimes covering them from head to toe, red dust clinging to running noses and festering sores.

Most of the houses are state owned since the nationalization of Portu-guese properties at Independence in 1975, their keys leased to residents by the nationalized state housing organization. The inhabitants are primarily merchants of South Asian descent, district-level Mozambican government functionaries and their relatives, a few foreign missionaries, Mozambican employees of what is now Mozambique Railway (CFM), other educated Mozambicans with access to money through formal employment or trade, and most rarely, Mozambican peasants who held onto their claim on colonial houses that had belonged to the Portuguese. Given twenty-four hours to evacuate the country, the former owners had fled on the eve of Independence, destroying as much as they could of the property and material wealth they were forced to leave behind.

Sampling, Secrets, and Other Detours

When I finally started formal research after having lived and worked in Mozambique for two years, things got off to a frustratingly unproductive start, as a journal entry from February 1994 after my first days of formal research reflects:

> This morning we have been walking door to door looking for pregnant women to see if they agree to be participants in the study. We have visited twenty-five houses and have only three potential participants. In one home a woman tells us that her pregnant daughter is not at home, but we can come back to talk with the girl tomorrow. Another young girl, clearly pregnant, on being asked if she would like to participate in the study, denied that she was pregnant at all! As we passed on to the next house, an onlooking neighbor watched us intently from over the hedge surrounding her house, and waved us over into her well-swept yard.
>
> "*Coitado* (Poor dear)! This is her first pregnancy, and she is living in her mother-in-law's house, right under her mother-in-law's foot! You cannot blame her for trying to hide *segredos da casa* (family secrets)." Without permission, she was not free to let out her secret. A third woman has agreed, but was very hesitant and would not tell us what month she was expecting. Javelina says that the fear of feitiço—sorcery—is very strong, even though the tradition is not as powerful as it used to be. "In the past," she explained, "one always knew who the feitiçeiros (sorcerers) were, and could identify them and keep clear of their path. These days, one doesn't know."

There was so much silence surrounding pregnancy in Mucessua that for a few weeks, I thought I might have to abandon the project altogether. My plan had been to go to each tenth compound across the five bairro cells until I could find a hundred pregnant women who would agree to participate in the study. But when my research assistant, Javelina, and I were met with such distrust and even fear, and I became aware of the unwanted attention we were drawing to women in Mucessua, I abandoned the strategy. I felt it would damage the sense of trust I needed to work on such a sensitive issue if we continued visiting house to house uninvited.

Since I had already scheduled focus groups with women in each cell of the bairro, Javelina and I decided that we would invite any pregnant women who showed up at the focus groups to participate in the study. This strategy gave women the option of exposing their condition if they desired rather than us exposing or embarrassing them. Bumping up against and, in fact, breaching the invisible social structures that made it taboo to publicly draw attention to someone's wealth and thus to their vulnerability, I fell back as I should have from the beginning on the formal social structure that mapped out a different but safer path to women's subjective experience—the government party structure.

Underneath its seemingly random and inviting dusty paths, the neighborhood of Mucessua was rigidly mapped along the lines of the socialist government party structure put in place after Independence in 1975. Following Independence, FRELIMO renamed Portuguese East Africa the People's Republic of Mozambique and implemented a multitiered government and party structure that reached from the national level to the provincial, district, and bairro or *aldeia* (village) levels, and then to the level of every ten houses (*dez casas*). While rural populations were encouraged to move, sometimes forcibly, into communal villages, the administrative centers and towns were organized into bairros. Invisible to my eyes, a map from the colonial anti-insurgency period hovered just below these collectivizing initiatives, causing some Mozambicans to note the irony that the proud socialist party structure was quite similar to the colonial structures that people had fought so hard to overthrow. In this complex social-political terrain I often found myself floundering—lost, looping in circles, stuck at abrupt dead ends, or pushing against invisible barriers.

Manica Province is divided into ten administrative districts. Each district has an administrative center, or *sede*, and is divided into administrative *postos* (posts), each made up of several *localidades* (localities). Each locality is divided into rural villages—*aldeias* or bairros—that form the boundaries of towns and cities. Appointed government officials direct government activities and services at each level. Bairros and *aldeias* are organized in a similar manner. Mucessua, one of five bairros making up the administrative post of the district of Gondola, is divided into four cells—*cellulas* A, B, C, and D. Each cell consists of a number of quarters or blocks called *quarteirões*. In each *quarteiro*, there are aggregates of households or compounds called *agregados*, which are often clustered around a common senior male family head. Individual families live on *talhões*, plots or compounds that make up the agregados.

Party organization in the bairro follows this physical layout. At the head of the bairro party structure, a party member is appointed to act as the bairro president, who represents the bairro at the level of the district and serves on both district- and bairro-level tribunals. The bairro president presides over the popularly elected Comité do Circulo do Bairro, the Bairro Committee Circle, which is headed by the first bairro secretary, who sits on the bairro-level justice tribunal.[5] Under the first bairro secretary is a secretary of organization and a secretary of information, mobilization, and propaganda. Just under these posts, also at the level of the bairro, is a bairro secretary of the Mozambican Women's Organization (OMM). In each cell there is another secretary with three assistants, a secretary of OMM, and one for the Mozambican Youth Organization (OJM). A *chefe* is elected at the quarteiro level and another at the level of every ten houses.

Working through the bairro secretary and with the mobilization of the OMM, women of child-bearing age were encouraged to take part in the focus group meeting in their cell. When one of my focus groups was to be held, the bairro secretary of OMM would contact representatives in the chosen cell to mobilize all women, especially pregnant women. On the morning of the meeting, usually about ten to fifteen women appeared. After explaining my study and asking general questions about pregnancy experiences and beliefs, I asked if any pregnant women would participate in the study. I offered no monetary compensation but said I would be as helpful as I could to the mothers who agreed to participate, for example, with transport when available. Some women would only volunteer discreetly, appearing later at Javelina's house to sign up.

In the end, eighty-seven women between the ages of fifteen and forty-nine participated in the research, though four women moved away before the end of the interviews. Most had very little schooling, averaging 2.6 years. Only one woman had completed secondary school. The majority of households were extremely poor, and household incomes were low and sporadic, and fluctuated seasonally. The average household income of 91,000 meticais (U.S. $9) per month was less than one-third of what the government estimated was needed to feed a household of seven for a month on top of adequate subsistence food crop reserves (MOH 1993). Only eight women reported having sufficient grain supplies to last until the next harvest. Women's positions in these households were especially precarious, as they usually did not have access to or control of cash needed to feed themselves and their children, while opportunities for them to earn income were limited. Two women were formally employed, both as domestics in government offices, and only one-third of the women reported earning cash that remained in their control, mostly selling extra garden produce. Most of the women had access to *machambas*, parcels of land cultivated with staple crops for family consumption and sale. About one-third had access to *matoros*, small vegetable gardens along riverbeds where they cultivated vegetables and fruits for home consumption, production of home-brewed alcohol, and sale in the market.

A View from *o Caminho* (a Footpath)

Entering Mucessua, one sees smaller, new houses of russet, sun- or kiln-baked mud-brick or wattle-and-daub construction with thatched roofs or roofs of corrugated metal sheets or blue plastic UN tarps. These homes vie for space near the colonial ruins and crowd the slopes down and away from the Corridor. For the first half kilometer away from the Corridor, there is a congested mosaic of wooden pole lean-tos; round and square mud huts rubbed smooth by women's hands with gray, white, and mustard clay; and brick and cement houses. Among these stand clotheslines, brilliant white squares of maize flour drying in the sun on empty relief aid corn sacks, thatch-covered latrine pits, garbage and ash heaps, and smoky cooking huts, along with avocado, tangerine, and breadfruit trees, and succulent flowering guava, bougainvillea, or passion fruit hedges. It is the vivid, impromptu beauty of such places that prompts privileged foreigners to make unfortunate comparisons between these "poor but happy" residents and the angry and unappreciative inner-city inhabitants of their own gray concrete cities, who, by comparison, may have many more material possessions.

Along the larger roads a few slanting kiosks made of wooden crates and poles tied together with twine sell tiny mounds of dried salt fish and shrimp, a few candles, packets of musty biscuits, and cooking oil in odd assortments of smudged recycled plastic and glass jars and bottles, pyramids of mostly green tangerines, tiny boxes of stick matches, and Life cigarettes, sold by the blood-red packet and singly to take the edge off hunger. Gradually the dwellings become sparse and the land covered by more and more tangled green as one reaches the southern border, marked by the distant profile against the sky of a state-owned eucalyptus plantation. The sandy footpaths link everything.

A Pregnant Silence

The first focus group that I conducted on pregnancy in Mucessua, in February 1994, further drove home the sensitive nature of my proposed work and the level to which women felt vulnerable to reproductive harm. I had expected ten or fifteen participants, but news had spread of a meeting being held with the *estrangeira* (female foreigner) for *mães* and *mães gravidas* (mothers and pregnant mothers), and the gathering under the huge shade acacia tree close to the three caving walls of Mucessua's roofless and doorless *escolinha* (preschool) grew throughout the morning to more than fifty women, many of them visibly pregnant. I was never able to clearly evaluate the power of the bairro party structure to compel or entice people to attend meetings. With the long tradition of community mobilization, from the anticolonial movement through Independence and continuing throughout the war of destabilization, one could say there was a culture of *mobilização do povo* (mobilization of the people) and town meetings. Perhaps in the end it was the tinkling of Coke and Fanta bottles sweating and glistening in their wooden crates that sang out to the neighborhood children, who ran the message home like a wire toy on the end of a stick.

In the meeting format that I had learned over the last two years in my work in the Ministry of Health, I began with a long ingratiating greeting and thanks to those gathered, an introduction of myself and Javelina (whom everyone knew but now saw in her new role as helper and translator to the *estrangeira*), and a presentation of my *assunto*—my issue. Shuffling through my carefully prepared focus group questions, I took a deep breath, set them aside, and asked the question that mattered most of all, the answer to which could render the rest of my prepared script—so American in its rude directness—and overall project irrelevant.

"Is pregnancy an acceptable topic of conversation?" Silence. "Would it be possible for me to ask you here today to talk about pregnancy and your experiences as women and mothers?" After more awkward silence, many heads looking away or down, mouths chewing on blades of dry grass, a very old woman rose slowly to her feet in a custom of formal town meetings institutionalized during the Mozambican war of Independence. Gnarled fist raised over her head, she croaked out, "*Abaixa* [Down with] . . ."

"*Abaixa!*" shyly repeated many of the women in the group, a few fists lifted to head level. "*O fome* [Hunger]!" The old woman's fist flung toward the ground. She repeated this call and response with the group three times, then ended with, "*Viva o povo do Moçambique* [Long live the people of Mozambique]!"

"*Viva!*" shouted the collective.

"*Viva!*" I joined in.

"*Muita obrigada* [Thank you very much]." Her voice trailed off. She stood a moment unsteadily and then spoke forcefully: "*Não têm perigo nenhum* [There is no danger whatsoever]." She stayed standing on wobbling legs, bare feet wide, their soles cracked and thick as shoes. She cast fierce eyes slightly clouded with cataracts about the large group, her expression defying anyone to challenge her. Despite her statement that there was no danger in responding to me, I suspected that she was speaking only for herself, a woman beyond child-bearing years, for no one else spoke up. There was more silence, in which the *velha* (elder woman) creaked down slowly and sat rearranging her cloth wrapper modestly on the bare ground, her strong, large hands, now in her lap, looking younger than the rest of her.

Somewhat desperately I began again: "Like some of you, I am pregnant, for the first time, and I am far from home. So I am hoping you will tell me what I might need to know for things to go well, *andar bem*." I tried to laugh casually, not suspecting how spectacularly foreign and crude such an act of personal disclosure was. On one hand, it was a shameless play for pity. On the other hand, without this revelation the project might have proceeded in a much different way.

I came to appreciate firsthand the "powerful vantage point that acknowledgment of the [reproductive] subjectivity of the ethnographer" allowed: "If in participant observation it is the person of the researcher which serves as the most central and sensitive instrument of research, it behooves us to be transparent, accountable and reflexive about the different modalities in which the self engages with others" (Wekker 2006: 4).

I went to Mozambique with my husband, and we lived and worked together at Mozambique Health Committee for nearly four years. We both conducted dissertation research on health-related topics, each in a different district. Our partnership sustained my heart and was helpful to my work in countless respects, but in one in particular. I was two months pregnant when I began in-depth research, and I gave birth in September. I wrote in my journal one morning a week and a half before the premature birth of our daughter:

> Not able to go to Gondola as planned today. Sent a note to Javelina and a sweater and booties to Raquela number two. There are now two babies named after me in Mucessua. Javelina says it is considered that my contact has been lucky to the mothers in the study, also that I have influenced more girls to be born. I am exhausted myself—a night of discomfort, anxiety attacks, moving baby and hunger. Ate cake and milk at 4 or 5 a.m. Dark outside. Went to check if the guard was awake. He appeared suddenly. I am losing energy and focus fast, although the work holds more and more interest for me. (September 9, 1994)

The fact of my pregnancy no doubt influenced not only my experience of the research, but also Mucessuans' experience of me. I learned quickly that my American way of approaching pregnancy was not only different from, but also dangerous in the context of, Mozambican cultural codes of pregnancy behavior. I was not prepared for the secrecy that surrounded pregnancy in Gondola. Yet, the fear and suspicion that fuels the concealment of pregnancy and at first confounded my attempts to enlist participants in my research project in the end helped cement a connection between many of the women in the community and myself.

As my pregnancy became known, I sensed that interest in and concern for my safety ultimately won me a place in the homes of many of the women in the case study group. As a woman pregnant for the first time and far away from my family, I was often met with sympathy. The older women, especially, took me under their wings to educate me in the ways of motherhood. My changing status made me more familiar with and respectful of the experiences and decisions I was asking women about. What others perceived as my need for knowledge lowered the barriers of a very strict code of personal modesty. I was treated first as a daughter, curious and perhaps vulnerable, and then as mother, initiated and more knowledgeable. It was more than fortuitous for me that my belly and then the name of my daughter went before me. After her birth, I was known only as *mãe da Solea* (mother of Solea). My pregnancy helped win me the intimacy and respect of women in the community. If I had had the good fortune to give birth to a son, it would have raised my esteem a little higher.

After the revelation of my pregnancy at the first focus group, the conversation took off energetically in a direction I had not anticipated. A second woman, Marta, spoke up to qualify the first statement by the oldest participant: "To talk with *you* maybe is not a danger. But one cannot speak of this in the bairro, because you don't know if someone who thinks badly towards you could arrange *drogas* [drugs; poison; substances used in preparations for purposes of witchcraft, sorcery] and make problems with the *parto* [childbirth or delivery]."[6]

A third woman, Tristeza, added, "If a person has problems in delivery, then they have to go to the curandeiro," an indigenous ethnomedical practitioner.

Something had shifted in the group. These statements, I would learn, were warnings. When the subject of sorcery and witchcraft was discussed, it was consistently claimed that foreigners were not affected unless they were African, or involved in a sexual relationship with an African. A light-skinned black person from the United States was an atypical category, and people were consistently unsure about my susceptibility, usually suggesting I play things safe and be careful. An extremely popular healer confided in me that her clients came from all over the region, including Zimbabwe and South Africa and *even* Europe. Like some people, some rules were not black and white. So play it safe I did.

Carefully sidestepping their own experiences or conditions, many of the women present proceeded to helpfully discuss the options for prenatal care in the bairro, options I had never seen. These women's stories and ideas also painted a picture of their precarious existence in a fast-changing world plagued by material need, as well as by social and spiritual dangers that threatened everyone, but pregnant women in particular. This meeting took place during the period of a ceasefire from the fifteen-year war of destabilization that had literally driven many of those present—minus a home, some minus a limb or one or more family members —to scratch a living from the edges of the Beira Corridor and the quickly diminishing lands available for subsistence crops. I, too, was there for reasons of safety, having chosen Gondola to locate the bulk of my research because UN convoys guarded the roads between it and the provincial capital and the region was believed to have been less heavily planted with antipersonnel mines than other areas in the province. Preparations for democratic elections were in the works, but no one really knew what that meant or whether the one-year-old peace accord signed in Rome would hold.

I quickly learned that as women recounted litanies of their troubles with infertility and general problems that occurred during pregnancy and childbirth, they were expressing anxiety about a wide range of disorders of human and social reproduction. Perceived reproductive threats posed by sorcery and *espirito mau* constituted a strong influence on women's strategies for seeking prenatal health care in Mucessua. This apprehension was exacerbated by congested living conditions and competition for scarce resources. Fear propelled women to seek protection for themselves during pregnancy and birth. Despite the wide coverage of women by the formal antenatal care clinic, a majority of pregnant women used alternative and additional sources of reproductive health care to defend against threats that originated in the social world of the living or the spirit world of the nonliving—threats best addressed in the nonmedical world.

Popular local healers and Apostolic church prophets competed for and sometimes played a role in diagnosing the common occurrence of sorcery- and spirit-provoked reproductive threats, using culturally acceptable idioms; churches and their healing specialists were increasing their dominance of popular reproductive health care delivery in the community. The formal health system did not have the priority, the resources, or the social currency to preside over socially acceptable responses to death and debilitation that Mucessuan women accepted as inevitable reversals of fortune resulting from the connivance of jealous neighbors or family, or from abandonment by angered ancestral spirits. Indigenous ethnomedical practitioners, curandeiros, were responding to this shift in popular preference by trading in the powers they once derived from clan spirits for the power of the Holy Spirit.

The first focus group meeting, lively and tremendously informative, lasted well past noon. Several more cases of sodas were purchased from the nearby market to accommodate the numbers and take the edge off the insistent midday heat that sucked up the cool from every spot of shade. But I went home worried about the folly of attempting to study a subject no one felt safe talking about. Nevertheless, I decided to persist. Women seemed anxious to talk about some things. This meeting would prove to be the first of many times that my research would tell me what it wanted to be, and what I really needed to be learning.

For the next focus group, fourteen women from another section of the bairro between the ages of twenty-one and sixty assembled. When I asked them how they felt talking about pregnancy, one woman responded immediately:

Mariana: No. We don't do it. It is a *segredo da casa* [family secret]. Among
   family you can say, to your mother-in-law maybe, or mother of your family.
   Friend or neighbor? No! Just as you cannot tell anyone where you leave
   the key to your house, or you will [come home to] find that a friend has
   arrived and taken everything in your house. [It is the same thing.]

Rachel: What might actually happen if you do tell someone?

Mariana: If you go tell a person outside [your family] even, you could get *uma
   aborta* [a miscarriage, abortion], since [the pregnancy and belly] are still
   little. Are you not going to feel shame then for flaunting it?

Yvonne: People never even think to tell a neighbor. It is the tradition since
   long ago.

Rachel: Does anyone know of someone who suffered from having spoken with
   someone outside the family about a pregnancy?

Theresa: Yes. It happened that a *senhora* walked around telling everyone, and
   [the pregnancy] grew so much. After that it disappeared suddenly with
   neither birth nor *aborto* [miscarriage]. It just ended. Nor can anyone ask
   questions about it for fear of being accused that they did the evil.

Within the "endangered collectivity" of the crowded bairro, reproductive
threats could also be drawn to the individual by naming that threat or by
having one's condition named, by being called, literally, out of one's name.
Hiding pregnancy is thus as much about not having one's vulnerability exposed as it is about not exposing oneself to others' afflictions (Sargent 1989:
65). Limiting contact with others is the best way to achieve both. From these
first near-disastrous field mistakes onward, I learned how anxious women
were about discussing pregnancy and the multitude of social threats they felt
exposed to and needed to protect themselves from on a daily basis.

Layers of Reproductive Vulnerability

Poisonous Words: The Power of Secrets, Gossip, Rumors, and Silence

As is true elsewhere in the world, in Mucessua talking about reproduction can be hazardous, because words themselves carry great power in their
ability to elicit either good or, literally, ill fortune (Sargent 1989; Das 1996;
Browner and Sargent 1996; Scheper-Hughes 1982: 274; Madhaven and
Bledsoe 2001; Stewart and Strathern 2003). Women feared for their own
safety and the safety of their unborn children, but they also feared the invisible harm both cast and magnetized by evil words. Gossip, rumors, and
curses are frequent sources of ill will that may lead one party to resort to
feitiço as revenge. It is partly the "untethered" and "signatureless" nature of

these "performative utterances from the shadows" that endows these kinds of spoken words with their destructive force (Das 1996). In Shona cosmology, the ancestral spirits are also said to be listening to the talk of the living, waiting to cut down to size someone whose words are bigger than their deeds (Gelfand 1992: 110–26).

So, in Mucessua, when a woman wants to inform her husband that she is pregnant, a silent, symbolic gesture replaces conversation between husband and wife. When a woman knows she is pregnant, she will inform her husband by passing him a plate on which she has placed a necklace of beads (*misanga*, Tewe). He will, in turn, inform his parents by presenting them with the same plate and necklace. These silent gestures reflect the power assigned to words and serve as an institutionalized reminder of the hazards of indiscreet social interactions, as well as of the dangers of information in the mouth of the wrong person. A sorcerer must call his or her victim's lineage name in an incantation to send a malevolent spirit to harm that person. This belief is one of the reasons why it is considered perilous to discuss pregnancy.

Growing awareness that one's fate becomes more intimately tied to that of complete strangers in the crowded bairro has contributed to an emergent conceptualization of reproductive vulnerability as a collective condition. Women fear that reproductive problems and loss are contagious, passed from mouth to mouth through the telling and retelling of *azar*, or misfortune. When such ill luck infects one member, the entire community is threatened, as words spread via gossip. The best way to avoid attracting misfortune is to keep one's fortunate and thus vulnerable pregnant state a secret.

This folk epidemiology is at work in a story I heard recounted several times in Mucessua. There was once, within recent memory of the storyteller, a woman who gave birth to an albino infant. In her distress she cursed every pregnant woman in Mucessua, vowing that they, too, should suffer such sorrow as she endured. In the following months or year, in one story six, in another seven, and in another eight more albinos were born in the bairro. Though I never encountered one albino child in Mucessua, I heard different versions of this tale from various sources. In another rendition, the woman gives birth to a deformed child; in another, the child is stillborn. In all versions, however, the same fate befell many other women in the bairro who gave birth after the first woman's tragedy. Her bad luck infected them through the curse. Javelina, age thirty-eight, explained: "In the past there were fewer problems. Now people ask, 'Where are these illnesses coming from? Without *tratamento* [treatment, in this case prenatal ritual and medicinal protection of pregnant mother and unborn child], children are not born well.' One explication is the accumulation of people. That provokes many problems for us Africans."

To make presumptions about the outcome of a pregnancy by concretizing it too early in words is also hubris. Insecurity about whether or not a pregnancy will "hold" (*kubata*, Sh.) leads women to hide their status for as long as possible from all but the most intimately involved, and to do as little as possible to give any evidence of their suspected condition. For example, women in Mucessua frequently attempt to bind their bodies under traditional cloth wraps in such a way as to diminish the protrusion of their pregnant bellies. They consider going to the maternity clinic an open act of bragging that might draw unwanted attention from a host of potentially harmful individuals, including jealous neighbors, resentful infertile women, female rivals involved sexually with a male partner, and prospective birth assistants. The first trip to the maternity clinic for prenatal services is also an investment of valuable time in a high-stakes gamble. This lack of public acknowledgment, however, like the waiting period of as much as a year or more before naming a child, is not a sign of maternal detachment, as might be inferred. On the contrary, it is a precautionary measure taken in an effort to move the poor odds of maternal and child survival closer to one's favor. Women's pregnancy management strategies expressed a cogent folk epidemiology that traced the distribution of reproductive crises not in terms of medicalized biological risk categories, but in terms of dangerous social encounters, often between kin.

Kinship and the Mozambique Shona Healing System

Mozambique Shona healing beliefs and practices are embedded in kinship relations that specify expectations and obligations between living and spirit kin, and these relationships form the basis of Shona cosmology. At the center of the Shona cosmology there is faith in the existence of a Creator God. Known by various names—Musikavanhu, Nyadenga, Chikara, or Mwari—it was the Great Spirit who brought into being all that is in the cosmos and heavens, both good and bad. The Shona God conceptualization attributes no form to this spirit, and it is generally felt that there is little or no direct or personal contact with this remote being as regards the everyday needs of humans.

Intermediaries to God are the spirits of the founders of the great Shona clans—the *mhondoro*. The *mhondoro* are responsible for the welfare of the clan, or of its extended lineage when it becomes large enough to constitute a subclan. The *mhondoro* spirits are concerned with the clan as a whole and take responsibility for the rain and in some cases the succession of kings (Gelfand 1992: 111–12). Their primary domain of power is the land and its fertility rather than individuals. These powerful spirits take the form of, or take possession of, young lions who roam the bush in their territory until they decide to enter a human medium. Through their medium they can be approached when drought or plagues of insects threaten the crops of their territory. They may even be approached when epidemic disease threatens the whole area, but more often sickness is the domain of family ancestral spirits (Bourdillon 1991: 255).

Family ancestral spirits—*vadzimu*, the spirits of the deceased parents and grandparents of both the father and mother—are directly responsible for the daily fate of their descendants. The family vadzimu guard the interests and welfare of the family nuclear unit or small lineages. In times of sickness or death of one of its members, the vadzimu must be consulted to see which one has withdrawn its protective powers and thus allowed evil to enter the home. Gelfand expresses this belief in strong terms: "In other words, no one should die. Man should live forever. Death is not natural. Even a very old person should not die and life is removed by the *vadzimu*" (Gelfand 1992: 114).

As Gelfand further describes, the kinship system rests on the importance of the "cult of the spirit elders." This means that the lives of the living are inextricably linked to the dead through the responsibility of the former to honor and oblige the vadzimu, and of the latter to protect the well-being of their living descendants. The head of the family is the intermediary between his family and the vadzimu, yet the will of the spirit elders is visited upon the living in the form of illness and ill fate, which can befall any family member. The incorrect behavior of one family member can as well bring trouble to the entire family unit until the wrong has been addressed to the satisfaction of the *mudzimu* (spirit elder) involved. The husband's vadzimu are generally believed to be able to influence the lives of any grandchild. However, a wife's vadzimu will be concerned only with her or her children, and not with the husband, because he is in a different lineage. An individual's vadzimu can attack only his or her blood relatives (Gelfand 1992: 116).

The greatest concerns of the vadzimu are the continuity of the lineage structure. Therefore, besides expecting to be remembered and to have their wishes carried out, the vadzimu are invested in a number of critical aspects in Shona daily life. According to Gelfand, these are:

1. the provision of bridewealth to all male cognates;
2. the Shona ritual by which a girl's maternal ancestors are remembered with a gift, formerly of a cow (*mombe youmai*, Sh.) and now of cash, for the girl's mother which must be included in the bridewealth;
3. the settling of a dead man's spirit with the proper ceremony;
4. the proper burial of the body of a cognate;
5. the creation of a serious incest offense should a man marry a woman of the same clan totem;
6. if a man leaves his family without informing the *vadzimu*, an offended spirit may demand his return so as not to weaken or break up the family;
7. care of the children of a deceased cognate's wife (The spirit elder may want

the husband to replace the mother with a sister. Thus sickness will be brought upon the deceased woman's house to alert him to the need to send another wife to his son-in-law);

8. *matongo*: a *dongo* is a vacant piece of land where a family once lived and it is believed that their *vadzimu* still hover. No one should disturb them by going to this place or changing the habitation by cutting a tree or plowing land. (Gelfand 1992: 119–20)

The central concept of Shona cosmology that informs the healing system is the belief that any of one's vadzimu may become angered for one of these reasons. They will express their anger by causing illness and death among their own kin and descendants. As Gelfand (1992: 121) explains: "If their protection is removed for any reason, [a person] may suffer any kind of illness, accident, tragedy, even death. It does not matter whether he is guilty in his own eyes or in the eyes of others. Any reversal in life may be due to a withdrawal of this protection."

This faith is a core foundation of the Shona healing belief system. To avoid angering the vadzimu, and thus to avoid misfortune, illness, and death, the ideal role of living kin is to exist in a balance of reciprocity and mutual respect with each other and with their deceased ancestors as determined by notions of seniority. Each younger member of the family or lineage must obey each elder. As they progress toward being the eldest living representative of the lineage, the elder members have increasing responsibility for their younger kin, charged with ritually remembering the vadzimu and addressing their wishes and concerns. Because this ideal is not always played out in people's lives, the world is not free of misfortune, illness, and death. Vulnerability can occur at multiple levels: between the individual and the natural world, between humans in the living world, and between the living and the nonliving in the spirit world. Pregnant women frequently perceived ruptures in relations with living and spirit kin to be the most significant reproductive threats. Women in Mucessua attributed the most serious pregnancy and obstetric complications to personalistic—human or spirit-induced—reproductive threats of witchcraft and sorcery.

The term "personalistic" refers to illness causality being assigned to "an active, purposeful intervention of an agent, who may be a living human (a witch or sorcerer), the spirit of a non-living human (a ghost, an ancestor, an angered or avenging spirit) or non-human (a deity or other very powerful being)" (Foster 1998: 112). In Mucessua, this category of reproductive threats includes the employment of *uroyi*, ChiTewe for witchcraft, sorcery, and spirit possession sought for the purpose of causing harm. The practice of *uroyi* in Mucessua is most often referred to, even by predominantly non-Portuguese speakers, by its Portuguese term, feitiço or *feitishismo* (fetishism). Feitiço is strongly believed to be untreatable in the biomedical sector, and widespread fear of feitiço is one of the strongest influences on prenatal care health-seeking behavior of pregnant women (Chapman 2003). In Mucessua, vulnerability to reproductive threats is thus frequently expressed as fear of feitiço.

Respect for feitiço is widespread among Shona speakers regardless of class or social station (Bourdillon 1991: 174). All types of misfortune are attributed to it, from falling in the path to losing employment, becoming sick, losing a child, or dying. As Bourdillon observes, belief in witchcraft does not necessarily contradict belief in natural causes. More exactly, natural causes which may determine *how* something happens are not accepted as an adequate explanation of *why* a particular victim is chosen. "When witchcraft is believed to be operative, it acts in conjunction with evident natural causes" (173).

Witchcraft

Across Manica Province, practitioners of feitiço are commonly called *feitiçeiros*, of which two large categories are identified. The first type is believed to be most frequently women who play hereditary host to the spirit of a maternal ancestor endowed with special powers to do evil, to cause suffering and death. The power to heal is always linked to the shadow power to harm. Therefore, much like a spirit diviner-healer, a witch is able to use "medicines" or poisons taught to them only by another witch or by their possessing spirit, perhaps through dreams. Only the witch knows the antidote to their personal medicines. Targets of witches may be their enemies—people against whom the witches hold a grudge or whom they dislike for some reason, or simply people in their paths, including family members, husbands, and their own children. Witches are thought to cause suffering for the pleasure of it, and to sate their naturally nefarious appetites, the most feared aspect of which is eating human flesh, especially the flesh of children. It is believed that witches cannibalize their young, and women who are childless or who have histories of reproductive loss are frequently suspected of being witches. This fear is a potent expression of collective awe of reproductive power and evidences the strict sanctions against women who attempt to control their own reproductive capacity. These beliefs fuel the accusations against and hostility and violence toward women who suffer from infertility or reproductive loss. According to Bourdillon:

> For this reason a barren woman, or a woman who aborts or whose children die young, is likely to be suspected of killing her children for the purpose of witchcraft. Human flesh is supposed to be the most powerful of a witch's "medicines." These "medicines" may be used [ritually] for socially acceptable purposes, for luck in gambling, for example, or success in business, or to

obtain good crops; nevertheless they are evil, and their use is held to convey an unfair advantage over others in the community. Power is always associated with the power to harm. (Bourdillon 1991: 175)

Importantly, both the indigenous and the often exoticizing colonial analytical discourses on witchcraft express a deep "dimension of insecurity" (Desjeux 1987: 178, qtd. in Geschiere 1997: 221) in peasant ability to control productive and reproductive processes central to their own continuity, for example, agricultural harvests, a rapidly fluctuating cash market, and human and animal fertility. Yet, rather than considering witchcraft only through a psychobehavioral critique of individuals and cultures, one must see witchcraft and sorcery discourses in Mucessua as connected to the erosion of the commons, those resources necessary to peasant survival. Like Taussig (1980), I see a credible parallel between women's interpretations of the connection between sorcery and reproductive vulnerability and critiques of capitalism's "magic" belief that capital is productive. Rather, the increasing presence of capital and capitalist relations in people's lives further and further endangers reproduction and thus community continuity. Comaroff's association of witchcraft activities with zombie workers and invisible plantations acknowledges the contradiction that "the goal of capitalist society is to transform life into the capacity to work and 'dead labor'" (Federici 2004: 16). Women of the Mozambican peasantry express a level of recognition of the contradictions built into capitalism's social relations—"the promise of freedom vs. the reality of widespread coercion, and the promise of prosperity vs. the reality of widespread penury" (Federici 2004: 17).

Sorcery

The second type of feitiçeiro acknowledged in Shona custom is most often a man. Anthropologists use the term "sorcerer" to distinguish this type of witch from a hereditary witch, for this type of feitiçeiro does not inherit his capacity to do evil from an ancestral spirit but acquires his ability to purposely harm others by buying powerful medicines (drogas) from a corrupted spirit diviner-healer, a herbalist, or another witch. A client can buy the services of such ritual specialists, who can manipulate magic to activate the spirit world, to harm someone the client dislikes or to gain some personal benefits to the detriment of another (Bourdillon 1991: 179). However, sorcerers are mostly thought to use their knowledge to increase their own wealth and power. Manica District of Manica Province was famous for a particularly potent type of Shona sorcerer able to control deadly lightning (trovuada) and strike down victims at will.

As in many African communities, precipitous accumulation of wealth in Mucessua is always suspected as being the result of dealings with the spirit world. It signals that one is a witch or sorcerer or has bought the services of a sorcerer to obtain potent *drogas*. Great success in generating extraordinary wealth through business, that is, through trade of a service or goods for money, is widely believed to require dangerous and expensive medicines involving sorcery and an act of abomination such as murder, necrophilia, cannibalism, or incest. A widespread belief holds that extraordinary material gain is always achieved at the expense of someone else. As Javelina explained to me, feitiço is about directly competing for resources on an uneven playing field on which some people are getting much more and getting ahead of you without trying. Whether neighbors or kin, anyone who suddenly experiences unexplainable good fortune or unexplainable loss in the current casino capitalist market is suspected of rigging the game. Thus, standing out materially makes an individual the focus of distrust and sometimes of outright accusations of being a sorcerer or having made a bargain with one. Talk of such a person is perhaps wrongly interpreted as general agreement that people do not like to see others doing better than they; jealousy and envy are most frequently cited as the main reasons for witchcraft or sorcery in the bairro.

However, as James Siegel (2006) found in Java, it is not so much being rich that generates hate and envy in Mucessua. It is the seemingly magical ability of people who have the same relationship and access to the means of production as others to generate more wealth than those around them. Crehan (1997) also found in Zambia that accusations of witchcraft clustered around kin who are doing well but who seem to be withholding their surplus from others who are in need. Sorcery is also suspected of someone who becomes consumed by envy and hate of others. Under these circumstances, feitiço provides a compelling discourse for interpreting reproductive threats.

In the tight quarters of the bairro, other reasons arise for distrusting neighbors. Arguments, fights, and conflicts, for example, over theft or land appropriation can escalate to the point of insult or accusation, and a kind of curse will be spoken. Revenge often takes the form of a verbal oath by the offended party that something will go wrong, that someone will suffer or die. As the most vulnerable in the family, the pregnant wife and her future child are immediately feared to be the targets. Congested living conditions and competition for scarce resources between strangers, on the one hand, and desperate relatives, on the other, exacerbate anxieties about personalistic reproductive threats. Anxiety about these threats steers women toward costly preventative and curative folk treatments.

The Shadow Side of Kinship

Despite the intense distrust women in Mucessua expressed regarding living among potentially malevolent and jealous strangers, they were certain that only ruptures in kin relationships can create the gaps in a woman's personal defenses through which reproductive threats from sorcery can enter. It was widely held that the machinations of feitiçeiros of any sort, however, are not likely to be successful unless the victim or a relative of the victim is indeed guilty of a crime against the aggressor, or unless a member of the family of the victim (dead or living) is involved in the aggression. When a spirit elder, a *mudzimo*, becomes angered or seeks revenge, this type of spirit is called *ngozi* in Shona, *mau espirito* in Portuguese, and *mfukwa* in Tewe (possibly from -*pfuka*, which means haunt, turn away from, leave in the lurch, abandon by an amiable spirit, Sh.) When angered, *ngozi* or *mfukwa* spirits can cause illness and misfortune among their descendants by withdrawing their protective powers.

Two types of *ngozi* are recognized. The first, *chikwambo*, is the spirit of a nonfamily or nonlineage person who has been murdered or maltreated during his or her life, for example, a traveler who was robbed and slain, a slave who was tortured, or an employee who went to his grave without being paid. This type of spirit will go outside its own family and return to punish the guilty party or descendants of the guilty party until the debt has been repaid. A *chikwambo* is considered the most vicious of spirits and is likely to cause illness and death among an entire family until its wishes are addressed. The guilty family is often asked to dedicate a girl to this *ngozi* as its wife (*mukadzi we mupfukwa*), as we will see; such a girl cannot marry and must remain in her father's compound.

The second type of *ngozi* operates against members of its own family, for example, a parent who was abused or struck by a child, an ancestor whose appropriate rites of respect have not been paid, or a relative who died without receiving assistance in a time of need. These *ngozi* are more likely to cause illness and misfortune than death among their descendants by withdrawing their protective powers. Ancestral spirits called *wadzimu* in ChiTewe were reported to operate against members of their own family, for example, the spirit of a parent who was disrespected. When this occurs, an unprotected person—a person outside the correct relations with dead or living kin—can become the target of all sorts of *azar* (ill fate, harm). Threatening the next generation by targeting reproductive health is a good way for angered ancestors to get the attention of living lineage members. By virtue of her physical and spiritual vulnerability, a pregnant woman is considered a prime target for spirit-induced illness.

Despite the distinctions anthropologists and others make between the roles of ancestral spirits, witches, and sorcerers, much of the perceived danger of witchcraft lies in threats very much of this world. People's firsthand experience with witchcraft involves human foes at the bottom of the elaborate cosmologies—disgruntled kin and neighbors who cause others bad luck because they are jealous, spiteful, or scheming. As practiced and addressed in Mucessua, feitiço speaks directly to the intensity and cost of social rupture and dissonance within households and exposes competing interests and divergent reproductive agendas.

Since social networks represent important access to limited resources, women evaluate pregnancy management strategies and prenatal health interventions in relation to their potential to cause or avert reproductive loss. In addition, however, births and reproductive losses are both weighed against a specific birth's capacity to solidify or endanger important social bonds and its potential to rend, maintain, or expand social networks (Pfeiffer 1997; Chapman 2003). Any imbalances in social and material well-being are communicated between generations as ruptures in good health, especially reproductive health of living female kin. As a result, women were fearful of feitiço-related reproductive harm that was directly or indirectly rooted in family conflicts over changing reproductive practices and intrahousehold competition for resources.

If a woman arouses the anger of her maternal ancestors, then she can expect to be punished through withdrawal of protection of her reproductive capacity (Gelfand 1992: 110–26). In cases of a child's unsanctioned union or unsanctioned pregnancy, parents may threaten to withdraw both material and spiritual protection from the child, an act that symbolizes the strain created by interruptions of intergenerational cycles of social and economic indebtedness and interdependence. Failure by grown children to make traditionally expected payments of respect, duty, labor, or material assistance to their parents poses a threat to women's reproductive health. For example, family disharmony frequently results from tension over unpaid, insufficient, or improper appropriation of bridewealth (*lobolo* in Tewe) or seduction fee payments (*masunggiro* in Tewe) that ensure the distribution of social and material wealth between generations of lineage and marriage-related kin.

These threats and fears of feitiço in Mucessua can be seen as attempts to manage insecurity that both expose and mystify the costs of reproduction. Accusations associated with feitiço also challenged and sought to influence the distribution of surplus among extended kin when relationships of reciprocity and obligation have broken down. Because kinship claims are so crucial to the distribution of surplus, kinship ties necessarily encompass an intense ambivalence (Crehan 1997: 205). Reproductive failure is thus ultimately a failure of social, and especially kinship, support.

Inside *o Quintal* (the Compound)

Everywhere on the paths are people—walking mostly, less frequently zooming by perilously on rattling bikes, and only occasionally creeping along in a dented, yellow pick-up truck, one of the few vehicles I ever saw in Mucessua other than the one I drove or was given a ride in by a driver from the Mozambique Health Committee. The yellow pick-up belonged to a man who had worked for Save the Children Norway for many years, and had amassed what was considered a small fortune, as demonstrated by his car and five wives.

Women walk the paths carrying almost everything on their heads, from a bar of soap or a hoe to a bucket of water, a tree trunk, a wide basin of cassava root or tomatoes, a huge stalk of bananas, or a 50-pound sack of dried corn. Women are always in motion—walking to or from their distant corn and millet fields or small riverbed vegetable, rice, sugarcane, and fruit plots; going to market with baskets of potatoes, pumpkins, butter beans, manioc roots and leaves, or cabbage to sell; walking to the public pump to draw water, greeting neighbors or crocheting while they wait to fill 10-, 24-, or 40-liter barrels to carry home on their heads. They pump the water, their whole bodies heaving, hauling it up in rusty buckets, then lean toward home with the water spilling from the pails onto their heads, mingling with the sweat running down their faces and necks.

Even in their homes and yards women are still moving, pounding or sifting corn or millet, sorting rice or sesame seeds, covering walls or floors with a fresh coat of clay. They braid hair or bathe, feed, or nurse children, babies and toddlers whom they carry in cloth slings on their back or hip. Children cry only when they are sick or injured, which is not rare. Women are always holding, kissing, caressing, soothing, bathing, nursing, feeding, bouncing, tickling, hugging, wiping, wrapping, rocking, suckling, running after, healing, lifting, calling, comforting, scolding, laughing with, and twirling children.

At the same time they keep stirring pots of thick cornmeal porridge, pouring tea, splitting firewood, planting flowers, chasing goats and chickens away from food or seed, selling bread on wobbling wooden chairs, serving meals to men, setting out mats to sit in the shade to cut greens for stew or to shell peanuts. With gourds or enamel cups, they scoop water cooled in tall or large round clay vessels or rusty oil drums into chipped enamel basins to wash a few dishes, cups, a pot, which they scrub with sand because there is no soap. With small basins of water they wash hands and mouth, clothes, terry cloth diapers, capulanas—women's cloth wraps in fading colors—scrubbed and slapped on river rock or stump or tub, bright rayon dresses sewn quickly by a neighborhood tailor, and secondhand pants from the used-clothes bazaar at the market. All the while, babies are on their backs, sleeping or watching, or on their fronts nursing. Women who are not moving are very old, praying, or waiting to be seen at the health center, the maternity ward, the home of an indigenous healer or prophet, or they are sleeping, or they are dead.

CHAPTER 3

The Nova Vida

In Mozambique, I am always caught off guard by the juxtaposition of contrasts. The way beauty and pain often resided side by side, or a scene of violence could give way to tenderness or, equally often, the reverse, evoked amazement mixed with despair, elation wrapped in dismay. I saw contrasts everywhere; in the profuse purple bougainvillea erupting from the lower windows of an abandoned and crumbling colonial hotel into the sun, where goats grazed on burnt grass by the entrance and in the cracks of the concrete walkway near once-grand marble stairs, now dislodged like loose teeth. Like the dry grass, persistent and unchallenged, families of deslocados have claimed the building over time; their sagging lines of dull laundry flap in the wind on the highest balcony like surrender flags, sun filtering in through the conceding, caved-in roof.

I am stopped in my tracks by the quick, balancing step and bulging neck artery of a barefoot woman straining under the weight of a gas stove on her head balanced atop a tightly coiled ring of reeds, who darts her eyes over and down as we pass each other to look at my clean feet and low-heeled sandals. I look back at her and realize she is trying to keep pace with a man walking ten feet in front of her in an ill-fitting suit and shiny, worn-down shoes, smoking a bent cigarette.

Contradictions greet me in the street, in the radiant smiles of two dust-covered boys outside a shop, their open shirts with one remaining button between them, trying to sell me a thin plastic shopping bag for one-third of a cent, while their reflections dance in the gleaming window of a store displaying two cherry red Mercedes-Benz scooters. They haunt the dark brown face of the young Mozambican man in a clean blue work jumpsuit, absently skimming the surface of a luxury hotel pool for leaves and frogs, his gaze smoldering as he watches a café au lait Mozambican girl wearing huge gold hoop earrings and a tiny red bikini who has never and would never see him, as she walks away hand in hand with a young French pilot. These contradictions are all part of nova vida.

On its glittering polished surface, the expression "nova vida" captures a wistful admiration for the burgeoning availability of imported luxury goods, and a longing for them as coveted status markers and fashion statements.

The term also encapsulates, however, a much more "entangled landscape" of power, desire, labor, and violence. Donald Moore uses the term to bring into play the complicated ways in which "multiple spatialities, temporalities, and power relations combine" (Moore 2005: 4). Just below and constantly shattering the surface of the nova vida is the predicament of exclusion of those without access to money or ways to get money from this new life of avid consumption. This predicament is the heart and the fruit of global neoliberal policies played out in Mozambique's postwar structural adjustment economy.

The nova vida is about a "contingent constellation of practice, milieu and materiality" of market fundamentalist policies and their effects, as I laid out in Chapter 1—increased privatization, introduction of fees for health care and education, monetization of formerly communal work exchange practices, intensification of women's workloads as subsistence cultivators, and increasing competition for land and jobs (MOPF 1998: 312). The desperation these policies produce is palpable and smells of twenty years of refuse left in piles around Mozambique's cities since Independence. The stench of abandonment casts its shadow over everything, even when most of the piles have been dragged outside the city limits into people's neighborhoods. Even though, or perhaps because, each year sees more stores and cars in the cities and towns, more deluxe resorts reopening for international tourists, more frequent commercial flights between the capital city of Maputo and provincial capitals like Beira, deepening inequalities are also more evident. It was not just the desperation that felt undoing; it was the constant merging of desperation with splendor, abundance intermingling with abjection.

Another layer of the predicament of the nova vida is increasing urbanization and the infusion of urban influences into peri-urban and rural cultures, including the fragmentation, dispersion, and nucleation of households. Common feelings expressed by Mucessua residents were despair over economic instability and distrust over increasing crowding. To the indignity of living in close quarters surrounded by strangers are added the tension of family separation due to dispersal and dislocation during the war and labor migration, competition for scarce resources, and the burden of long treks to family agricultural plots far from town. Most of all, however, women in Mucessua described their vulnerability to poor maternal health and frequent pregnancy and infant loss throughout their fertile years. Women's reproductive bodies are thus also entangled landscapes in Mucessua, where the effects of national and transnational economic austerity policies are localized in the condition of reproductive vulnerability, the daily experiences of pregnant women, and their strategies for seeking reproductive health.

To contextualize the layers of women's reproductive vulnerability in the nova vida, it is necessary to examine them within the broader context of social and economic restructuring at the household, community, and nation-state levels. How women live and how they make a living in a community of shifting size, ethnic makeup, social organization, and distribution of resources are key aspects of the local dynamics that influence the patterns of reproductive health seeking and pregnancy management in Mucessua. By examining these features of precolonial and colonial Shona life, it is possible to broadly characterize earlier sociocultural patterns of the Tewe in Mozambique. A comparison of these earlier patterns with current sociocultural formations reveals "a trajectory of social change" (Pfeiffer 1997: 137); as the political and economic environment of Mucessua shifts, reproductive behavior reflects the deep and growing vulnerability of an already marginalized population. Such an excavation project must be attentive to the ways that "historically sedimented processes" and "situated struggles" are assembled in place (Moore 2005: 2).

In this chapter, I examine the historical development and transformation of gendered relations of production and reproduction in Gondola and the surrounding region. Shifts in economic and social organization have resulted in the erosion of women's sources of material subsistence and social support networks and have intensified intrahousehold inequality, distrust, and conflict. To grasp the effects of these transitions requires an understanding of long-standing Shona social institutions.

History of Hope, Legacy of Inequality
Identifying the Inhabitants of Mucessua

The district of Gondola lies within what was once the territory of the Tewe kingdom. As Virtanen (2005) has pointed out, in the academic literature on Mozambique, ethnic identity has been traced through language (do Rosário 1999: 68–69; Firmino 2002: 110–11; Magode and Khan 1996: 81–82). As ChiTewe language, together with ChiManica and ChiNdau, has been classified as part of a "dialect continuum" with the Bantu language ChiShona, the ChiTewe-speaking peoples are usually classified as an ethnolinguistic subgroup of the Shona. "Shona," a label that came into use after British colonization of Zimbabwe, has been applied to all Shona-speaking groups across contemporary Zimbabwe and Central Mozambique (Bourdillon 1991: 6–7).

The Shona inhabit a large area covering most of Zimbabwe and extending as far as the coastal areas of the Indian Ocean in Mozambique. According to official statistics, ChiShona speakers constitute the majority in Central Mozambique, comprising about two-thirds of the population in Manica Province (INE 1999: 51; cf. Firmino 2002: 93). While the Shona include various subgroups and do not represent a unified political community, according to most scholars they share (in addition to language) a common historical identity and certain cultural traits, such as an adelphic collateral system of succession (Beach 1994: 23–42; Mudenge 1988: 8–30; Virtanen 2005: 227).

Historically, the most inclusive term for the Shona was "Kalanga" or "Karanga," used by the northern and eastern Shona by 1506 and by the western Shona by at least 1727. The language-culture cluster to which the Tewe belong is now classified as eastern Shona. Even before 1700, however, the eastern Shona usually referred to themselves by the names of their kingdoms, such as Tewe or Manyika, and this practice became common among the central Shona as well (Beach 1994: 31). The majority of current inhabitants of the Gondola District area identify themselves as Tewe and their language as ChiTewe.

Several ethnic groups make up the population of Mucessua today, though no official data give a formal breakdown. According to the first bairro secretary, the majority of bairro residents are still Tewe, and the principal language spoken is locally called ChiTsakara, a mixture of the Shona-related languages ChiTewe, ChiSena, ChiManica, and ChiGorongosiana. Most of the pregnant women with whom I worked most closely identified their ethnic background or *raça* (race) as Tewe and their *lingua materna* (mother tongue) as ChiTsakara. The next largest group was Ndau, followed by Sena, Nyungwe, Gorongosa, and Barue, and one speaker each of Shangana from Gaza Province, Shona from Zimbabwe, and Sua (from ChiMucessua, like ChiTsakara). In discussions about life in the bairro, the difficulties of living among strangers from different ethnic groups figured prominently, compounded by witchcraft, adultery, robbery, and disease.

Constructing an ethnohistorical account of Mozambique Shona presents at least three major challenges. First, although a common language links the numerous subgroups of the Shona, significant historical, cultural, and linguistic variation distinguishes them. For example, in recent history, the colonial boundary between western Mozambique and Zimbabwe, while artificially dividing the eastern Shona groupings, has provoked meaningful social, economic, and political differences (Virtanen 2005; Ranger 2002). Second, while an extensive body of ethnographic and historic literature has been generated about the Shona on the Zimbabwe side of the border, few detailed ethnographic documents focus on the peoples of Central Mozambique in either the colonial or postcolonial periods. Third, where descriptions of earlier periods exist, "our knowledge of past realities is dependent on past observers whose cultural lenses may be unclear to us," in the words of Micaela di Leonardo, who quotes Louise Lamphere: "In some sense we really will never know what it was like to be an Iroquois woman in the sixteenth century or a Navajo woman in the eighteenth" (Lamphere 1987: 24, qtd. in di Leonardo 1991: 30). We may never know much of what it was like to be a Shona woman in precolonial or early colonial Mozambique.

Nonetheless, taking into account the weaknesses, biases, and political agendas of colonial anthropological accounts of African life, useful information can be drawn from the Zimbabwe Shona material.[1] This material, bolstered by limited and equally problematic Portuguese and British accounts of the Manica and Sofala Province regions, underscores the ethnohistorical specificity of both gender and health systems in contemporary Gondola.[2] Decades and even centuries of population movement and the transformation of political and economic relations have contributed to the current context and deepening impoverishment of already marginal communities and vulnerable groups, disrupted long-standing social formations, and reshaped gender relationships.

Mapping Shona Gender

Scholars of precolonial Shona life and history generally agree that while subordinate to men in some spheres of political power, women held central roles in social, cultural, and spiritual life, and especially in utilizing and conserving the natural environment (Mazarire 2003: 41). The recurring theme of female fertility, rainmaking, and environmental powers that emerges from the cosmology, myths, totems, and art of Shona subgroups, which has been called the "Shona fertility complex" (Matenga 1997), supports the assertion that precolonial Shona women held spiritual and ritual political influence due to their role in sustaining both human and agricultural fertility (Mazarire 2003; Ranger 2001; Schmidt 1992). It has been proposed that this power and perhaps the more matrilineal and matrilocal orientation associated with these forms of female power were attenuated and eventually subsumed under male hegemonic political and spiritual power. This shift likely resulted from changes in traditional religion due to external factors such as conquest and the adoption of a "new cult ideology" that led to a "masculinization of ecology religion" (Ranger 2001: 99; see also Phiri 1997 on Malawi).

Mazarire has called this the Shona "cult of male superiority" and suggests that up to the present, women's exploitation and subordination in the Shona social order stem directly from their fundamental roles in human reproduction and fecundity of the land. That is, male political claims to and struggles over land have always been played out through power in and over women and women's fertility. Mazarire writes of precolonial Shona society in general and Chivi Zimbabwe in particular that "female fertility . . . was also associated with the fecundity of the land, so that control over this vital resource also determined whether people would eat or starve. Therefore, control over women indirectly meant control over the environment" (Mazarire 2003: 42).

Archeological evidence from the precolonial period and oral literature suggests that the organization of production and division of labor increased male access to wealth accumulation while reinforcing a division of labor that tied women to unpaid subsistence food cultivation (Young 1977). Growing Iron Age communities' heightened dependence on cultivation may have contributed to defining women's roles in terms of subsistence agriculture and biological reproduction. These same forces are presumed to have bolstered men's potential for wealth accumulation through the ownership of cattle and the participation in external trade markets. These strategies, in turn, may have offset an unreliable agricultural base or helped gain the bride-price for women in an increasingly stratified society (Beach 1980: 30).

The Scramble for Mozambique

Portuguese Influence

Portuguese arrived on the coast area of what is today Mozambique as early as 1500. The main impact of the early Portuguese presence on African polities in the region and in particular the Tewe kingdom was to shift control of coastal trade networks away from Muslim traders, who subsequently were often forced into the role of agent for the Portuguese in the interior (Beach 1980: 110). The Portuguese presence increased until the middle of the seventeenth century, especially through the establishment of *feiras* (centers of trade) and *prazos* (land grants) tied to European occupation throughout the Tewe and Manica kingdoms. These settlements contributed to the constant reconfiguration of intra-African polities, as regional rulers struggled for a foothold in the new trade alliances.

In relation to women's status, two observations are important. First, the overall increase in the volume of trade due to Portuguese expansion in the area, especially of ivory, may have bolstered male but not female economic opportunity. For example, as Young (1977: 70) points out in her discussion of the impact of increased trade on the gender division and male-female opportunities in southern Mozambique during the same period:

> The complementary relationship in sharing products resulting from an equal division of labor, with men providing meat through hunting and herding and women providing grain crops and vegetables from cultivation, was fundamentally altered as a result of trade. For from this point onwards men's hunting activities no longer yielded purely internally shared and consumed products, but produced ivory and horns of value in trade which could produce additional prestige goods and investment in cattle. These could be further reinvested in more wives and thus supply men with cumulative power which women could not gain from subsistence food production through cultivation.

Second, the Shona economy was quick to respond to new mercantile opportunities spawned by Portuguese expansion in the area, especially Portuguese demand for food supplies (Newitt 1995: 51–52). These forces, argues Bhila (1982: 250), contributed to the "peasantization" of local communities during this period, that is, the involvement in trade relationships of independent agriculturists who cultivate in the hopes of profit (Beach 1977: 56). Women, as primary cultivators, probably played an important role in cash crop production and expanded food crop production. Underpinning this process, Portuguese documents attest, was a strong market for imported commodities gained through distant trade. The drive to acquire imported goods, especially cloth and beads, fueled the economy of the entire plateau and lowland area as well (Bourdillon 1991: 9). Exploitive Portuguese and Muslim traders sold African goods for much more than the value of commodities they gave their African suppliers. In their role as primary subsistence cultivators, women today bear the brunt of impoverishment in a region whose economy has deep roots in the inequity of these early trade relations.

From the mid-eighteenth through the nineteenth century, the rise of the trade in slaves in response to the demand for labor in Brazil transformed Mozambique into an international labor reserve (Isaacman and Isaacman 1983: 16). By the late nineteenth century, male laborers had begun to migrate to neighboring Rhodesia and to the mines at Kimberley and Johannesburg in the Republic of South Africa. The forced removal of the most productive members of Mozambique's indigenous societies through the slave trade, like the unequal terms of external plateau trade relations, "intensified the process of underdevelopment and impoverishment" (18), a process that was given further momentum by later colonial policies of *chibalo*—internal and exported forced labor—and labor migration (Isaacman 1996).

In the latter half of the nineteenth century, the Portuguese reintensified their effort to establish sovereign territories in Mozambique. Already weak ties were further threatened by the encroachment of other foreign interests, especially the British on the coast and in the Manica highlands, the Sultan of Zanzibar, and the revolt of the Afro-Portuguese and Afro-Goan *prazeiros*. The Portuguese foothold in Mozambique was further diminished in the scramble for Africa during the 1880s. Rulings of the Congress of Berlin denied Lisbon's territorial claims to Mozambique and made abolition of the slave trade, pacification, and effective control of territory minimal prerequisites for international recognition of Portugal's right to colonial rule.

Portuguese pacification of Mozambique was a thirty-year process entailing an unprecedented use of Portuguese military force bolstered by the heavy recruitment of indigenous support through coercion, by playing upon historical divisions, and by offering substantial economic rewards. African resistance was also weakened by internal conflicts resulting from either popular opposition to authoritarian rule or cleavages within the ruling class. As Isaacman and Isaacman summarized: finally, "the strategic role of collaborators, the technological advantage of the Portuguese military, and the failure of Africans to unite permitted imperialism to triumph and set the stage for formal Portuguese rule" (1983: 25).

Early Colonial Rule

The lack of capital available to the Portuguese crown drove and shaped early colonial policies, a dynamic that continued throughout Portuguese dominion in Mozambique. In an attempt to compensate for its financial weakness, Portugal came up with two strategies. The first was to cede direct administrative control of large areas of territory in the center and to the north of the colony to foreign concessionary companies. The second was to develop labor legislation that effectively transformed Mozambique into a cheap reserve pool of migrant workers whose labor was to be utilized in the development of colonial enterprises or rented to neighboring countries. A three-tiered administrative structure of Portuguese officials extended its control over the territories of the new colony in areas under direct Portuguese rule. The colonial regime was greatly aided by the manipulation of African collaborators (often royal family members, called *regulos* in their colonial capacity) who collected taxes, arbitrated minor disputes, recruited labor, and maintained public order (Isaacman and Isaacman 1983: 29).

In areas under direct Portuguese rule, a highly structured, centralized system of governance was installed to carry out the expropriation of labor, production, and raw materials that was to characterize Portuguese occupation of Mozambique until Independence, in 1975. By the 1890s, local populations faced heavy taxation in the form of a hut tax (Newitt 1995: 407). The burden of taxes, payable only in European currency, combined with the artificially low prices paid for peasant-produced commodities, was designed to generate revenue as well as to steer local workers into low-wage jobs in the capitalist sectors of the colonial economy. The overall effect, however, was to push male laborers out of Portuguese territory in pursuit of better opportunities. Migrant labor, whether in clandestine forms to evade taxation, conscription into "volunteer" state work forces, or as part of formal recruitment agreements with neighboring South Africa and Southern Rhodesia, created serious labor shortages in the colony itself. To stem this flow and to address growing internal labor needs, the forced-labor system, locally called *chibalo*, increasingly depended on the use of "unbridled coercion" (Isaacman 1996: 23).

Based on the 1899 native labor codes, *chibalo* was the result of a pact among colonial administrators, the Department of Native Affairs, and European capitalists who wanted cheap labor. According to Isaacman and Isaacman (1983: 23), the system worked in the following manner:

European planters, agricultural companies, factory owners, and local merchants who were unable to meet their labor needs through volunteers, as well as state officials overseeing public works projects, would petition the Department of Native Affairs, which in turn would notify regional administrators. They would then order local administrators (*chefes do posto*) to conscript men for six-month periods. Each *chefe do posto* would then send out African police (*sipais*) to contact designated chiefs, who used either the *sipais*, or their local retainers to round up peasant recruits.

The labor recruitment tactics used on Mozambican peasants were brutal. Men were often captured from their homes at night, bound, and marched sometimes long distances to be delivered to their new nonpaying employer. Local police and administrators had complete discretion in their choice of workers, without concern for the men's activities or their families' economic security (Isaacman and Isaacman 1983: 23). As long as they supplied the labor demanded of them, local administrators and police were free to—and likely encouraged to—prey upon the local population.

This situation had a particularly cruel impact on women and girls, who were often the target of police brutality in the form of sexual coercion. Isaacman and Isaacman quote one elder who had fled to Southern Rhodesia in 1917: "[The *sipai*] have been ravishing young children who are too young for a man to sleep with. Many girls were very ill and had to be sent back. One *sipai*, Nyakatoto, actually cut the girl's private parts so that he could penetrate her" (1983: 31). Another striking example appears in the report of a British official, who wrote in 1912 of the *sipais* in the territory of the Nyasa Company in the northern third of the country: "The tax is collected by the simple expedient of sending out the native soldiers from the post at collection time to round up all the women on whom they can lay their hands. The women are brought to the posts and kept there until the husbands and fathers rescue them by paying taxes" (Livingston 1857: 637, qtd. in Isaacman and Isaacman 1983: 37).

A 1924 report by a U.S. sociologist on the employment of "native labor in Portuguese Africa" further exposes the ways women suffered under *chibalo*:

Women, even pregnant or with a nursling, are taken for road work by *sipais*. In out-of-the-way places the Government builds little barracks to house them. No pay nor food. According to the circumscription the term is from one week to five but women may be called out again in the same year. Others in the village bring food to them, in some cases a day's journey away. Girls as young as fifteen are taken and some are made to submit sexually to those in charge. They begin work at six, stop for an hour at noon and work until sunset. There are some miscarriages from heavy work. (Ross 1925: 40, qtd. in Isaacman 1996: 24)

As Isaacman observes: "This combination of forced labor, terror and sexual abuse would become a hallmark of the forced cotton regime twenty years later" (1996: 24).

Concessionary Companies and Gondola

In the Sofala region of Central Mozambique, and in what is now Manica Province, where the town of Gondola and Bairro Mucessua are located, the imposition of the colonial political and economic agenda was mediated by the administrative control of the oldest of the concessionary companies to be established by the Portuguese in Mozambique, the Companhia de Moçambique (Mozambique Company). Founded in 1888, the Mozambique Company was originally intended to develop the infrastructure in the region to further exploit the rich mineral deposits and timber in the area. Dominated by French and British interests, the firm neglected to invest in local infrastructure. The company's investors were happy to reap huge profits from stocks, taxes, forced male labor on wild rubber and coconut plantations, forced female cultivation of cotton and other cash crops, which the company purchased at depressed prices, and the sale of conscripted labor to neighboring settler estates (Isaacman and Isaacman 1983: 36). Under the company's administration, the forced-labor policy and other abuses by local administrators, who supplemented their low wages by pillaging local populations, became so intolerable that a significant proportion of the local male population migrated illegally to nearby Southern Rhodesia to work at the mines. Conditions in the company territories led to many forms of resistance on the part of Africans, including major uprisings in Barue in 1902 and 1917.

The Mozambique Company also set up several subconcessions, including the Beira Railway Company (BRC) which was leased to Cecil Rhodes and his associates. In 1989, BRC finished construction of a line from the port of Beira to Southern Rhodesia. Revenues from the port of Beira soon became the company's most important asset (Newitt 1995: 369–70). When construction of the railway was complete, the company leased estates on both sides of the line to Portuguese and other European companies and individuals. This arrangement formed the basis for later settler farms in the colonial administrative districts of Manica and Chimoio, which included the current Gondola District. Even before the completion of the railway, the company had encouraged colonial settlement in the region and by 1911, fifty-one farms surrounded the town of Chimoio, and forty-six around the town of Manica (Bannerman 1993: 4). Although this settlement led to land appropriation, many locals were not forced to move from their lands since there was great interest in maintaining them as a source of cheap labor. According to Portuguese documents, the African population in this region at the time was more concerned with taxes than with the loss of their land (5). The administration of the Mozambique Company lasted until 1941, when its charter expired.

The presence of the Beira Railway Company was particularly important to the development of the Gondola administrative center, Gondola Sede. According to local oral history, the railway was built over a dirt path made by ox-drawn carts, and soon the trains were spewing fire and smoke. The Gondola station was at first no more than a stopover where mechanics from Zimbabwe and Beira changed shifts. The stop consisted of a large warehouse near the railway station, a mill, a police station, and a farm and orchards run by Greeks who grew oranges, bananas, guavas, peanuts, and beans for export. In exchange for fruit from the orchards, local Africans brought in loads of wood used to build crates for shipping the Greeks' crops.

The railway company built the area's first hospital for its workers in Vila Gondola and to either side of the train stop; a neat row of tiny company houses, Bairro dos Trabalhadores, sprang up next to the track, along with a cluster of larger railway administrators' offices and dwellings. To cater to this growing community there followed more stores, bars, a boardinghouse, and even a sports club. Only much later did the Portuguese construct a small hospital near the central train stop for whites and *assimilados*—beginning in 1927, a legally defined status for Africans who could speak Portuguese, had abandoned their African way of life for European behaviors, and earned income from an occupation in commerce or industry. A smaller unit treated *indigenas*, non-Europeanized Africans, at the entrance to the Vila. The facility evidently treated only a tiny portion of the African population, most of whom depended on indigenous healers for treatment of their illnesses. Franciscan missionaries who ran a small boarding school maintained a mission hospital in Amatongas for the priests and their students, to which pregnant women would sometimes walk great distances before they were due to wait for delivery; there, local people remember, the nuns who served as nurses took in, fed, and cared well for local rural women.

As a group of Gondola's oldest male residents recalled in a May 1995 interview with me in Vila Gondola, by about 1942, only one store remained in Gondola—a Portuguese-owned barbershop where one could also trade food crops for goods such as much-desired cloth for women's wraps. The only currency used was English until 1949, when it is said the first Portuguese currency, *escudos*, appeared. In those days, 1 escudo bought two cakes, 5 escudos bought two drinks and a chicken, and 25 purchased a whole goat. At that time it cost a man 10 escudos to court and become engaged to a girl, and 50 to finalize a marriage negotiation. If the girl was *sika*, the daughter of a chief, bride-price would cost from 100 to 150 escudos.

In many ways, the early colonial period represented a significant rupture with the past, as rural social structures were forced to adapt to shifting relationships of production and reproduction. The imposition of a cash economy and the increasing number of men engaged in waged labor contributed to the prevalence of cash being used as the currency for loblolo, or bridewealth payments. This process, in turn, allowed young men to become increasingly independent from a kinship obligation—the generational debt to elders normally incurred in the transference of lineage wealth between families in the form of cows or hoes in marriage agreements. At the same time, colonial requirements of forced labor and taxes supplanted local systems of authority based on patrilineages and tributary relationships with local rulers (Pfeiffer 1997: 87). Local rulers enlisted by the Portuguese who did not cooperate with colonial demands were replaced or undermined. Domestic organization adjusted to the increased absence of men.

The Salazar Regime and Labor Reform

In 1926, a right-wing officers' coup overthrew the Portuguese parliamentary regime and in 1928 installed Antonio de Oliveira Salazar as minister of finance. In 1932, Salazar became prime minister and Portugal entered forty years of fascist rule, the Novo Estado, which implemented important changes in colonial policy. To increase profits from the colonial territories, during the Novo Estado state control in the colony increased, as did the number of Portuguese immigrants to Portuguese East Africa. Many of these Portuguese settlers were issued large landholdings in the areas of what are today Manica, Sussendenga, Chimoio, and Gondola. Although *chibalo* was officially abolished under the Novo Estado, new legislation was enforced that required most African men between the ages of eighteen and fifty-five to work at least six months a year to pay taxes. Formalized in 1942, this labor policy in practice legalized the forced-labor system until 1961, when international pressure forced its final abolition.

During the later period of Portuguese occupation, the entire colonial economy became increasingly dependent on compulsory male labor. Families were separated, often permanently, as members were sent to neighboring countries or as far away as Brazil and Sao Tome. A related form of labor expropriation developed around the forced production by women of cotton and rice cash crops on familial landholdings. Food production became increasingly the domain of women. These changes had a significant impact on the central region, although male labor migration was more common in the North and South, and cash cropping, especially of cotton, was most intensive in the North. In Manica and Sofala Provinces, between 10 and 28 percent of the population was engaged in cotton cultivation. In these areas, where state and the concessionary companies' policies deprived rural communities of male labor, cotton production fell disproportionally to rural women (Isaacman 1996: 83).

To assure the availability of male labor for wage and forced labor, colonial policies reinforced the increasingly sharp gender division of labor. This system intensified women's roles in nonsubsistence production while maintaining the community's dependence on women as the primary providers of food and child care. Where these two roles competed for women's time, rural families bore the social and economic costs. As evidence of this dynamic, Isaacman and Isaacman report, seven thousand women in Sofala went on strike in 1947 and refused to accept the government's cottonseed for forced cultivation. They complained that with their men absent to do forced labor on local sugar plantations, they could not both meet their cotton quotas and feed their families. In the end, local administrators exempted pregnant women and mothers with more than four children from forced cotton production (1983: 66).

Independence

Opposition to the Portuguese colonial presence took many forms and involved various levels of organization and participation. From individual flight to avoid labor duties or taxes to group work slowdowns or organized strikes and armed resistance, which occurred as late as 1917 in the Barue kingdom (Isaacman 1996), Mozambicans throughout the region resisted their plight as forcibly colonized peoples. By the 1960s in the Portuguese colonies, as in many places all over the African continent, Mozambicans within and outside the colony, influenced by nationalist struggles, began to organize for Independence. The Portuguese government in Lisbon made changes in relation to the colonies after World War II, through the fifties, and into the 1960s, including increased expenditures on rural development, commitment to the abolition of bound labor and forced crop cultivation, the official end to the use of the distinction between *indigenas* and the rest of the population, and repeal of the 1928 Labor Code, but the efforts were too little, too late. Forged from several nationalist organizations in 1962, FRELIMO began an armed campaign for Independence in the North in 1964. Ten years later, after protracted armed struggle, as an impoverished, war-weary Portuguese government fell in Lisbon, Mozambique won its independence on its own terms, officially becoming an independent state in 1975.

The flight of the Portuguese on the eve of Mozambican Independence reflected the severe nature of Portugal's occupation, for so long extracting profit from Mozambique's mostly rural population through forced labor, forced production, and unfair terms of trade while investing little in the country's social infrastructure. When the majority of Portuguese fled following the coup in Lisbon in 1974, sabotaging what technology or material wealth they could not carry with them, FRELIMO, the new socialist government of Mozambique, faced what seemed insurmountable obstacles to rebuilding the nation. Within the first years after Independence, however, policies were instituted that had important impacts on women and whose legacies continue to affect their lives today.

Stephanie Urdang (1983, 1989) and Kathleen Sheldon (1994, 2002) provide the most vivid and comprehensive accounts of the ways in which Independence has affected the lives of women in Mozambique. At the time of Independence in 1975, women had few opportunities for education. While the overall illiteracy rate was 90 percent, the rate for women was even higher. Besides forced cash crop production, the only other area where Mozambican women were gainfully employed in wage labor was in the capital's thriving prostitution industry, based on the patronage of South African tourists and foreign seamen.

Upon independence, FRELIMO immediately abolished forced labor, coerced cultivation, and the tourist trade in prostitution. Education was nationalized and expanded. In five years, the national literacy rate fell from 90 to 75 percent overall (Marshall 1989), but unevenly, with women at 85 percent and men at 59 percent. Women fought to be trained in all types of work, and where they were allowed to enter the workforce, they succeeded. The Mozambican Women's Organization (OMM) was made an arm of the government, a national women's organization of the FRELIMO party, with official status and funding to implement the integration of Mozambican women into the country's social and economic life at every level (Sheldon 1994, 2002).

Communal Villages

One FRELIMO policy with important implications for women's productive and reproductive lives was the creation of communal villages, *aldeias comunais*, the primary rural development strategy of the new government (Roesch 1986; West 2001; Pitcher 2002, 2008). The goal of this policy was to mobilize rural people to resettle in planned villages as a means of concentrating the rural population. Villagization, the often-forced resettlement of rural people into collective villages (Pitcher 2000; Newitt 1995: 549; Manning 2002: 59; Alexander 1997: 4–5), was considered a necessary precondition for rural development and the socialist transformation of the countryside. Otto Roesch, author of the single existing ethnographic study of communal village life in Mozambique, explains the thinking behind the plan: "Only through the villagization would the peasantry be able to overcome the isolation and obstacles which dispersed settlement patterns entailed: and only through villagization would it be financially possible for the government to make the necessary economic and social investments for developing rural productive forces and raising the standard of living for the rural population" (1986: 91). Through villagization, FRELIMO aimed to collectivize agriculture and extend basic infrastructure, including primary health care, sanitation, educational, and social services, to remote areas. The plan was also a vehicle for incorporating the peasantry into the national cultural and political life of the country.

More than 1.5 million people—15 percent of the entire rural population—were moved into more than 1,500 villages. The goal was to have the majority of the rural population voluntarily resettled by the end of the 1970s (Urdang 1989: 114). Communal villages were set up throughout the district of Gondola. Around the town of Vila Gondola, five distinct bairros or neighborhoods were organized using the same principles as for the communal villages. Each bairro had its own party structure organized from the bairro level, down through bairro cells composed of blocks, or *quadrões*, which consisted of a number of individual compounds called *talhões*. Mucessua encompasses five cells containing a total of nineteen *quadrões*.

The communal village arrangement influenced women's lives in several ways. Though his work focused on a communal village in Gaza Province in southern Mozambique, Otto Roesch (1984) observes that in general ways, villagization in Mozambique brought about a substantial improvement in women's social and political, if not economic, conditions. In economic terms, villagization may have increased work for women because they were farther from their fields and sources of wood. Village infrastructure had to be maintained on top of subsistence farming. On the other hand, the smaller village household, or *talha*, compared to the traditional patrilineal compound, or *muti*, and the presence of several wells in every neighborhood meant considerable savings in time spent cleaning and procuring water. The child-care functions of schools also saved women labor (Roesch 1986).

Socially, women's position in the household, as well as in the wider social context reportedly improved in the villages. Because of the close proximity of households, domestic violence decreased through the intervention of neighbors and relatives. The closer proximity of living spaces also favored the development of non-kinship-based forms of community support and cooperation. This development was especially helpful to older women without any close living relatives, who, in more isolated rural conditions, would not have received the assistance often lent them by neighbors in the village. Publicly, women had a voice and a formal institutional role as *responsaveis*, or those responsible for the running of their community, that they had not had before. There were probably more female *responsaveis* in the villages than men (Roesch 1986). Villagers also elected their own local assemblies and justice tribunals, often choosing women for these positions. The OMM also became active in the new villages (Urdang 1989: 114).

Other evidence suggests, and women in Mucessua told me, that the creation of communal villages also prompted a swell of social ills, especially increases in the incidence of communicable disease, adultery, theft, and accusations of witchcraft (Roesch 1984). From her study of political power in Sussundenga District, Alexander (1994: 41) concludes that the rise in post-Independence perceptions of the practice of witchcraft was not just the result of FRELIMO policies that suppressed redress against it by banning all "obscurantist" practices. It was also a result of tensions introduced by people living closer together, in conjunction with other profound economic and political changes. What has been overlooked so far in the work on communal villages in Mozambique is that women's unprecedented if superficial expanded role in village politics, and the increase in their unsanctioned sexual unions in the communal villages, signaled a decline in the ability of traditional institutions to control relations of reproduction. Witchcraft accusations in this context may have been more than a response to increased jealousy and illness resulting from close contact; they could also have represented heightened tensions over control of women and reproduction, as well as women's expressed greater sense of reproductive vulnerability and power.

In the later war of destabilization, the communal villages were primary targets of attacks by the insurgent army, the Mozambican National Resistance (RENAMO). Inhabitants of rural villages in the district moved closer to the towns and to the Beira Corridor to avoid violence. Many of the women who participated in this study moved from rural dwellings to Mucessua as a result of the war. Some of the same dynamics of the villages may have held true for the peri-urban bairros, where more and more displaced families resettled as the war went on.

Because the sexual division of labor within the house remained unchanged, women's possibilities for increased leisure, education, and work outside the home remained limited (Cliff 1991: 20).[3] This situation was reflected in the lack of equal representation of women in all levels of government and decision-making positions (Urdang 1989: 28). It was also reflected in the absence in the Land Law of 1979 of any reference to traditional land tenure systems or any other statement that would establish, clarify, and reinforce women's rights to land (Kruks and Wisner 1989: 164). Despite its progressive mission statements, OMM, as the institutionalized voice for women, ultimately failed to play an active role in affecting the direction of the new country's development policies in ways that prevented the marginalization of women (Urdang 1989: 25–26).

> Despite the important gains for women, . . . certain conditions effectively blocked women's complete integration at every level of society, thus impeding the process of liberating them from economic and social exploitation. Women are encouraged to take on men's roles in every sphere. They are made equal in the law and in the constitution, and are engaged in diverse tasks that were previously regarded as men's domain. But when it comes to perhaps the most fundamental issue—the sexual division of labor within the household—little change can be perceived. (ibid.: 24)

While the vanguard vision of the young nation's leaders was to harness local participation to produce social change and to integrate women into all levels of the social, political, and economic life of the country, early policies worked against this vision in critical ways:

> FRELIMO's own radical attempts to create not only a centrally planned and managed economy but a command society soon alienated large portions of the Mozambican population, particularly in rural areas. Increasingly these populations reverted to historically effective strategies of exit, as FRELIMO's ever more heavy-handed intrusiveness (further aggravated by wartime conditions) reawakened and reinforced long-established assumptions about the state's detrimental presence. (Alinsky 2001)

Heedless of its proclaimed social agenda, the government favored state-sponsored programs for agrarian reform that gave priority to cash cropping and state farms over the family sector and male workers over female workers (Kruks and Wisner 1989). State farm work, the only source of wage labor in most rural areas, went primarily to men. As Urdang predicted, a result of the direction of early policy was that the gap between women (as family farmers) and men (as cash croppers) grew rather than shrank, and women have been increasingly marginalized from national production (Urdang 1989: 26).

The Health of Independent Mozambique

Indigenous Medicine

Under the colonial regime, health services for the majority of Mozambicans had been almost nonexistent. Thirty percent of the colonial health budget and two-thirds of the trained health personnel were concentrated in the hospital in the country's capital, Maputo. For a population of ten million, only seven antenatal clinics existed, all in urban areas (Cliff 1991: 19). Yet 90 percent of Mozambicans lived in rural areas, and only 70 percent lived within the reach of formal health care (Walt 1983: 2).

It was the goal of the FRELIMO government to restructure Mozambican society using their model of "scientific socialism." According to this vision, "traditionalism" was the main barrier to the creation of a modern, nontribal, nonracial, and equitable nation. As part of the strategy to rapidly transform the country's economy and society, FRELIMO tried to abolish such practices as bridewealth, polygamy, initiation rites, and land tenure, as well as indigenous healing practices. It created a Department of Traditional Medicine within the Ministry of Health to identify and record indigenous ethnobotanical knowledge and to research the efficacy of plants used in indigenous therapies.

These developments notwithstanding, indigenous healers, spirit mediums (called *ngangas* locally or curandeiros in Portuguese), and religious leaders were discouraged and frequently suppressed as purveyors of "obscurantism" and "superstition," and as private practitioners. Many continued to practice clandestinely outside the villages. Others continued to exercise power informally, as did many local chiefs and other indigenous political leaders who FRELIMO stripped of official authority (Green 1994: 7). It has been argued that this alienation of traditional and ritual leaders and healers was a significant factor in FRELIMO's ceding political control of most of the geographical area of Mozambique to RENAMO during the war of destabilization (Hanlon 1984). It has also been suggested that the government's imposition of centralized national health policies and program planning undermined self-reliance and fostered dependency (Green, Jurg, and Djedje 1994: 7).

Since the mid-1980s, a growing awareness within the Mozambican government of the failures of certain strategies to win the support of the population has led to a series of reassessments of policy aimed first at religious practice and indigenous healers, and most recently at traditional chiefs, political leaders, and land reform. Since the late 1980s the Ministry of Health has made efforts to develop a collaborative relationship with indigenous healers, particularly in the areas of childhood diarrhea and AIDS/sexually transmitted infections (Green, Jurg, and Djedje 1994).

The Nationalization of Health Care

Two of the first policies FRELIMO implemented following Independence were the nationalization of health care in 1975 and the implementation of socialized health services in 1977. Through the construction of rural health posts and the training of community heath workers, the goal of the nationalized health plan was to extend primary health care to the rural population. The health program emphasized the benefits of preventive health care, especially vaccinations and improved sanitation through the building of latrines. A vaccination and health education campaign began in 1976 and swept the country. Between 1975 and 1982, the number of rural health posts went from 426 to 1,171, giving many more rural people access to primary health care (Cliff 1991: 20).

At the time of Independence, women and children were identified as the groups most affected by poor health and lack of health care. Women often bore children from an early age until menopause. This factor, combined with poor nutrition and insufficient and inadequate care in early pregnancy, made women of childbearing age extremely vulnerable and maternal mortality rates due to complications in pregnancy and childbirth quite high (Walt 1983: 11). In response to these realities, in 1977 the FRELIMO party platform prioritized improving maternal and child health, and some improvements were put into place: the number of maternity beds in the country increased by 39 percent by 1986, and the number of midwives trained rose from 457 in 1980 to 971 in 1986. Mothers' and children's clinics were integrated so that a single visit could serve the needs of both a mother and her child. Expansion of the prenatal care program resulted in its use by more women. Antitetanus vaccines and family-planning campaigns met with great success. By 1981, national data showed that almost 50 percent of pregnant women attended antenatal clinics. New legislation gave women the right to two months paid maternity leave and encouraged breast-feeding (Cliff 1991: 20–22).

FRELIMO's commitment to improved maternal health conditions and emancipation of women did not go so far, however, as to give women ultimate control of their reproductive capacities. By carrying over from the colonial period legislation making abortion illegal, the state denied women the right to safe, affordable pregnancy termination, a policy decision that forces many women into life-threatening circumstances. Though data on maternal mortality in Mozambique are scant and rely mostly on hospital or statistically estimated figures, it has recently been calculated that at least one in every fourteen Mozambican women of reproductive age dies of maternal causes, and attempted abortions in unsafe conditions contribute to at least 9 percent of those deaths occurring in a hospital. It is possible that these numbers represent just the nose of the hippopotamus, as many women die outside hospitals and complications resulting from abortions often go unregistered because of the social stigma and the legal aspects of abortion that prevail in the country (Granja 1996: 6).

Women, Health, and the War of Destabilization

Soon after Mozambique gained Independence in 1975, Ian Smith's Rhodesia formed and financially supported an anti-Communist movement calling itself the Mozambican National Resistance (MNR), or RENAMO, in an effort to destabilize the newly independent country. Bringing together disgruntled Mozambican groups that did not get their due in terms of power following independence from Portugal, this guerrilla force was mobilized with the participation of Mozambican political dissenters to undermine Mozambique for its role in supporting Zimbabwe African National Liberation Army (ZANLA) and providing a rear base for African National Congress guerrillas' anticolonial movement in South Africa. When Zimbabwe won its independence in 1980, South Africa took over funding RENAMO with assistance from the United States.

In 1982, the campaign of destabilization intensified, driving Mozambique into a period remembered as the Emergency. Through the early 1980s, roads were unsafe for travel, as mines and ambushes greatly restricted peasant access to markets in urban centers. People were unable to cultivate their fields for fear of attack, and many left their homes seeking refuge in administrative centers such as Gondola and all along the Corridor, where there was a greater military presence. In the wake of mass migrations, the populations of towns and urban centers doubled, placing extreme pressure on available land, water sources, and services, for which there was intense competition. Drought in the early and mid-1980s heightened the scarcity of food, as did the halt in subsistence farming in much of the country, increasing the toll of malnutrition and starvation among the population.

Until the ceasefire in 1992, RENAMO continued its destructive course, targeting the economic infrastructure of the country, the civilian population, and any visible signs of government success in health and education initiatives and especially the communal villages (Hanlon 1984). In the end, some four million people were displaced within Mozambique and more than 1.7 million refugees sought asylum in neighboring countries. More than one million Mozambicans died before the conflict ended in 1992.

According to Julie Cliff, who documented the impact of this war of destabilization on women in Mozambique, women were direct and indirect victims of the war:

> A function of young girls and women is to provide sex for the (RENAMO) combatants; . . . these women are required to submit to sexual demands, in effect to be raped, on a frequent sustained basis. . . . One of the frequent refugee complaints (verified by medical workers in some refugee camps) is the level of venereal disease which this practice proliferates. Severe beatings are inflicted on young girls and women who resist sexual demands. Such punishment may also be inflicted on the husband or father of the female who resists. Such punishment reportedly can include execution in some circumstances. (Cliff 1991: 22)

Women's health was further undermined as health facilities were targeted, reducing access to maternity units for delivery, which "undoubtedly increased maternal deaths from hemorrhages, infections, eclampsia, and anemia" (ibid.). When the war displaced rural populations and made cultivation impossible, women left behind by men who had migrated and those who depended on women for food lost their livelihoods and homes. Fleeing the violence, women were separated from children and lost their husbands. The violence and dislocation suffered by a majority of civilians during the externally driven civil war after Independence in 1975 intensified these dynamics (Cliff 1991).

Structural Adjustment and Health in Mozambique

In addition to the suffering caused by the war of destabilization, Mozambique faced an economic crisis resulting from several factors other than the cost of war: a dependency on primary product exports in an inequitable world trading system, an extreme shortage of managerial personnel, and early agricultural policy errors that gave priority to state rather than family farms (Cliff 1991: 24). South Africa, while funding RENAMO's antigovernment insurgency, had undercut the Mozambican economy by diverting traffic from Mozambican to South African railways and ports (Cliff 1991: 24). In an effort to win favor with U.S. policy makers whose intervention was critical to negotiating an end to the war of destabilization, Mozambique initiated a series of changes in its economic policy. Under pressure from the United States, which had openly sponsored RENAMO until 1987, Mozambique joined the IMF and World Bank in 1984 and in 1987 announced an economic austerity program of structural adjustment—the *Programma de Reforma Economica* (PRE), that is, Program of Economic Reform.

Mozambique's structural adjustment program involved a major devaluation of the Mozambican currency and government cuts in public spending, most severely in health and education, along with the introduction of fees in these sectors. An end to subsidies in staple foods, rents, and utilities led to steep price increases. FRELIMO's version of economic reform investment was still directed to the productive sector; foreign trade was regulated and few government enterprises were privatized (Hanlon 1996: 18).

As theorists Saskia Sassen (2003) and Isabella Bakker and Stephen Gill (2003) have argued, the politics of international debt have had the greatest effect on the sphere of social reproduction and thus on women, while amplifying patriarchy. Austerity programs necessarily target poor, rural women, whose lack of access to good land and small chances of intensifying production limit their ability to benefit from the new market conditions created by adjustment (Cliff 1991: 26). Without ways to boost their incomes, women, in particular those responsible for feeding families, suffered the hardships caused by inflation and rising prices as subsidies and price controls were dismantled. It has also been proposed that under structural adjustment, pressures on women, already responsible for extensive agricultural and domestic labor, would intensify in the "stabilized" economy, as government programs focused on family-sector production without taking measures to raise women's productivity (UNICEF 1991: 33).

Women's positions in impoverished households grew especially precarious, as poor women usually did not have access to or control of cash needed for food and other necessities for themselves and their children. Under these emergent conditions, the exigencies of migrant labor flows in regional economies like Mozambique's have accentuated this "super-exploitation" of rural women who are already overburdened in the work they do in the areas of childbearing, health care, and care of the elderly, injured, and disabled (Bond 2007: 188). This gendered pattern of superexploitation is part of a broader global trend of "the reprivatisation of social reproduction" outlined by Isabella Bakker and Stephen Gill (2003: 136). This trend includes:

+ household and caring activities are increasingly provided through the market and are thus exposed to the movement of money;
+ societies seem to become redefined as collections of individuals (or at best collections of families), particularly when the state retreats from universal social protection;
+ accumulation patterns premised on connected control over wider areas of social life and thus the provisions for social reproduction;
+ survival and livelihood. For example, a large portion of the world's population has no effective health insurance or even basic care.

Indeed, in Mozambique, the negative effects of structural adjustment policies have undermined the status of women in ways that continue into the present moment. For Mozambicans, as for many Africans, the costs are high: "the denial of access to food, medicines, energy, and even water is the most extreme result; people who are surplus to capitalism's labor requirements find they must fend for themselves or die" (Bond 2007: 188).

Still Bearing the Burden: Shifting Economy and Gender in Mozambique

Women's agricultural labor in family-sector farms continues to be the cornerstone of both household subsistence and national food production, though their dependence on men for access to money has not decreased. Most of the efforts to improve rural production have failed to reduce women's workloads; indeed, there is evidence that women's workloads have intensified (MOPF 1998: 312) while indigenous forms of social support for women, and women's access to cash and land for growing food, may be eroding (Pfeiffer 1997; Chapman 1998). Meanwhile, inflation and increased commoditization of the local economy require that women have access to money. These contradictions and vulnerabilities expose the gendered features of what Parson (1985) has called the life of the "peasantariat"—people who have been drawn systematically into the labor market but must still depend on nonmonetized agricultural production. Survival turns on what land one has rights in and what ways one is connected to others with rights in land.

Precolonial Land Allocation and Production

In the Shona ethnolinguistic continuum, one can describe oral histories as kincentric; that is, history is told through and known primarily in reference to kinship links, and kinship is narrated in relationship to specific land, land features, and landscapes (Salmon 2000: 1328–29). In turn, the land inscribes and conditions kinship through people's relationships with it through agricultural production and through their movement across land over time. History, land, and agricultural production mutually sustain and inform kinship and political structures (Bourdillon 1991: 67). For example, until the colonial period, land was not considered private property but was held collectively by the patrilineage and intimately associated with the history of a chiefdom, with the ruling chief or *mambo* (Sh.), and with ancestral spirits who lived on the land (ibid.). Theoretically, in the name of his patrilineage, a *mambo* (later called *regulo* in Mozambique under the Portuguese colonial administration) has sovereignty over a geographical territory called a *nyika*, which was subdivided into wards or *dunhu*, ruled over by subchiefs or *sadunhu* (all Shona terms), who are usually kin to the *mambo*. The *mambo* has domain over the land as the senior living representative of the land's ancestral spirit guardians, and it is within the authority of the chief or one of his ward *sadunhu* (headmen) to allocate land to followers, or even on occasion to persons from outside the *nyika* (Bourdillon 1991: 73). Rights to cultivate land are normally permanent and not revoked unless a landholder has left the land uncultivated for a long period, seriously damaged the land, or committed a grave offense against the local community. In Shona areas, these rights in land, once given, customarily pass through the male lineage from a landholder to his sons (MAARP 1995a: 58).

From the late colonial period until recently, a woman gained access to land for cultivation through her husband, who received his allocation of land on behalf of his family from the *mambo* and was expected to allot separate portions to each of his wives (Ranger 2002; Bourdillon 1991: 72; Holleman 1952: 7). The wife was then expected to raise enough crops to feed herself, her children, and her husband from her plot, called a *munda* in Shona or a *machamba* throughout Central Mozambique. This is how women became the primary agricultural producers in this region, as produce from their plots supplied the bulk of food for home consumption as male labor was constantly drawn away from home cultivation (Isaacman and Isaacman 1984).

Wives maintained some autonomy over their individual plots, generally cultivating grain and subsidiary crops. Produce from men's fields (*zunde*) was more often for ritual use, guests, trade, or sale. A husband would also be expected to share his stock with a wife whose stock had become depleted (Bourdillon 1991: 73). Wives in polygynous households worked on their own plots, helped in each other's plots, and worked in their husband's fields. If a man had only one wife, the couple usually jointly cultivated one field on which they raised staple crops with the help of their elder children (Holleman 1952: 9). Through their husbands, women were also allocated access to their own lowland riverbed plots, called *matoros* in ChiTewe and *baixas* in Portuguese, to produce winter maize, vegetables, sugarcane, and fruits like bananas, mangoes, oranges, and pineapples (Bourdillon 1991: 74).

Although a household's members performed most of its daily agricultural and domestic work, there are frequent instances of long-standing collective work practices in which members of several families or of neighboring villages work collectively in rotation on each other's fields. A more limited form of work exchange, called *majanggano* in Shona, involves members of several households coming together to arrange a schedule of reciprocal aid for specific tasks, for example, clearing, ploughing, weeding, and harvesting. The compensation for such work exchange might be the day's meals.

Nhimbe is a more extensive form of collective labor in which a large number of neighboring villagers work in rotation on one of their fields (Holleman 1952: 10–11). Central to the *nhimbe* work party is the distribution and consumption of homemade beer or spirits made for the event by the host of the work party. Through these social mechanisms, men and women both were able to cultivate more land than they could have managed with the aid of their families only (11). Being able to mobilize collective labor in these ways was no doubt especially valuable to women, whose concentration on producing food for home consumption might otherwise have kept them from increasing or even maintaining that production during the long periods men were absent from the household, a common occurrence throughout this area during much of the colonial period.

Gender and Production in Contemporary Gondola

The colonial political economy was characterized, as we have seen, by large-scale land appropriation for commercial and settler use, forced male and female labor, widespread male labor migration, and forced cash cropping, all of which the peoples of the region strenuously resisted. In the contemporary period, the bulk of agricultural production in the family sector in Gondola is for home consumption, and the work is backbreaking. Land is still cleared in phases by ax and fire. Crops grown on machambas in Gondola are mainly maize (called *milho* in Portuguese and *magwere* in ChiTewe), cassava, and sorghum. Millet, sweet potatoes, and pigeon peas are also common.

Besides these staples, women in Mucessua plant peanuts, rice, groundnuts, tangerines, pineapples, and pumpkins in upland machamba plots. In their riverbed matoro plots, they commonly plant sugarcane, bananas, rice, and beans—mostly kidney and butter. Crops of tomatoes, sweet potatoes, large tubers called *madumbe* and *nyam*, rabe, onion, cassava, cabbage, garlic, lettuce, tangerines, potatoes, and oranges were also reported. When the winter months of July, August, and September come around, it is time to burn the machamba fields and prepare them before the October rains. (Although necessary for the machambas of newly planted maize, the rains often flood the riverbed matoro plots, making them difficult or impossible to cultivate.) Next comes the time for weeding the machamba, and the cycle is renewed.

Most women have between half an hour and half a day's walk to their machamba. If her machamba is distant, a woman may spend several days in a row working in her plot of land, sleeping in a small, temporary hut (*palhota*), her nursing infant with her, her weaned children at her bairro house in the care of a female relative or older child.

Women and Land Access

In the nova vida, changes and uncertainties in land tenure have hit poor households hard in Gondola (Alexander 1994). Some trends, however, mitigate especially against women subsistence farmers' access to fertile land. Among the forces that have undermined women's bargaining position in their households, diminishing their control over their own and their children's lives, are, for example, weaker traditional systems of land allocation, less community and lineage-based support for land clearing and land access, more commoditization of land access (e.g., rent payments or land purchases), and continued land alienation (Pfeiffer 1997: 156).

The assumption is that women have gained access to land through men within the strongly patrilineal kinship organization of Shona villages since the late precolonial and colonial periods, as noted earlier (Ranger 2002). A woman derived rights to land from her husband through marriage, and a woman who left her marriage could access land through her natal lineage. After Independence, when the vast majority of Portuguese colonists fled Mozambique, abandoning many farms and rural properties, the Mozambican government nationalized all land. A provincial report summarized the status of the family sector in light of contemporary land laws in 1995:

> The family sector household does not require authority to occupy land when it is outside protected zones (for example National Parks etc.), or planned agricultural development (e.g. commercial farms, state farms etc.). However, the land must be free from other occupants. If families have suitable lands, housing etc. they can apply for title. If the land is abandoned for more than two years it can be forfeited. Nevertheless, the regulations dealing with the family sector do not appear to give family sector households sufficient protection in the Manica, Gondola and Sussundenga Districts, as many family households are residing on farms, upon which they, or their forebears,

have always resided, but for which they have no legal rights. (MAARP 1995a: 55)

Land allocation practices in Gondola reflect competing claims by state, private, and long-standing indigenous institutions. Influences on the customary system of land allocation over the last hundred years include Western ideas regarding private ownership, the alienation of land under the administration of the colonial concessionary companies, the post-Independence policy of land nationalization, and the establishment of agricultural cooperatives and state farms. In spite of these influences, however, some customary methods of land allocation have survived (MAARP 1995b: 57–58). In Mucessua, one can still acquire land in much the same way as described by customary law, but in towns and their bairros, government functionaries have taken over the conflict resolution role of headmen or *regulos*, who resolved land disputes based on traditionally inherited land rights:

> When someone needs land for a machamba, they must approach the person who is *dono* (master, owner) of the land, whose parents lived and died there. If the *dono* is not able to clear the land himself, he will contribute it to another person. It depends if the land has plants that are his family's or his. Others hand [the land] over. The *dono* can. When people arrive in a [rural] zone, family of the *regulo* continue [to have power] there. Whoever wishes to sell a *mashamba* has to give testimony before the family of the *regulo*. The *regulo* is *dono*. [The transaction is finalized by] a verbal declaration. Fruit trees mark [the boundaries]. (Ibid.)

Parallel systems of allocation, however, are undermining traditional claims on land. As the first bairro secretary of Gondola told me in a 1995 interview, while family-sector farmers are seeking land in one arena, commercial and foreign interests go through different channels to seek land rights in the same area. As traditional and local government authority is superseded by higher-level Ministry of Agriculture policies, smallholding family farmers are losing out: "Foreigners [seeking formal access to land] must go to [the Ministry of] Agriculture. It is on maps where there were farms since long ago. The [district] director of agriculture goes and tells the people [that land has been leased], and the people have to get out of the way."

This pressure for land has led to competition and conflicts. By 1995, all the fertile riverbed matoro land in the Mucessua area was occupied, except that thought to contain landmines. As the traditional system of land acquisition collapsed, an illegal market emerged in response to demand for the land from rich purchasers who, rather than apply to the state for a lease, "buy" land from peasants desperately strapped for cash.

The direction of land access disputes created a new area of uncertainty in terms of women's social and economic security, and in the emerging land market, women with little access to money were not influential players. In the current cash economy, even land that was traditionally distributed through lineage males to wives and daughters on a need basis is now increasingly bought and sold in a formal and informal land market. As land shortages increase for the fast-growing peri-urban populations like Mucessua (Bannerman 1993), women without capital cannot compete.

Among the women I worked with, 80 percent reported they had access to a family cultivation plot, or machamba. Of the 20 percent who did not, most reported that someone else in the household had access to land for cultivation. Only two households reported no access to land for a machamba. Twenty-five women said they did not have personal control over production since they worked in another family's plot. Access to matoro or *baixa* river-bed plots in Gondola is even more restricted, which has particular implications for women. Matoros are key resources because of the constant water supply and the relative fertility of the alluvial soil. Every family in Mucessua strives to get access to a matoro in the same way families seek to own cattle in other parts of Africa. A matoro means prestige, as well as cash income. In Gondola it is frequently lamented, "If you do not have a matoro, you are not a man" (Shumba 1995). Women without their own matoros were greatly disadvantaged. Their families had no personal source of food to diversify the family diet and would have little opportunity to generate cash. As these lands with irrigation potential are often the prime sites for commercial agricultural ventures, conflicts over matoro land have become the critical land tenure question (Shumba 1995). Sixty-five percent of the case study women I worked with had access to matoros.

Market Infrastructure in Gondola

Until 1993, Agricom, a state company, provided institutional support and structure for larger-scale rural trading. The company purchased families' surplus produce at government-set prices, transporting it to central markets for resale at subsidized prices (below buying cost), and supplying agricultural inputs like seeds, plows, tools, and fertilizer for sale to rural producers. Agricom's fixed prices, provision of transport, and input supply all bolstered rural family production. When the company failed financially and ceased to function between 1993 and 1994 (MAARP 1995a: 144), a trading crisis ensued (MAARP 1995a: 127). As rural family farmers lost their access to protected prices and transport to markets, and as many rural input outlets closed, market incentives for rural family production sank (Shumba 1995). Following Mozambique's increasingly capitalist orientation under IMF economic reform, private traders offering depressed prices stepped in to fill the gap created by Agricom's collapse, as intended by the structural adjustment program.

These independent private buyers, known as *comerciantes ambulantes*, represented a new private rural trading nexus directly dominated by large commercial interests based in Chimoio, Beira, and the national capital, Maputo (Pfeiffer 1997: 158). With no alternatives, family farmers were forced to sell their surpluses at discouragingly low prices.

The lifting of other kinds of state price controls under structural adjustment has worsened terms of trade for family farmers generally, and women family farmers in particular, in other ways. From 1993 to 1995, the first period of this research, while prices remained stable in the Gondola markets for some locally produced foods, the government abolished price controls for staple goods like oil, maize flour, rice, bread, and sugar. The price for twenty kilos of maize meal shot from 5,000 meticais to 20,000 meticais, and the price of sugar, wheat flour, bread, and rice tripled. In the inflationary economy, the cost of most manufactured goods also skyrocketed. The price of a bar of soap more than doubled, from 4,000 meticais to 10,000. At the same time, the market price for vegetables grown locally in matoros and sold by women—tomatoes, cabbage, sweet potatoes, and cassava root—stayed almost level. As I followed exchange rates, household budgets, and market prices for only a year and a half, women producers suffered especially in this quickly changing economy as their purchasing power for household staples declined.

The Gender of Opportunity

Since Independence in 1975, internal and international forces affecting male labor migration in Manica Province have changed considerably, also shifting the employment and opportunity structures for women. The end of colonial forced labor, the closing of the Rhodesian-Mozambique border in the late 1970s, new economic policies in post-Independence Zimbabwe, and the exodus of Portuguese settlers from commercial enterprises on the eve of Mozambican Independence—all of these reduced male labor migration from Manica Province (Pfeiffer 1997: 160). In time, new state enterprises in Mozambique made up for the jobs lost by creating state farms in place of private farms or plantations. The ostensible goal of cooperative and collective farming strategies, usually associated with communal villages, was to acknowledge and support women's roles in food production and social reproduction (Kruks and Wisner 1984). However, in the state farm sector, where government economic programs concentrated their resources, the labor force was mostly male. Women continued to function mainly as domestic food producers. FRELIMO, the government of Mozambique immediately following Independence, thus largely reproduced the gendered rural labor division that existed under Portuguese colonial rule.

The war of destabilization further disrupted patterns of employment. State-sector enterprises were attacked, and private enterprises were also often forced to stop production. Military service took many rural men from their homes. The breakdown in rural production and trade and the lack of cash resources, combined with recurrent droughts from 1979 on and especially in 1992, forced many rural families to depend on emergency food rations. In the wake of the ceasefire, the people of Gondola talked of emerging from crisis: elections were held, and 1993 and 1994 brought the first promising harvests in many years.

Though the overall absence of men from Gondola in 1994 was less than it had been even ten years earlier, 30.5 percent of the male partners in the households of the women in my group were absent for short or extended periods, sometimes for paid labor. According to the first secretary of Bairro Mucessua, most Mucessua residents were subsistence farmers. He estimated that 80 to 85 percent of the male population was otherwise unemployed, because of the war and the recent influx of immigrants.

The sporadic nature of employment, as well as the cultural penchant for guarding information regarding wealth and assets, makes reliable information on income generation in a peasant economy difficult to obtain. Of the seventy-two women who reported employment and household income, 52.8 percent reported that someone in the household had a job in the formal sector. Fifty-eight percent reported that someone in their household made some cash in the informal sector by selling commercial grains for export; from the small-scale sale of fruit and vegetables at local markets, homemade alcohol, secondhand clothes, homemade bread, hand-made baskets, or herbal medicines and charms; or from running a church. Eleven households (15.2 percent) reported both formal and informal income sources. Twelve women reported selling produce occasionally at the district market.

Formal-sector employment in Vila Gondola was dominated by state, parastatal, and private institutions, which employed mostly men. While the biggest employers in Gondola were the Mozambique Railway—Caminho de Ferro de Moçambique (CFM)—and Avibela, once a state-owned and then a privately owned poultry and egg commercial wholesaler, only two households I worked with reported a family member currently employed by CFM and only three reported one at Avibela. Other types of formal employment among the case study group included guard, teacher, police officer, mechanic, mason, shopkeeper, agricultural extensionist, cook, electrician, carpenter, motorist, market-stall seller, member of the military, and nongovernmental organization employee. With the exception of two women employed in the public formal sector, all reported formal-sector employment was male.

Information about men's income was especially hard to obtain, as most women claimed they did not know their husband's salary or the total amount cash earners in the household donated to household expenditures. From the limited data I gathered, two significant patterns emerged: men's sources of income, first, were more regular and, second, on average brought in higher cash earnings than women's. Of the twenty-seven men whose incomes were estimated, nineteen (70.4 percent) were derived from formal employment and eight (29.6 percent) from the informal sector. Reported male incomes ranged from 25,000 to 500,000 meticais, although the one high number reported might have reflected the total sales of produce over several months rather than a steady monthly income.

Women's patterns for generating cash income were very different from men's. For the sixty-three women in the case study for whom it was possible to estimate income, forty (65.2 percent) reported they earned no income themselves. With the exception of the two women formally employed, all other women's income was generated from the informal sector. Only twenty-two (35 percent) women in the sixty-three households with cash incomes reported having their own source of cash income, which came from the sale of produce, homemade foodstuffs, or alcohol, and in one case used clothing. One woman was a domestic in the administrative office of a foreign nongovernmental organization. Two others had jobs at the district level with FRELIMO party mass mobilization organizations (OCM, the Organization of Continuers of Mozambique; and OMM, the Mozambican Women's Organization), though budgetary problems had led both women's subsidies to be cut for the duration of my work in Gondola. None of the women reported earning cash by working seasonally on others' fields. The small number of women who reported monthly earnings had incomes from 1,000 to 300,000 meticais (+U.S. $0.10–$30); the highest incomes derived from selling alcohol, running a small market stall in the bairro, and selling produce. In the six cases of reported incomes over 100,000 meticais, the respondents shared their work with a male family member, usually a husband or brother, and did not control the income independently. The majority of incomes were less than 50,000 meticais (+U.S. $5). All the women said that their incomes were sporadic and tended to fluctuate seasonally.

All but two of the women I followed through pregnancy worked at subsistence cultivation and domestic labor for their own household along with any other productive labor in which they were engaged. Of the two who did not work in subsistence farming, one was a recently married seventeen-year-old who was living temporarily in her mother's house while her young, educated husband searched for waged labor in the provincial capital. The other was a recently married eighteen-year-old who had been brought to live in the household of her husband's brother, in which five members were gainfully employed in the formal sector.

Farming in this area is a year-round occupation, and the requirements of access to both a machamba and a matoro make it difficult for women to undertake nonfarming activities. However, during the dry season, many women make and sell homemade fermented millet, sorghum, or corn mash beer called *ndoro* or spirits called *nipa*. *Nipa* is distilled from the juice of fruits, especially bananas and mangoes, as well as sugarcane. Some households that do not produce sugarcane or bananas themselves often buy the ingredients, as selling *nipa* is said to be a lucrative business. Five women earned income from brewing alcohol.

While selling homemade alcohol has increasingly become a means for women subsistence farmers to earn money, as has elsewhere been observed, not all the consequences are positive. In a 1995 study of land-use issues in the Gondola area, researchers found that residents made a connection between the high consumption of *nipa* and the high number of stillbirths in the community (Shumba 1995), although more comprehensive data are needed to follow up these observations. In a broad study of women's health in East Africa, Raikes (1989) suggests that beer brewing, while an important source of income for women, reinforces their subordination: in many settings where homemade beer is sold, the drinking leads to greater physical and verbal abuse of women and children.

Such alcohol-related abuse may be linked to changing economic relationships, with men refusing to accept their responsibility for household food crop production yet unable to find other regular work. Without affirming roles in the family or the labor market, men take refuge in the patriarchal household, and women pay the price in their own compromised nutrition, as well as physical and psychological violence. Male beer consumption and other activities associated with drinking, including the consumption of food and sex, also drain family coffers of cash needed for household expenditures (Raikes 1989: 453). How beer brewing redistributes cash between men and women and between households and what impact these transactions have on individual and community-level health and gender status remain open questions.

Women's Economic Vulnerability

The government, NGOs, and research scholars agree that the levels of income women in Mucessua report fall well below the minimum required for bare subsistence (MOH 1993: 43). These are not even the wages of poverty; they represent an extraction of women's productive and reproductive capacities that goes unmentioned in many studies and reports. Only three of the women in the eighty-three households reported earning enough cash to sustain a household of seven, the group's mean household size. Based on the patterns of unemployment in Gondola, salary levels during my research, and Ministry of Health calculations for cash requirements that fail to take into account categories such as housing materials, clothing, medical costs, household items or agricultural inputs, or firewood, the monetary income of most households I worked with was too low to cover its members' basic nutritional needs.

Women without access to or control of money and collective labor also had difficulty getting help on their agricultural plots, especially for clearing and harvesting, as generally people would work only for cash. In the increasingly monetized economy, only women with cash at their disposal are able to mobilize labor outside their immediate domestic unit. In most cases, women must depend on their husbands, or in some cases brothers or mothers-in-law, to make cash available to pay for short-term agricultural labor. Unable to generate their own income, most women did not control cash until they controlled the labor of their children who earned cash. Women's economic marginalization was thus linked to changes in household structures and expectations—in other words, to kinship.

Changing Relations of Reproduction and Conflict

Shona Kinship, Households, and Social Organization

Kinship and the rights, rules, and responsibilities of kinship-based social relations are at the heart of Shona social organization. The Shona household is part of a larger corporate lineage group on whose perpetuation and health households depend for their continuity and well-being (Bourdillon 1991: 27). As the basis of a society organized primarily around kinship relations, the Shona kinship system meets two essential requirements, according to Holleman (1952: 30):

a. it provides a definite pattern of social order in which any two persons or classes of persons of the same sex, closely or remotely related by blood or by marriage, are placed in a position of relative superiority or subordination;

b. it regulates the reproduction of unilineal and exogamous kin-groups, with due respect to native conceptions of incest, and the existing social order referred to [in (a)].

While traditional structural functional anthropology looks for and posits coherent social patterns of static, self-enclosed social relationships, my observations in this case suggest a much more complex and fluid social organization connected to both colonial and international influences. How does such a system get disordered, and what are the implications for gender and health?

In cultures where there is a strong emphasis on lineage, "[the lineage] is seen as a descent group reaching infinitely far into the future. Only a small proportion are alive at any time. Yet, that extension into the future should be the central concern not only of those now alive, but also of their dead ancestors" (Pearce 1995: 198). What Pearce observed among Yoruba households in Nigeria holds for Shona social organization as well: it is the role of women to produce a suitable number of offspring to preserve the strength of the patrilineage through the next generation, as well as to supply enough workers to ensure the survival of the living. In the patrilineage, the birth of sons to carry on clan names was also paramount, and many births might be required to produce an acceptable number. In Shona cosmology, spirits of the dead, especially ancestors, would punish lineage members who shirked their responsibility for the welfare of the lineage group (Bourdillon 1991: 233).

The control of a woman's fertility was not, thus, a personal or family issue alone, but a concern of the lineage. Within the Shona extended patrilineal compound, a woman frequently lived with her husband's parents, with his siblings and their wives, and where polygyny was common, with co-wives of her husband. Control over fertility was maintained by male and female senior members of the patrilineage through marriage arrangement, payment and residence rules, organization of domestic units, gender and seniority division of labor, and the upholding of the value placed on children, levirate—the social practice of marrying a widow to a sibling of the dead spouse—and polygyny. Through forms of social pressure from gossip to divorce, from threatening sorcery to using intimate partner violence, social control of women's reproductive functions was embedded in these community institutions. Many aspects of these patrilineal kinship structures that traditionally managed the fertility of women remain powerful.

In her discussion of Nigerian women's use of contraceptives, Pearce (1995: 198) aptly points out that in regard to the social, political, and institutionalized nature of social control of women's reproductive functions, the patrilineage health metaphor has long been in use: "Women's reproductive behavior was conceptualized in terms of the present and future spiritual and physical health of the lineage. Again, since their own social standing within the lineage was dependent on the production of children, women's physical, mental and social health was strongly linked to prolific childbearing. This linkage was made quite clear by the harsh treatment accorded to barren women."

While no claim can be made here as to whether or at which historical points in the Shona political economy "prolific" childbearing has been the ideal (Beach 1980), it is clear that for the Central Mozambique Shona, women's social status as well as their physical, mental, and social health are tied to their ability to bear children who survive. The frequently harsh treatment of childless women in Shona culture, as well as the great lengths to which women in contemporary Mucessua go to avoid and cure infertility speaks to the intensity of the society's pronatalist pressure up to the present period.

Contemporary Kinship and Social Organization in Gondola

The general kinship-based living patterns just described have changed for many people in the Gondola area, but only in the last two or three decades. Life histories of women in Mucessua revealed that most grew up in small, rural, extended patrilineal compounds of two or three generations, typically including their father, mother, and siblings and some combination of their father's other wives and children, their father's parents, and their father's brothers' families. According to local oral history, in the late sixties and early seventies, the Portuguese colonial administration in Gondola moved local people into *aldeamentos*, small villages, a move that some locals understood to be a means of controlling civilian movement and preventing villagers' contact with the guerrilla liberation soldiers. Many of the longtime residents of Mucessua had been moved to the central Vila area by the Portuguese. FRELIMO's villagization policies in the early 1980s further disrupted rural living patterns, but it was the war of destabilization that pushed the majority of people into the crowded bairros of Mucessua seeking safety.

The general trend today at the level of household organization is toward smaller households and weaker kin support networks. The primary evidence of this attrition is that, in contrast to the extended patrilineal family structures of the previous generation, called *chisvarwa* in Shona, households in contemporary Gondola are increasingly nuclear and neolocal. Rather than moving into a husband's or husband's father's compound, new couples were moving to a location separate from both husband's and wife's natal lands. Of the eighty-three households, only 18.3 percent reported patrilocal living arrangements; that is, they lived in a compound with their husbands' kin. Only five of these fifteen households resembled the multigenerational, patrilineal *chisvarwa*. A greater percentage, 24.4 percent of all households, resided matrilocally, with the wife's kin. Many of these households included single mothers and young mothers who were not living with their partners. The majority of households, however, 57.3 percent, lived neolocally; they had set up their household apart from the kin of either partner.

When I asked women, "Who is the head of your household?" only five (6.1 percent) identified themselves as single female heads of households, though seventeen were not in a partnership with the father of their child. A male partner's parents were household heads in only 11 percent of the households, and the pregnant woman's parents in 19.5 percent. The woman's male partner headed the majority of households, 58.5 percent, but in almost a third of these families, he was intermittently absent from the home, mostly due to labor migration. In the remaining nine households, the male partner was reported absent for an extended period due to work or travel. A male partner was present in fifty-six, or 68.3 percent, of households.

When I asked them what had changed most in their lives since the period when they grew up in their mother's *imba* (house, Sh.), the women responded that while they did much the same tasks, conditions had worsened, because women today lived farther from family than their mothers had. They also lived in smaller compounds and had less help at home and in their fields than their mothers had in their extended households. As thirty-eight-year-old Javelina complained one day: "For me everything is harder. In my mother's time, she had help. Even one task is very hard for me."

In these smaller nuclear households, the collapse of social capital was evident. Women's support networks were limited, and social support in the form of material, domestic, agricultural or material help for women who were pregnant was minimal. In the formal interviews, of the fifty-three pregnant women who gave information on social support they received during their current pregnancy and in the two weeks preceding the interview date, 71.7 percent reported receiving help. The sources of help, however, were mostly immediate family members—usually the women's own children, followed by male partners or husbands. This help from family members did not tend to increase during pregnancy in recognition of the women's increased physical burden, and only a few reported this help as greater than help they received when they were not pregnant. They received little assistance, especially material contributions of food or cash for food, from either patrikin or matrikin (28.3 percent). Fifteen pregnant women (6 percent) reported receiving no help from anyone during their pregnancy.

Another major change in social life organization that contributed to the erosion of women's everyday social security was the decrease in formal marriages and in the number of polygynous compounds where one man lived with multiple wives. Women pointed out this trend, complaining that many men still establish several "small houses" or *casas pequenas*—geographically separate nuclear households—with *mulheres d'esquinas*, "around the corner" or "other" women. Because of neoliberalism, unemployed and underemployed men on the margins of the shifting economy found it ever more necessary to support themselves by relying on the unwaged, socially necessary labor of women across several households.

In this informal type of polygamy, women fear they are competing for men's emotional and sexual attention as well as for material resources, especially cash incomes, with women they frequently do not know and may never have seen who might try to harm them and their pregnancy with sorcery to steal their man completely. Sexual rivals were frequently suspected of targeting each other's reproductive health, since a man often divorces or abandons a woman who cannot produce children for a more fertile partner. Thus, women perceive that personal reproductive threats derive primarily from the breakdown of social networks and kin relationships. They bemoaned not having the agricultural and domestic help their mothers had from sisters-in-law, aunts, and even co-wives, especially during pregnancy.

Several lifelong inhabitants of Gondola recalled their experiences of the changes in living patterns in the area since their childhood. The shrinking distance between compounds and increasing presence of strangers from ethnically different and distinct groups were common themes, as was a sense of eroding social cohesion:

> When I was small our neighbors were four, even five kilometers [away]. We drank from the same well. We [dug the well together] (*cavavamos*). Yes. Now we are linked, each touching the other. We know each other, but there are confusions [*confusões*, problems] between neighbors. (Adelaide, age thirty-two)

> [Here in the bairro] there were big boundaries [between houses]. It wasn't too far away. We knew our neighbors, but it was different because the houses weren't so very close together. In your courtyard it was suitable for a big vegetable garden. This changed in 1976 with the accumulation of houses. Many people needed to live near the city. Many were hoping/waiting [*esperava*] to enter the houses [of the Portuguese who fled]. (Javelina, age thirty-eight)

> In those days in the bairros of the city [Gondola], there was no tradition [sorcery]. People didn't speak badly of others. They were all Tewe. Now we are between all different races—Ndau and Gorongosa. (Joanna, age twenty-five)

> [Neighbors in the bairros set up by the Portuguese in Gondola] were close during the colonial period. [People] lived in the village, as close as they are now, only different. Here there are small houses of deslocados. Back then it was well organized. We knew our neighbors and trusted in them. Now it is different. Then, when you were with your neighbor it was like a sister. Now we live alone and isolated. People used to help those who needed help. Here they don't help. (Anita, age thirty-plus)

Despite these changes in domestic organization and the eroding sense of place, kin relationships continue to be central to determining patterns of health and illness in Mucessua, especially women's reproductive health. In these struggles over land rights, employment stratification, privatization of public services, and advancing rural/urban disparities in spending and infrastructure, global and national policies intersect with local processes of reproduction and reshape households and communities. These local economic and sociocultural transformations are the backdrop against which women's reproductive health choices in Gondola must be analyzed. Women in Mucessua make choices for the social management of biological reproduction with less and less control over the reproductive and productive labor central to their daily lives.

CHAPTER 4

Reproducing Reproducers

"It was so hard to conceive. It was my first husband who couldn't conceive. We searched for treatment as far away as Zimbabwe. I finally conceived a child with another man after my family counseled me to leave and divorce my husband. I always loved that first man, but he had always blamed me [for the infertility] and never accepted treatment himself. I did not make any promise to stay with the second [man]. That was only an experiment to see whether it was I that couldn't conceive. [The second man] went off to the military, and I bore the expenses myself for the child. The child—she was a girl—died at three years with fevers. She was living with my mother then." Jacinta, a lively and stunning twenty-six-year-old, fell silent as she sat with Javelina and me outside the small house where she lived as the fifth wife in the compound of her husband, Senhor Bartholomeu, some years her senior.

A longtime employee of Redd Barna, Norway's Save the Children, Senhor Bartholomeu was the only person I knew in Mucessua who owned a car. Each wife had her own small mud-and-pole house and either cooked outside or in a shared cooking hut. Jacinta's house was the only structure in the compound with a plate glass window, of which she was extremely proud. Her account of hardship with infertility was not unusual. As she described the intimate details of her ordeal, her story conveyed the longing, insecurity, competition, and pressure, as well as the fixed determination, of many women in Mucessua who have difficulty becoming mothers of children who survive. More than anything, she longed for the company of a child, and the sweetness of having someone to tend to and nurture every day.

The double standard for male and female infertility always lays the blame on the woman. In fact, there is no word in the Shona language for a man who is infertile. A woman who suspects that it is her husband and not herself who is unable to conceive can attempt to hide the problem by becoming pregnant secretly by another man. Discovery, however, holds only shame for the woman.

"There are women who don't want to destroy the secret of their house [*segredo da casa*]," Javelina joined in, referring to women covering for men's infertility by going outside the marriage to conceive. "Others divulge the secret. But if you divulge, the shame is for you. People will say you are a woman of *má vida* [bad life], a prostitute and adulterer. Men could learn of it and then arrange to wash their face [of shame] by fighting." Javelina shook her head in sympathy and affinity.

"Eh! My first husband had four other wives. Some of them had [children by other men]. The first wife always lost her children. In our tradition"—Jacinta turned her attention, dazzling white teeth, and flawless complexion to me—"if you make a child outside [your marriage], you must arrange medicine for the child not to die when it encounters the other man. The second wife also had children outside, but they lived because she treated them [with appropriate protective medicines]. The third and fourth wives did not arrange [to get pregnant] outside. The third left when she discovered his secret. We others stayed because he was treated with drugs for women to always love him. His sister was a curandeira [indigenous healer]. I did not know he was drugged. When my family made me leave him, I was treated to not think of him anymore. I was given *medicamento*, a type of flour to put in food. It took one year of this treatment to separate [my heart from his]." She tells this story with a dramatic flourish, clutching at her heart, and Javelina and I rock with laughter. Despite what seems to be a constant parade of challenges, Jacinta is fiery and full of fun.

As the fifth wife of another older man who brought her from her family's home in another district to live with him and his four other wives in Mucessua, Jacinta once again has had a hard time getting pregnant. She finally conceived while being treated by a prophet in a church other than the church where she was a member. Once she became pregnant, problems began to crop up in her church and between Jacinta and her four senior co-wives.

"This time I was treated by a prophet so that I could conceive for my husband. The second wife spoke of this with her friend, who told the wife of the evangelist [of my church], who told her husband! He asked to know, 'Who is going around saying the church does not treat its own people?' During mass the evangelist told everyone not to listen to this rumor.

"All this came about because the evangelist's daughter cannot conceive. The wife of the evangelist said to him that they should send their daughter to the prophet who treated me, and she sent their daughter to ask me the prophet's name. I refused to say! I said that I had only been blessed in our church. When the wife said that they should send their daughter to this same prophet, the evangelist did not like it. He wanted the people not to leave his church [to go to the other prophet]. [For his daughter to seek help elsewhere] is a disgrace. It is saying he does not have *força* [force, strength, potency]. But people think that treatment from outside is better.

"When this got back to my husband, he threatened to beat the second wife and her friend who gossiped. Now the second wife is threatening me and still talking with other people. She was beaten for it by my husband." Jacinta came to this point with a look of ripe fruit satisfaction poked through by little wormholes of worry. Who knew the route the second wife's revenge would take next time, or for how long the infatuated old man would reach out to protect her from the other wives? Jacinta's greatest worry was that jealousy would drive one of her older co-wives to use sorcery to make her lose "hold" of her pregnancy. Her security in her new marriage depended on first producing a lineage son who would protect her social, spiritual, and material rights in her husband's extended family compound and lineage land rights, and whose future wife and children would serve her. Then she wanted, in her words, a "*comboio das meninas,*" a train of girls whose hard work and, later, bridewealth payments would sustain her in old age, even if her husband died. Unmarried daughters would fill her house with laughter and beauty, helping with everyday chores in her cornfield and in the compound, even selling vegetables for her at market. Married daughters, she dreamed, would continue to nourish her heart and hearth down the road with visits, gifts, and maybe a special grandchild to dote on, to spoil with favorite foods and attention. This special *neto*, grandchild, would honor her in life by bearing her name and waiting on her as an elder, and in death by attending to her memory and wishes as a spirit ancestor.

To interpret the shifting reproductive strategies of women in Mucessua, I situate their experiences within a larger, culturally defined reproductive cycle that includes all aspects of biological reproduction, as well as the social reproductive processes by which communities envision, organize, and attempt to ensure their continuity through children who survive into adulthood, as Kaler and others have pointed out. "Human fertility, a power that is biologically the property of the young and the female but is also a necessity for the social power of men and elders, is inevitably implicated in symbolic and material struggles across gender and generation," according to Kaler (2000: 678).

Reproducing Womanhood in the Nova Vida

Reworkings of Geertz's now classic analysis of religion as a cultural system (1973), such as Carole Delaney's book *The Seed and the Soil* (1991) and Pamela Feldman-Savelsberg's article subtitled "Fear of Fertility in the Cameroonian Grassfields" (1994), have convincingly suggested that beliefs about reproduction, like religious beliefs, project ideal versions of cosmic order and its disruption onto human experience (Delaney 1991: 9). Because reproduction "is both the material conditions under which new human beings will be born and a durable metaphor for the survival of societies" (McDaniel 1996: 84), the expressions of reproductive beliefs and agendas are key symbols in a culture, encapsulating and specifying how the world should work and what threatens it. In Mucessua, this cosmic order involves notions of gender, kinship, age and lineage seniority, and social differentiation. In that sequence of signification, the reproductive cycle is a socially constructed political process that unfolds over time and spans a woman's life. The symbolic values assigned to reproductive norms, however, and the variety of meanings they acquire depend on the social location of the actors involved (Kaler 2000: 704).

For example, norms by which a society influences levels of fertility are all based on well-defined aspects of the reproductive cycle—the stages of courtship, the initiation of sexual activity, the time of marriage, appropriate sexual and marriage partners, the start and duration of the reproductive period for men and women, the number and preferred sex of children, the eligibility for contraception, the meaning of menopause and infertility. However, the specificities of local reproductive practices do not recreate a "fixed, traditional residue" but rather project a constantly changing set of notions reflecting and reinterpreting new circumstances (Geschiere 1997: 222) and reflecting different subject positions. As Susan Greenhalgh notes, "micro-power" and "micro history" are crucial dimensions of reproduction; reproduction "is political in that relations of power within a society both shape reproductive practices and are in turn shaped by them. It is dynamic in that the social management of the family begins prenatally, with the manipulation of marriage and birth control practices such as contraception and abortion, and continues long into the postnatal period, through infanticide, fosterage, adoption, and a myriad other means" (Greenhalgh 1995: 15).

A growing feminist literature has rightly critiqued the frequent focus on African women primarily as reproducers and bemoaned the absence of representations of the full range of their experiences and behaviors from sexuality to selfhood and other intersections of gender, race, class, and gender politics (Hodgson and McCurdy 2001; Shefer and Foster 2001; Mikell and Skinner 1989). When addressed, the construction of African women's reproduction through discourses on pathological sexuality (normative male and deviant or marginal female) and fertility "always already" carries the burden of "systemic and epistemic violence enacted on black female sexual bodies" (Wekker 2006: 77). This absence constitutes a "gaping wound" in social scientific studies of women of African descent (Wekker 2006: 76; see also Gilman 1985; Hammonds 1997).

Aware of this history, I had hoped that through my writing about Mozambique I could contribute to a literature of African women's lives other than one on motherhood and reproduction, and yet here I am. The fact remains that as de facto heads of vulnerable households, many African women must take on a widening range of social and economic responsibilities for themselves and often for their children, leading some scholars to claim that African women's roles as reproducers have been further entrenched in their subsidization by the new economic order (Demble 2002; Avotri and Walters 1999). I could not ignore that for many Mozambican women, bearing children who survived continued to be the most central sign of female and maternal lineage health and of evidence of female competence, and the main route to female social status and material security. Fertility is important for Mozambican men and women both, but it epitomizes Mozambican woman-hood. As in most other African settings, fertility is a driving principle of social life in Mozambique, mediated, of course, by geosocial position. As I explore in this chapter, the cultural importance of female reproductive capacity finds its reflection in the emphasis on the gender socialization process of girls that prepares them from a young age for their roles in reproduction.

The enormous pressure on many African women to bear children is evident not only in high fertility rates, but also in the harsh treatment of women who cannot or will not take up expected gender, reproductive, or sexual roles; women who are infertile; or women whose offspring do not survive (Oboler 1986; Pearce 1995; Bledsoe 2002; Sargent 1989). Women's angst about reproductive "mishaps" (Bledsoe 1998) or "awry-ness" (Jenkins and Inhorn 2003: 1832), such as infertility, miscarriage, and stillbirth or infant death, also evidences their reproductive stress.

Anthropologists listening carefully to women from Tanzania, Cameroon, Mali, Gambia, and Mozambique note that women's perceptions of the social contexts that threaten their fertility and reproductive health differ considerably from actual outcomes, as well as from official definitions of maternal health risks employed by international and national health policy makers. These competing interpretations of risk also expose social, economic, and political threats that women experience at the community level and that influence pregnancy management in unexpected ways (Allen 2002; Feldman-Savelsberg 1994; Randall 1998; Bledsoe 2002; Chapman 2003).

There is intense social preparation of girls as reproducers, and males and senior women in patrilineal and patrilocal kinship structures maneuver to assert control over women as reproductive resources (Kaler 2000: 695). Every phase of the reproductive cycle receives great attention, as limited routes to female social and economic self-determination and high maternal and infant mortality define the contours of women's reproductive vulnerability. Their vulnerability is not static, however, and in this chapter I focus on the livelihoods and lifeways through which women navigate their social positions during their life cycle and that of their hearth-hold (Cornwall 2005: 5). I follow transnational feminists such as Wekker and Alexander, who have sought "to theorize from the point of view and contexts of marginalized women not in terms of victim status or an essentialized identity but in terms that push us to place women's agency, their subjectivities and collective consciousness, at the center of our understandings of power and resistance" (Alexander 1990: 148, qtd. in Wekker 2006: 171).

It is impossible to ignore the effects of the nova vida on the power and agency of women in Mozambique. Within the current context, especially as community and institutions are transformed and reproduction is commoditized, women in Mucessua struggled in rather small ways to exercise control over their own and sometimes others' reproductive labor. They worked to maintain and occasionally to subvert the social relations of reproduction at different points in the life cycle. These processes increasingly involve transformative work, "the tiniest slivers of human agency" that might get overlooked or be presumed to be built into the local setting rather than produced by shifting forces internal and external to the actors and the stage (Mullings 1995: 123). While the observation that African women are under great pressure to reproduce may be old news, paying attention to the microtransformations of everyday reproductive practices reveals that the constellation of pressures on Mozambican women to bear children is quietly, steadily shifting (Steady 2001; WHO 1985b; Bolton et al. 1989; Alexander 1990; Hartmann 1987; Morsy 1995a).

Raw, Hot, and Spoiled Girls

Early Lessons

Very early on, boys and girls in Mucessua are expected to take up subject positions in relation to the biological and social reproduction of the household. Girls learn the tasks of their mothers and are as involved in domestic chores, child care, and agricultural labor as their physical coordination and responsibility allow. Girls buy and sell in the market, pound and sift corn, light and tend cooking fires, fetch water or cut and carry firewood, wash clothes or dishes, bring food, offer water to men or guests for washing or drinking, and pick up and distract, carry, and feed an infant as soon as they are physically able. Boys sometimes engage in these practices, but if a group of boys and girls are playing together, it is usually a girl whom adults will ask to stop to help with chores unless only an older boy can handle the responsibility. As in any culture, a gendered and age division of labor is part of play, and parents positively reinforce even the youngest children's efforts at gender role-play. Girls still learning to walk practice carrying small items on their heads and skillfully wrap cloth around themselves to carry dolls on their backs in imitation of their mothers and other women. Girls as young as three and four carry a younger sibling on their backs. A young woman is expected to take over more and more responsibilities in her family, and by the time girls are fifteen, they may be expected to be able to run the entire household (Jules-Rosette 1980: 395).

The time when a girl begins to develop breasts (*kubudza*, Sh., Tewe) is considered a significant point in her social development, and as older women hinted to me, she then must be watched more closely. The Portuguese term for this budding adolescent girl is *donzela*, and *mwana mwakura* in ChiTewe (grown child). As nineteen-year-old Sandra explained: "*Donzela* is a girl already ripe—already going into the phase of *senhora* [Mrs.; a woman, not a virgin] and learning how to treat her body." Now aspects of etiquette and manners are stressed, for example, how girls should sit in the presence of men, elders, and strangers, and how they should give and receive anything with their hands. The carriage of rural preadolescent girls is usually introverted and sexually modest, and it is reinforced that they should never look directly into the eyes of men, elders, or strangers. When they greet such a person, they should bow or kneel and lower their gaze to the ground as they clap cupped hands (*kuvucira*, to clap hands in deference to one's superior, Sh.). This is in contrast to the way males, depending on the social hierarchy of those involved in the greeting, may incline slightly or kneel to the ground and clap, fingers extended, pointing out. A girl is taught to receive anything handed to her in this same lowered position, which offers respect to anyone with seniority by gender or generation. After clapping, she should rest one hand on the opposite upper forearm while whatever is given is placed in her outstretched hand. She claps again after receiving it to show thanks, her eyes downcast.

Pulled Out of Childhood:
Female Preparation for the Nova Vida

Coming-of-age practices in Mucessua—what anthropologists frequently refer to as "initiation rites" in many African contexts—are called *kupanga masikana*, or *preparação* (preparation), and involve preparing girls to be sexual partners, mothers, and wives. When a girl is beginning to develop breasts or even earlier, her sexual education begins. The first step is the manual elongation of the labia minora so that they are visible outside the labia majora, a procedure whose purpose a girl may or may not be told. She may be sent away from her home suddenly to live with a trusted elder female family friend or relative to begin her preparation. Women of different ages described the steps involved in this part of preparation in detail, all speaking from experience:

> When you complete twelve years you have to prepare sexually. There is a proper tool to treat the sex—*resino*. You burn it, put it in a flask, and use it every day to pull the vagina to grow it. The oldest woman in the family or a trusted woman is responsible for teaching this. (Justina, age thirty-seven)

> At ten years you prepare for rites of initiation. You learn to burn this plant and how to utilize it until you are fifteen years old. At fifteen it is explained to you how to live with a husband. Some girls refuse to do it. Others accept.

Why do some refuse? We don't know. *A vida nova* [the new life]. (Dona Rosa, age fifty-plus)

There is this education. A girl, when there are signals for her breasts to come out, ten, eleven, twelve [years], must initiate this education. Long ago one had to arrange medicamento [traditional medicine], and pull the sex. [Now] just *resino* is mixed with this medicamento, a type of sweet potato, very soft. You burn them together. These roots you burn apart, then put with *resino*. You burn this. Put it in the hand and do a massage until it becomes a type of oil. In the church they use *pomade* [face cream], green or white oil which is given to the *mãe pastor* [wife of the pastor] to bless. Churches also bless cooking oil. (Regina, age forty)

When the phase arrives when you are already grown—eleven years old—you are going to initiate the preparation to be an educated woman. You use in this education *resina*, which is put in the sun. When it dries, you burst it open. It has two shells. You burst the first and peel off the second. The white part [of the seed inside] you burn until it becomes black. Rub it fine between both your hands, and then keep it in a jar of *pomade*. Use it each day about four o'clock in the morning. You go out to a place outside behind the house, sit and begin to take it and pull [on the labia]. At first it hurts, and then you begin to like it. Other times girlfriends who are already educated can show you, or your grandmother. (Maria, age twenty-eight)

When Anita, then thirty, was eight years old, her preparation began: "[I learned] how to treat a husband's parents, brothers-in-law, and husband from my grandmother. My father's sister, when I was eight, began my sex. [It is] education for when you are going to make love [*namorar*]. I was to do this under my blanket each morning and each night. I stayed at her house one day. Children today and yesterday are different. What was explained for me to do, I fulfilled."

Joana, age twenty-two, was much older than the frequently reported age of eleven or twelve when she began her preparation: "My aunt taught me. I was sixteen. I stayed at her house, my father's sister, for six months. But [initiation] is useless these days. It is over, that [practice]. They are things from long ago." During the interview it was clear from Joana's discomfort and silence that the subject was awkward for her and difficult to talk about. At the end of the interview, however, when I was about to leave, she offered abruptly that it was her older sister who had taught her much about the elongation process. She added: "I liked it, but I felt ashamed to do it."

Though several women were shy or embarrassed when discussing their own initiation, most wanted their own daughter to go through it. Older women clearly articulated their views that the rites played an important role in controlling girls and keeping peace in households, something younger women were beginning to openly challenge. Only younger women expressed shame or disdain for the practice. Javelina, age thirty-eight, explained to me that times are changing, and girls are resisting the codes that shaped their mothers' and grandmothers' lives. Families feel they are losing control over their daughters, she said:

> Today many girls already know [about initiation]. Other girls already told them. This causes problems, because you go to explain this to them, and they already know. Others don't use it, and it causes divorce. "What type of woman is this?" a husband will ask. In Maputo it is different. They want a woman who knows of love, not just of vagina. Every region has their tradition. But, after Independence, FRELIMO said you could not separate [boys and girls] and that you could not control a girl. The problem is that girls go with whatever others until they decide to stay with one only. They can go freely. And then when they start saying they know it all . . . eh, when before it was not like this. To do or not to do [rites] depends on the family, but others don't depend on their family.

Although Signe Arnfred (1988: 13–14) found that girl's "initiation" in the northern Mozambican province of Nampula was meant in part to instruct girls how to please themselves in sex, this was not the narrative recounted to me in Mucessua. Women agreed that the stretching process was meant to make women more sexually attractive to men—the sight of the elongated genitals pleases and arouses men. Nineteen-year-old Sandra was initiated by her grandmother and sisters: "It was explained to me that some husbands don't like it when you don't have this material." Women further explained that the state of having been prepared in such a way also communicated to a man that a girl had been well trained to be a wife. It was a sign that she was an obedient woman who wanted to please, and that she was trained with good housekeeping skills, knew the secrets to keeping a peaceful household, and was versed in the arts of male sexual pleasure. She was domesticated.

Most of the women I spoke with did not recount feeling physical or erotic benefits from the process. However, some women by accident discovered it could be quite pleasurable. As women related their experiences of initiation—the sudden, furtive journeys to a feared or beloved elder woman's house; the strangeness of familiar, secluded settings transformed by clandestine acts; the loneliness of being away from home; the still, dark mornings or nights awakening surprising feelings of pleasure and shame entwined—there emerged a common narrative of childhood awe at the sense of mystery and secret sharing of these homosocial, if not homoerotic, rites of womanhood that sometimes bonded young girls and much older women and consecrated intimate camaraderie between older and younger sisters or best friends.

The benefit of preparation for women was most often discussed in terms of avoiding humiliation later in their lives. For example, a woman could be disgraced if, when bathing in a stream or river with other women, it was revealed that she was "*não formada*," literally, not formed, but with the added connotation of being unschooled. Women used words to describe a woman who had not undergone the process of labial elongation that translated into Portuguese as uneducated (*não educada*), wild or raw (*cru*), or unprepared (*não preparada*). Such a woman would be seen as unsocialized, even antisocial. As one woman explained, it was the duty of elder women to make a girl respectable by teaching her to inscribe or forcibly inscribing on her body the evidence of her socialization by her family. A good family, it was implied, would force a girl to submit to *ritos* (rites) for her own good, even if she resisted, as Marida, age twenty-seven, explained: "Someone really stubborn might be grabbed by her grandmother who takes a small piece of pottery, and takes and pulls [the girl's labia] until it hurts. Afterward they say that [if we don't do it] tomorrow [when we have sexual relations] we will be ashamed. One would seem like a person without family." The broken clay pot, once used for cooking food or holding water, gets recycled as a tool for transforming the raw girl into the cooked.

The seed of the *resina* plant was the ingredient most often mentioned in relation to this part of the girl's preparation process. Javelina brought the seed from this plant for me to see, a red-brown seed the size of a chestnut enclosed in a spiky green casing, like a horse chestnut pod. As the casing dries, it becomes brown and hairy, swells, and then pops open suggestively when ripened in the sun, revealing the shiny inner red seed. *Resina* may be the seed of the castor-oil bush, which Gelfand (1979: 19) found to be the seed used for this purpose by Shona women in Zimbabwe (*pfuta*, Sh.; *Ricinus communis*, Latin). *Resina* might be supplied by mother or grandmother, guardian, girlfriend, or older sister. It was reported that in northern areas of Manica Province, a girl's lover might provide her with the powder. Another ingredient mentioned in the stretching process was *moseku*. A preparation used more in the past but still available was made from the labia of a zebra (*mbidzi*, Tewe), which is used to provoke coughing (*kuparapara*, Tewe). A young mother of four, Marida, age twenty-eight, told me that coughing makes pulling the labia easier by pushing it out:

> The zebra has a vagina like a woman. Hunters, when they kill a zebra, cut [the labia] to dry it well and save. They sell it to elder women. When someone comes [to buy it] they cut a piece. This piece you must put in

the fire and burn to ashes. The ashes you put in water. When you drink it makes you cough. As this makes you cough, it makes your sex push out. If you take too much it can make lots of water come out of you. There is a correct measure. The elder women have to watch and control it.

As older women might control the substances used to prepare girls and younger women, they might also be controlling those younger women. Kaler (2000: 700–703; 2003) writes extensively regarding the important role that older Shona women played as "gatekeepers" in the control of fertility and sexuality of younger Shona women in Zimbabwe. The ability of older women to "direct the fertility of their sons and daughters-in-law" is, indeed, a source of power that they were reluctant to give up by sharing the sources and doses of traditional or indigenous means of fertility regulation. From making up for the losses due to war to protecting one's daughters from the burden of heavy childbearing, elder women expressed a wide range of reasons for restricting women's access to fertility-limiting knowledge, preparations, and practices. Kaler documents the protracted negotiations with and resistances to this power relationship that younger women discussed with her and the corresponding secrecy of young women's strategies to "seize control of their own means of reproduction" (Kaler 2000: 702–3). Among the women in Mucessua, loss of control over younger women was a well-worn theme in older women's narratives of gender, which they often couched within the retelling of a recent past or tradition in which younger women were better behaved than today's girls of the nova vida.

The second stage of a girl's preparation involved lessons in how to move her changed body to please a man and help him achieve sexual satisfaction. One technique involved showing the girl how to move her hips while lying on her back, lifting them above a pillow that had been stuck with something sharp that would prick the initiate should she tire and let her hips gyrate too low. A girl's mother never carried out this education because her teachings would inappropriately hint at secrets of parental sexual intimacy. Instead, an older and trusted female neighbor or relative taught this lesson, as Javelina described:

At fifteen I was sent to the house of a *senhora* entrusted by my aunt. I arrived and swept the courtyard. She did the education of the movement to help on top [of a man], *como movimentar* [how to move]. The Ndau are more involved in this than the Tewe. The Sena even instruct the boys how to do [it] when they get a girl. How to take *resina* for their future lovers to do [preparation]. In Tanzania, whoever does not know how to help [a man] is not a woman. *Maunyu* is Ndau for help in bed of a woman for a man. Lack of this respect to the husband is the cause of much divorce.

A girl's paternal aunt often serves in this role of *madrinha* in Portuguese, or *samkuru* in Tewe, acting as a guardian who teaches a young girl other lessons about how to maintain a happy *lar* (literally, hearth in Portuguese), including how she should wait on and interact with her in-laws and what her duties will be as a wife. A madrinha often plays an ongoing role in a girl's life. For example, when a girl is sent to live with her *padrinhos* (like godparents, the madrinha and her husband), her virginity is entrusted to them for safe-keeping. After inspection establishes that the girl is a virgin, it is the task of the *padrinhos* to make sure that nothing happens to threaten the payment of the seduction fee and bridewealth to the girl's parents. The madrinha is frequently involved as a go-between in courtship rituals, engagement ceremonies, and marriage arrangements, or acts as a counselor should problems arise in her charge's natal or marital home. She will often be called to witness the in-laws' inspection of a bride's virginity to determine the bride-price payment. In exchange for this responsibility, a madrinha can expect to receive a gift of respect, *respeito*—often a capulana, a cloth wrap, with money on top—as a show of thanks when a girl's education is complete.

"Break Your Mother's Back": Menstruation, Fertility, and Coming of Age in Mucessua

Shona ethnography represents menstruation in Shona culture as a powerful, and sometimes dangerous and harmful state (Gelfand 1992 [1973]: 170). Menstrual blood itself possesses potentially destructive or creative properties; because it is such a potent substance, it is a necessary ingredient in indigenous contraceptive methods, curses against other women, charms for attracting lovers and securing a partner's fidelity, and infertility treatments. According to Gelfand, in Shona culture "a menstruating woman is regarded as being in a dangerous state and should be separated from others until the cycle is finished." A woman who is menstruating is not allowed to hold another woman's baby and should not touch strangers, especially children she does not know. Gelfand also documents a prohibition against sexual intercourse during menstruation, the breaking of which causes illness to both the man and the woman (Gelfand 1979: 6). In past times, he notes, a menstruating Shona woman was given a hut on the periphery of the compound where she could remain until the end of her cycle, signaling either her right to seclusion, her potential danger to her family (Gelfand 1992 [1973]: 171), or perhaps both.

In Mucessua, sexual intercourse with a postmenopausal woman was believed to be fatal if engaged in without proper ceremony to protect the man from the *sujidade* (dirtiness) of menstrual blood trapped in the woman's body. While it has been suggested that menstrual blood in this part of Mozambique is "an agent of contagion," such a claim overlooks assertions by local healers that for women, menstrual blood is a source of cleansing from certain illness conditions (Green 1999: 143) and ignores local practices in which women use menstrual blood to control fertility or create love charms to secure a lover or keep a lover's attention and loyalty (Chapman 1998). In Mucessua, the menstrual symbolism articulated a range of constructs to "manage and control the mobility and sexuality of female bodies" and established the appropriate parameters for women's bodies and sexuality (Mupotsa 2008). While women did not mention ritual physical seclusion of menstruating women, they reported obeying many prohibitions that constrained their movement and created a psychic spatial seclusion. For example, until a certain number of days after they stopped bleeding, six being most frequently mentioned, menstruating women were prohibited from stepping over people, especially children and pregnant women, as well as over food, water, or cooking pots.

Without exception, the women saw sexual intimacy with menstruating women as taboo, and they spoke openly about their husbands seeking the beds of co-wives or other around-the-corner women during their own menses. Through sex with a menstruating woman, a man would draw *sujidade* (dirtiness) through his penis into his abdomen. There, the blood would coagulate and prevent him from urinating. This condition could be fatal if a cleansing treatment was not undertaken that involved putting hot sand into water and drinking it. Like birth, death, sexual intercourse that is adulterous, or a woman's first experience of intercourse, the first menstruation is generally believed to cause an imbalance in the body. The body becomes hot (*quente*, Pt.; *mwiri kupisa*, hot body, Tewe) as it is infused with ceremonial power and in need of a counteracting ceremony or treatment to restore balance. Being in a state of ceremonial imbalance is potentially dangerous not only to the ceremonial heat bearer, but also to whomever he or she comes in contact with.

Mhandara is the Shona name for a girl when she reaches adolescence and her breasts have developed. When a *mhandara* menstruates for the first time, she tells her mother or more often her grandmother, who informs her mother. This communication is important, for, if a daughter becomes fertile and sexually active without her parents' knowledge, the secrecy may lead to indiscreet sexual behavior that will disgrace the family and possibly lose them a portion of the material value of her reproductive capacity. Male payments for parental approval of and rights to sexual access to girls, in whatever currency, are commonly said to be "eaten" by the girl's parents. Thus, if a menstruating girl does not make the proper ritual acknowledgments of her potential fertility to her parents or guardians, or if a daughter has sexual relations before marriage, it is held that any food she cooks for them will poison them, and they will become critically ill with back pains and bloody diarrhea.

"Menstrual ideas do not exist in isolation, but rather occur within religious, political and reproductive contexts. Thus situated within a wider framework, they manifest culturally specific understandings of female creativity, health, leisure, gender relations and empowerment" (Buckley and Gottlieb 1998: 51). In the context of a lineage-based social organization that reinforces seniority across generations, most ceremonially caused illnesses are, at some level, about ruptures in kin obligations. Ruptures in the duties between child and parent are potently symbolized in the relationship between mother and infant. When children fail to conduct the proper ceremonies, the parents, especially the mother, suffer.

To avoid causing illness to her parents, a girl is given special medicine called *mutyorwa* (Sh.), which she secretly puts in her parents' drinking water when she has finished menstruating. "Once is enough," Gelfand also reports of this long-standing careful attention paid to menstruation in Shona social life. "She throws away any that is left over. In former days, when a girl first began to menstruate, she put a smoldering ember into her father's special plate and took it to her mother, indicating what had happened" (1979: 18). The ember burning on the father's plate and the potential to inflict deathly gastrointestinal poisoning on one's parents are effective means of signifying a daughter's filial duty not to "spoil" her parents' meal or break her mother's back/belly. The mother's back and belly signify, by extension, her husband's patrilineage—all offspring of all *wamai* (mothers of lineage sons, Tewe).

This belief is expressed in a Tewe proverb: "*Ukatama kudya mutombo, unorwara msana*" (If the correct medicines are not prepared, the back [spinal column] will hurt). The back or spine (*msana*, Tewe) is the locus of women's pain from a pregnancy, labor pains in childbirth, and the weight of carrying a child once born. The localization of pain in the back (*msana unohwadza*, the column hurts, Tewe) caused by the omission or incorrect performance of a ceremony made me wonder about the origins of a jump-rope song I grew up singing in suburban and urban northeastern United States: "Step on a crack, break your mother's back."

The onset of the first menstruation figured in many women's life histories as the moment at which they were considered to have passed from girlhood to womanhood, and these events were ritually marked.

> [I was considered a woman] from fourteen years on, from the day that menstruation appeared. You have to be instructed that way. Even before [you menstruate], they explain it to you. Other families only give medicine after the first menstruation. The medicine is meant to keep your legs shut [to lovers]. I did not keep mine shut. I walked hot paths [*caminhos quentes*, had sexual relations that make one ceremonially hot, meaning impure]. Maybe this is what made me not conceive. (Javelina, age thirty-eight)

[I was considered to have become a woman] in 1987. I was fifteen. I had to put salt in the fire. In Gorongosa they put medicamentos [traditional medicine] in the fire. Others eat [the medicine]. This was so my mother would not get sick when I cook for her. (Joanna, age twenty-two)

I don't remember [how old I was]. There was a ceremony. All this took place at the house of my husband. I went to my mother-in-law's house when I was small. The family of my husband *tratou medicamento* [took care of or arranged the traditional medicine] to go to my parents' house. At my first menstruation. Father and Mother stayed at home. I made porridge with *musekesa* [a branch from a certain tree] and dropped it at their door. Father came out first and stepped on [the branch]. Second, Mother stepped on it. I could go in then. Then everyone sat. I pretended to feed some food [which she had prepared with special medicine] to my father but then threw it away. After, I gave him food to eat. I repeated this gesture with my mother. I don't know the medicine, but the parents eat all of this, while other people eat other food. This is for the parents not to become sick with dysentery, diarrhea with blood. Many neighbors watched [the ceremony]. If this ceremony is not done, you cannot cook for your parents. As soon as you would put in salt, the salt would spoil your parents' food. (Anita, age thirty-plus)

When I was fifteen was my first menstruation. I told a friend. My friend said that I had to tell my *mbiya* [grandmother, also the woman who assisted your delivery, Tewe; in this case, Marida's father's first wife]. When I went to tell my *mbiya* I had to stay three days in the house, and I couldn't see my parents. Because we were [followers of the prophet] Johane Marange, I got blessed water and made porridge with this water. My parents ate it. (Marida, age twenty-seven)

These ceremonies accompanying first menstruation emphasize the girl's new position of responsibility and capacity to labor and to be sexually active. Until she is married, and the payment of bridewealth transfers rights in her labor and offspring to her husband and his lineage, a woman is expected to labor to support her own parents. This she does through cooking for and serving them, and through protecting their investment in her productive and reproductive use value by behaving correctly (see also Jules-Rosette 1980: esp. 394–96).

Mukadzi, Wife

Men and women in Mucessua both described the ideal wife as physically attractive, round and smooth like a well-made pot. She should have undergone appropriate preparation to be an obedient wife and sexual partner. She should know how to prepare tasty dishes, keep a house neat, treat her husband with respect, and sexually gratify him. She should have good personal hygiene and not get into squabbles with others, especially her husband, in-laws, and co-wives. She must be hardworking and uncomplaining, with all her efforts aimed at keeping a good "hearth," that is, a full cooking pot, a house full of children, and a peaceful home. Extra industriousness can make up for lack of desirable physical attributes, and is a quality especially sought by in-laws in their selection of an appropriate wife for their son. Special cooking skills are also a bonus. Being a superb cook can give a woman an edge in the competition she may be in with her co-wives in a polygynous household where the husband rotates eating at a different wife's house each night or week, his literal meal followed by a carnal meal that the wife also has a right to enjoy (Bourdillon 1991: 48). As Feldman-Savelsburg (1994: 464) found in the Cameroonian Grassfields, in Mucessua a good cook may share more meals of both kinds with her husband than she would otherwise be eligible for, thus improving her chances of becoming pregnant with the much needed, if not desired, preferably male child.

Over the years, as the family moves through its developmental cycle, a wife's power to control her life and the lives of others changes significantly. In the beginning of her married life, despite the traditional prestige derived for the wife-giving lineage over the wife-receiving lineage in a customary Shona marriage transaction, a Shona wife enters her husband's extended household as its newest and therefore lowest-status member. Even a baby daughter of her husband's lineage has seniority over the new wife. Traditionally, she was not allowed even to establish her own home and have her own cooking fire separate from those of her mother-in-law until after the birth of her first child. Following the tradition of patrilocal marriage residence, the new wife is expected to show respect, serve her husband's kin, and do the most despised chores. This subordinate position, which is extended to all her female kin group, is expressed in the term *vamwene* (owner, Sh.), by which she must address all women of her husband's family, according to Bourdillon, who suggests that "the inequality between women in the two families is partly explicable in terms of the residence patterns according to which the young wife is an inexperienced foreigner to the group in which she has to live, and partly in terms of the transference of bride-price cattle: the marriage of the *vamwene* theoretically provided the cattle with which the new wife is married" (1991: 38).

In the new social and economic context I observed in Mucessua, in which more families are increasingly neolocal and nuclear, some of these dynamics were attenuated. While women were losing some of their traditional standing with relation to their position in their own extended patrilineage, they might also acquire some degree of social and even economic independence that improved their relationship to their husbands. In Mucessua, for example, in the absence of any of their husbands' kin to be subordinate to, and with their husbands often away from home as migrant laborers, women had greater de facto control in their own households than they would have in a traditional extended patrilineal compound. It is also possible that some women have lost women's time-honored standing without gaining status in their new, more isolated situation (Bourdillon 1991: 57). Bourdillon has described the same contradictory shifts in kin power relationships for Shona women in Zimbabwe (51).

As women in Mucessua have become further immersed in a monetary economy, and the nature of lobolo payments in marriage transactions shifts, women's status may suffer further. The conventional form of lineage-based marriage with bridewealth in a peasant economy guaranteed a woman's right to access land through the marital lineage and some autonomy over its cultivation. A woman also maintained close contact with her natal family and could return to her own lineage if a marriage did not work out. Her status within her own lineage derived from her ability to provide cattle from her own lobolo payment for the marriage of her brother (Holleman 1952: 66). Historically in Gondola, in acknowledgment of a sister's value, a brother was often assigned as a special guardian to one of his sisters (*cipanda*, cattle-providing sister, Sh.) to protect her virginity and influence her to make a prosperous marriage choice, as her bride-price would determine how much would later be available to pay out in bride-price for his own marriage.

When a man earns monetary wages, however, his sisters lose their traditional status over his wives and children because his lobolo payments come from his wages rather than from his sisters' marriages. Cash payments of lobolo interrupt the circulation of the lobolo fund, and a sister can no longer claim that her marriage made her brother's marriage possible (Thompson 2000; Bourdillon 1991: 51). In Mucessua, parents are also increasingly unable to support a woman's bid to leave an unhappy marriage, as they frequently cannot repay the cash they demanded for lobolo and have long since consumed. Furthermore, as couples more frequently live apart from either partner's extended family, the guarantee of a woman's access to fertile land through her husband's inheritance no longer holds.

According to Meekers's survey study of the institution of bridewealth among Zimbabwe Shona, the erosion of social control of the lineage associated with "socio-economic development" is leading to a greater prevalence of what Meekers called "irregular marriages." In Gondola, frequently no bridewealth was paid, and many unions were not arranged between families. Meekers's study also showed that without the payment of lobolo, men frequently denied responsibility for children they had fathered. In these cases, women had to turn to their natal families for support. Since lobolo seems to have provided a strong social incentive for men to take responsibility for their children, the erosion of long-established marriage transactions may also increase the vulnerability of women as sole primary caretakers in families in which they and their children are economically at risk (Meekers 1993). These same patterns of vulnerability were apparent in Gondola in the mid-1990s and were still hot topics of discussion in 2008. At a gathering with a handful of women whom I had worked with in Mucessua since 1993, I asked about lobolo:

> Rachel: When I first interviewed you in 1994, each of you told me that if you had a daughter, you would ask for lobolo, even though most of you said that lobolo was a bit of a burden for you, because to be paid for, you ended up under pressure and indebted to your in-laws. Are you asking for lobolo for your daughters, or does this system even exist anymore?
>
> Rosinha: It is happening. The question of lobolo never ends. Ten million [meticais] . . . [more than four hundred dollars].
>
> Javelina: Umm.
>
> Rosinha: Ten million!
>
> Javelina: Three?
>
> Rosinha: Three, five, four, ten. It depends on the amount needed.
>
> Odete: This amount never actually gets paid . . .
>
> Marida: If it happens that the guy works [it does].
>
> Rachel: But do people here actually succeed in paying all this?
>
> Odete: They don't pay it!
>
> Ilda: They don't pay. Only you run the risk of charging this money, then your child [daughter] goes off there, does not study, does not go to school. That man does not work, makes babies, everything disgraced!
>
> Odete: [Your daughter] returns home again, comes to give you more expenses in your house.
>
> Ilda: This is creating a lot of prejudice, especially towards the girls.
>
> Etelvinha: The types of people who charge really high prices, do you think they are going to be able to repay it? [clicks her teeth]
>
> Ilda: Then, if you go and say, "Look, you can't do this [charge lobolo]," a thousand times people say, "Ah! You want to teach children prostitution. I want my child to get married!" Now, is marriage preferable to studying? To working? To having your daily bread, paying your own way instead of being handed over to someone who himself does not have anything to eat, or wear, does not work, does not do anything?
>
> So, you hand over your daughter, he gives you two million–disca-disca. [brushes each hand once, as if washing her hands of a situation] Hey, I don't know [shaking her head] . . . You end up with no recourse. Then when those children are born, [your daughter] comes and sits back in your house, everything lost, because you ate the five million [meticais paid for lobolo].
>
> There is a case in this zone where the grandfather said, "Hey, I don't

want to know about it, I don't want to know [about the potential problems of lobolo]," so he hands over [the girl] to this man. The guy births five children, but he does not do anything—nothing. When he goes out drinking, comes back home without anything, pronto, it comes to blows. He has to give something to eat, has to sustain those five children. I am seeing that having a real husband, there is no advantage whatsoever.

Representing Women's Reproductive Health

Calming the Snake, Plowing the Field:
The Ethnophysiology of Pregnancy in Mucessua

Conceptions of reproductive ethnophysiology in Mucessua reveal further detail of the layers of women's reproductive pressure and vulnerability.[1] Evidence of this is largely derived from linguistic usage. The Shona term for uterus, *chibereko*, builds on the root *–bereka*, which means to carry on the back, to bear offspring, to produce. In use, *chibereko* seems to carry less of the clinical, anatomical meaning of the English "uterus" and more reference to the place of woman's productive, cradling, creative essence expressed by the term "womb." Each woman is believed to possess a womb—in Portuguese, *criador* (creator)—which from birth has its own nature and the potential to bear children. Cleansing by menstrual blood is critical to the proper functioning of the *chibereko* in procreation, and only human interference through witchcraft, sorcery, or adultery can interrupt the menstrual cycle.

In Mucessua, the *chibereko* is related to, and sometimes conflated with, the Shona term *nyoka*, which refers to an invisible snake that inhabits a person's body from birth and regulates diet and digestion. In Central Mozambique and other societies for which there is information, according to E. C. Green (1997: 92), nyoka

> appears to be a force that requires cleanliness and purity of body; reacts to the introduction of "dirt" or impure, spoiled foods by provoking variously bodily discharges such as diarrhea and vomiting as well as grumbling in the stomach; guards the body against impurities or what Shona healers called "contamination"; and requires clean external surroundings. [The] internal snake is conceived as a protective life force when perceived as invisible under all circumstances; it is an ethnophysiological concept when related to digestion and stomach disorder when it is conceived as a worm (less often, a snake or grown-up worm) that becomes visible outside the human body.

Women and indigenous healers in Mucessua used the term "nyoka" in relation to pregnancy in reference to the dysfunctioning of the womb. For example, in a discussion of causes of infertility, the term was used when I asked Senhor Quingue, Javelina's neighbor and an herbal healer, for an explanation of the phrase *comeu sujidade* (ate dirt or impurity): "*O homem que juntou com voçe deu doença, sujidade que cobra* [nyoka] *não gostou. Mentruaçāo appareceu cedo—nzoni*" (The man that joined with you [had intercourse] gave you a sickness, impurity that your snake (*cobra*, Pt.; *nyoka*, Sh., Tewe) did not like. Menstruation appeared early—cramps). *Colicas nzoni* are menstrual cramps caused by the introduction of impurity (for example, a venereal disease) into the nyoka, which rejects it. Thus, a pregnancy introduced into the womb in an impure way or by an impure (infected) person will not seize, or catch hold (*kubata*, to seize; *kubata mimba*, to become pregnant, Sh., Tewe). *Nyoka* was alternately translated as *uter* (uterus), *receptor* (receiver, receptacle), or *concebedor* (conceiver). Treatment is necessary to cleanse a "polluted" womb and return it to proper functioning. As Green hypothesizes, this conceptualization of infertility as pollution-related illness "tends to be roughly coterminous with diseases biomedically classified as contagious" (1997: 83).

Some innate (congenital) problem with the nyoka also may cause primary infertility. The potential, at least, is implied by the use of the term by an indigenous health practitioner describing an infertile woman: "*Hana nyoka ye kubara munhu.*" The speaker rephrased this in Portuguese as, "*Não tem cobra, criador que recebe o spermo do homen*" (She does not have a snake [womb] that receives a man's sperm). There is also treatment for this kind of infertility.

Evidence of the ethnophysiological connection between womb and nyoka turns up in other reproduction terminology; for example, in another description of the treatment process for infertility, the first phase is *kurapa nzoni* (Sh., Tewe), translated as *calmar nyoka, cobra*—calming the "snake." The second phase is cleansing, *kusuka* (Sh., Tewe), and the third phase is conception, *kusimika* (planting, Sh., Tewe). The phrase *nyoka dzirikuruma* (literally the snake is biting, stinging, gnashing teeth) can mean "he/she has [abdominal] pains," although these could be stomach pains, abdominal pains that are a symptom of pregnancy, or labor pains. Among Shona procreative beliefs, according to Gelfand, is that life begins as a snake (nyoka) or worm in the mother's womb (1992 [1973]: 175n5).

Impurity caused by sexual transgression also causes reproductive risk during pregnancy and childbirth. Such illicit activities as incest, sex during menstruation, adultery, and witchcraft used, for example, by a jilted lover, can cause the womb to eat dirt—*comer sujidade* (dirt, impurity). These actions and conditions compromise the normal functioning of the womb, which becomes blocked by impurity. The resulting spiritual state of imbalance manifests as physiological irregularity symptomized by abdominal bloating (perhaps a description of swollen lymph nodes that accompany some genital infections), inability to urinate, cessation of menstruation, pain during urination, or severe pre-menstrual cramping. If untreated, these conditions result in infertility or even death. Adultery on the part of the husband can also kill his pregnant wife: if the woman with whom he has had the affair comes near the wife while she is in labor, the wife will begin to sweat and then die.

Not surprisingly, Mucessuan women's approach to their reproductive health reflected and sometimes mirrored their approach to the natural environment on which they depended for their livelihood. Like the prescription for a good agricultural harvest, a woman's fertility is generated not only from the potential of her body as rich soil, but by the constant careful attention of the individual cultivator, and by the maintenance of harmonious and respectful social relations, especially with living and spirit kin. Images of fertility and infertility frequently involve metaphors for bodies and sexual relations that draw on women's central role in families' subsistence agriculture—seeds planted or wasted on the ground; pots covered or uncovered, full or empty, round or broken; fields planted or transplanted, sowed or lying fallow, well watered or dry; and water flowing, still, or collecting in drops on a blade of grass.

Threats to fertility take natural and personalistic forms, from malaria, poison, or droughts to witches, jealous or avenging kin, disgruntled ancestors, or hostile neighbors. In the case of infertility, for example, a woman who is not able to bear children is called *mhanje*, the Shona word for a barren animal or a field that has been plowed but not sowed. To be made barren or to have prolonged labor by means of magic is *kusungwa*, from the Shona verb root *sunga* that means to bind, fasten, tie, or arrest. However, in keeping with more general local beliefs about health and illness etiology, and the integration of the secular and spiritual, laypeople and folk healing specialists in Mucessua assumed that most fertility problems were not physiological in origin but were signs of social and spiritual problems posted in the form of ill health, which the sufferers and their caretakers would ignore at their peril.

The treatment for infertility, therefore, was not likely to be found—if it could be found at all—only in a biomedical setting. To treat infertility, women turned most often to churches and indigenous healers who specialized in evoking and addressing the social causes of illness and ill fate. The cost of infertility was so high, however, that women who could not conceive, had difficulty carrying a pregnancy to term, or lost an infant or child used any accessible means to find a solution, including biomedicine. Women's fear that they might experience one of these reproductive hazards was itself a condition in need of treatment, so protecting oneself against such fate and fear was a critical facet of many women's reproductive health-seeking strategies.

Until the last two decades in Mucessua, indigenous healers provided most nonbiomedical treatment for reproductive problems like infertility. Indigenous health practitioners are more accessible than the formal health care system for the majority of Mozambicans. A preliminary census in Manica Province in 1990 suggested that there was approximately one indigenous healer per 200 people (Jurg, Tomas, and De Jong 1991), an estimate comparable to those made elsewhere in Africa. The physician-to-population ratio in Mozambique is approximately 1:50,000, with about 52 percent of all doctors concentrated in the national capital, Maputo (Green et al. 1994: 8). In 1991, the Ministry of Health began a public health program to work collaboratively with a professional association of traditional healers in Mozambique, AMETRAMO, in the areas of childhood diarrhea and sexually transmitted diseases, including HIV/AIDS (Jurg, Tomas, and De Jong 1991). AMETRAMO has representation at the provincial and district levels, although a budget pinch limited association activities during the period of my research. In Gondola AMETRAMO functioned most visibly in its role of registering practicing healers and setting fee guidelines for traditional therapies.

Mucessua is home to a wide range of indigenous healing specialists. The general term for a healer is the Shona term *nyanga*, or *curandeiro* in Portuguese. A female *nyanga* is *nyahana*, and a male *nyanga* is *chiremba*. The two main categories of Bantu healers are most common—herbalists and spirit mediums. A *dhota* is an herbalist who works mainly on symptoms with herbs and suggestive magic for curative purposes. A *makangeiro* is a medium who works with both spirit possession and herbs as a diagnostician and healing specialist. Usually inherited through lineage spirit elders (vadzimu), the healing powers of a *makangeiro* can be used to either cure or harm others; corrupt *makangeiros* might even send a spirit to someone to ensure themselves of a client. Though I heard of a few older women in the community known for having special skills as midwives, they were more often sought for their expertise as some other form of healer, mainly herbalist, spirit diviner, or faith healer. Although in the past, I learned, curandeiros were paid based on the outcome of their treatments and accepted both labor and payment in kind, more and more frequently they demand significant cash payments based on services rendered, regardless of treatment outcome.

Indigenous healers' approaches to infertility varied but usually involved first a *consulta*, or consultation, with spirits and living family members to determine the possible cause of the problem. A diagnosis follows, and the proper medicine is prepared based on the individual case—often a series of preparations. The first preparation is often a cleansing mixture that provokes diarrhea for a brief time. During the next period, three months, the woman ingests a prescribed tea made from a paste of leaves and roots. To protect the pregnancy once conception has occurred, another tea with sugar was sometimes given. For example, when Javelina, who had been successfully treated for infertility by an indigenous healer, felt labor beginning in her fifth month, she first went to the maternity ward, where she was admitted for observation but given no treatment. She asked to be released so that she could pursue treatment at her home with her neighbor, Sr. Quingue, the herbalist who had helped her conceive. He gave Javelina another medicinal tea, and the pregnancy "stayed" until term.

President Chissano formally lifted bans on churches in Mozambique in 1987, and in the aftermath of war and in the midst of economic change, Pentecostal and African Independent churches (AICs) influenced by Pentecostalism have rapidly spread throughout Central Mozambique. The AICs, which include Zionist and Apostolic movements with historical roots in South Africa and Zimbabwe, have found fertile ground among the poor, recruited primarily through prophetic healing. Other churches more directly identified as Pentecostal have had similar success in attracting new members through offers of healing, including manifestations of the Assemblies of God, the Apostolic Faith Mission, the Universal Church–Kingdom of God, and the Full Gospel Church. Because of overlap in central tenets and practices, and in spite of some important differences, scholars generally view AICs and Pentecostal churches as constitutive of a broader Pentecostal movement. They are similar in their incorporation of key tenets of Pentecostalism, including belief in the healing power of the Holy Spirit, the authority of New Testament Scripture, ritualized speaking in tongues, ceremonies of baptism, and spiritual explanations for misfortune and illness (Pfeiffer 2003).

Both groupings of churches in southern Africa trace their histories to the same early Pentecostal evangelists. However, some of the Pentecostals have international links to global networks, while AICs are linked only to regional groups and are often founded locally. AICs also use prophet-healers to communicate with the spirit world in the healing process in ways that are often described as "syncretistic." Mainstream Pentecostals frown on this prophet healing, which recalls African traditional healing. Pentacostal pastors instead heal through prayer (summoning the Holy Spirit) and the laying on of hands. However, key characteristics of both Pentecostals and AICs suggest that social capital may be especially important in their influence on the HIV/AIDS-related health behavior and choices of their members. The churches are noted for their significantly greater involvement of poor women than other faiths, members' intense and frequent church participation, and active mutual aid support systems, especially among women.

A "revival" of churches in Gondola, which continues to flourish, began in the mid 1980s, Senhor Moyo, the Gondola District secretary of churches and president of the Gondola Organization of Churches, told me in Vila Gondola in May 1993:

> During the colonial time, the Portuguese government did not want
> Pentecostal churches. They were prohibited from the city. If you were caught,
> you were sent to prison. There were Catholics, Swiss Baptists, American
> Methodists, and Anglicans from England—whichever church had a mission.

During colonial times Johane Malanke and a Zion church also existed, hidden in the bush, and the Jehovah's Witnesses had a small group in Beira. During that time, the acceptance of churches by the local people was low.

In 1978 FRELIMO closed the churches. You couldn't congregate. You had to come to one central church, each faith at a different time. They sent police to overhear the messages being preached.

The position of the churches had suffered from this persecution. Some people gave up [church]. Others continued. Members of government left the churches. The Assembly of God maintained its believers, the Church of Apostle's Faith Mozambican Mission, and the African Assembly of God. During that time, about 1984, that they were oppressed by FRELIMO, there was much acceptance of the churches—actually, a kind of revival.

In 1986, church leaders from around the country were called to a meeting with then-president Chissano in Maputo. Moyo was among those summoned. At that meeting Chissano promised that religious persecution would end and officially rescinded the ruling that barred the building of churches. Since then, Moyo has seen a continued revival of religious worship in the district of Gondola. By 1990, a flood of churches had opened their doors, both foreign missions and local independent churches. When congregations of either type get too large, or conflicts between church authorities begin to surface, discontented groups split off from older congregations and a new denomination springs up. These small, independent churches commonly claim to treat any affliction, including reproductive problems, using the laying on of hands. Pastors are frequently asked to preside in cases of difficult births at home deliveries and even occasionally at a rural health post. In cases of extreme complication or illness, an entire congregation may be called to offer collective prayer for a woman.

Most local churches run a weekly class for churchwomen, advising them how to treat their children and husband and how to wash, clean, and be hygienic. Common themes in these classes are monogamy and sexual fidelity in marriage and the requirement that women give in to men's requests for sexual relations even before the traditional period of postpartum abstinence is over to keep husbands from looking elsewhere for sexual satisfaction and straying from the marital bonds. Pastors' wives are frequently described as able to work with the power of the Holy Spirit, *espirito Santo*, to heal and save, especially churchwomen. They are frequently called on to direct prayers for women experiencing problems during pregnancy, and to assist in difficult home births. After a woman in the church gives birth, the pastor's wife organizes other women in the congregation to help with sweeping, getting water, and supplying cooked food. In the case of a death, the churchwomen help with the funeral preparations and raise money for church members in dire situations to cover costs and expenses.

These social aspects of the church, common among the mission and independent churches in Mucessua, take on special importance in the context of changing domestic organization and diminishing kin networks. One of the most significant attractions of these new churches and their prophets, however, is their acceptance of traditional beliefs in the power of spirits of the dead and in the power of witchcraft and sorcery—*feitiço* (Bourdillon 1991: 295). Through prayer and salvation, they offer cures for these familiar problems that do not, unlike indigenous healing therapies, depend on the involvement of the extended lineage.

In the spring of 1995, forty-seven churches were officially registered with the Gondola District Organization of Churches, established in 1989. Moyo estimated that as many more unregistered churches surely existed in Gondola District alone. The 1997 Demographic Health Survey (DHS) estimated that 60–65 percent of people in Gondola District participate in churches other than the Catholic Church. Among the women I followed through pregnancy, fifty-seven (69 percent) were affiliated with one or another of fifteen church congregations. The majority of women attended the Catholic Church, one of the long-standing faith-healing Pentecostal mission churches, or an offshoot of the independent Zionist "spirit-type" churches.[2] These churches grew out of the Zionist movement in South Africa, connected to similar movements among African Americans and ultimately traceable to Zion City, Illinois (Bourdillon 1991: 292). Central to the workings of the Zionist independent churches is faith healing.

Religious Diviners: Prophets

In Mucessua, twelve of the forty-seven government-registered churches, usually those identified as stemming from the Zionist church tradition, had prophets who performed divination and healing treatments. The prophets I interviewed were usually called to their profession by the Holy Spirit through a dream or vision as a result of serious illness or fasting and praying. Two of the most common practices among prophet-healers are diagnosis using divination and the calling forth and exorcising of spirits or demons in the name of the Holy Spirit. A third common practice of prophet-healers is the administering of sacred waters, sometimes combined with other ingredients (such as black tea leaves, butter, milk powder, salt, and oil) in healing liquids called *taero*. Taero are administered by mouth and as enemas. Other techniques used by prophet-healers included laying on of hands, incision, steam baths, charms, prayer, fasting, baptism, injection, and sympathetic and suggestive rituals. Across the board, prophets prohibited the use by their church members and followers of "traditional medicines," including preparations made from indigenous plants.

Community churches represent serious competition for indigenous healers and biomedical facilities in terms of gaining access to women, who represent the opportunity for material gain, social control, or both. Unlike curandeiros, who often professed to be expert at healing a specific set of illnesses, prophets in Mucessua claimed the ability to heal any illness or problem a client brought to them, though many admitted they had specialties for which their services were most frequently sought. Prophets' specialties included demon exorcism, male impotence, female infertility, anemia, sexually transmitted diseases, problems in the home, and problems at work. The most consistently reported specialties were treatments for social and reproductive problems, including abortion. Payment for treatment was requested only in some cases, although most patients gave offerings at a designated time in the treatment ritual and many treatments involved the handing over of cash as part of the ritual process. Rather than paying a one-time fee at the time of diagnosis or treatment as is now required by indigenous healers, the members of a church regularly brought small cash or food offerings to their church and always made an offering when asking for a pastor's or prophet's intervention. Church offerings were also gathered from members at each meeting, and some pastors and prophets made membership in their church a condition for treatment.

Thus, while the churches cater to the needs of the community to manage loss and eroding family structures, they also extract their fees, but more painlessly than do their competitors, the indigenous healers, who increasingly charge cash for services rendered. I was often told that most churches treated sick people free of charge; however, the institutionalization of the offering, or chipo (gift, Sh., Tewe), guaranteed a constant flow of cash into the pockets of the pastors and prophet-healers.

In describing an elaborate treatment for infertility she had received from a well-known Zion City prophet outside her own church, Jacinta recalled:

> I did not pay for my treatment. Some churches charge and others don't, but they make sure you stay and pray with them. Normally they only treat members of their church, and so you must say that you are going to comply and stay in that church. This prophet is treating many people. From as far as Pipeline they are coming for treatment. It is filling with cars there. She has a farm and helps many people. Since she treats me without charge, when I go I bring soap, fish, or sugar when I have it. She does not charge and does not ask. Chipo is a type of gift that you offer in church and during treatment. At the time of saying your problem, you offer whatever you can. When you arrive, you sit at the table. You take out your money to ask for succor. [The prophet] is listening to the most important points and then begins to prophesize what are your problems. With the cost of living today, eh! I give what I can.

There was general agreement by laypeople, healers, and prophets that faith-healing churches have surpassed indigenous healers in popularity as sources of treatment for reproductive problems. The gift of prophecy and healing through the power of the Holy Spirit is a feature that attracts many members to the independent Zionist churches in Mucessua. While other independent and mission churches offer the material advantages of extended social networks and supposed healing powers of their leaders, there are significant parallels between prophets and traditional Shona spirit mediums. Important ritual similarities exist in both diagnosis and treatment.

Treatment for infertility by a prophet, for example, was repeatedly depicted in three distinct phases that correspond to both the procreation/cultivation analogy and the personalistic reproductive illness etiology. The first phase is a cleansing process called *ku-diridza*, meaning to water or irrigate. The second phase is *kufemba*, the process of removing or calling forth the malevolent spirit that has manifested its presence and displeasure in the form of illness or blocked fertility. The third and last phase—treatment of the patient once she has been cleansed by the first two steps—is called *kurapa kugadzira*, which can mean to apply or administer medicine, to cure, heal, or repair, to settle the spirit of a dead person, or to castrate. These representations reflect the inextricable association between the land, the body, and social relations.

Churches in Mucessua also depended heavily on the effects of fasting to make the supplicant fertile for receiving the power of God. As one woman who had been treated for infertility while a member of the Zionist Evangelical Church Assembly of God said: "You cannot plead with your stomach full. You must plead hungry." Two types of fasts are common at this church—a half-day fast from morning to evening, and a twenty-four-hour fast from one evening until the next evening's meal. Church-related treatments for fertility problems also included individual and group prayer, internal and external cleansing regimens, casting out demons, laying on hands, building altars, and multiple uses of blessed waters.

Ilda explained to me: "Curandeiros don't have much acceptance with people any more, because they come to see that there as no advantage in it. There are certain things that a curandeiro cannot do, that can only be done in the hospital or the church. We see that curandeiros can't give someone blood. A curandeiro can't put water in someone [intravenous rehydration]. A curandeiro can only have something to do with spirits, things that are traditional, not things that are official."

But the growing pull women feel toward churches and church prophets in Mucessua suggests that something more than "official" biomedical technologies were important to those seeking healing for themselves and their children. Javelina, with her amazing skill at drawing people out, and always tuning into the questions she heard me hovering around, had this conversa-

tion with Louisa, her niece, at the end of an afternoon social visit at Louisa's
home in September 2008. Louisa had been talkative but, I noticed, preoccupied and somber. Her smile never stayed for long on her lips. As we got up to
leave and the two said their goodbyes, Javelina took Louisa's hand gently, and
asked: "Alright then, I don't know if there is anything else you wanted to add,
my daughter?" I knew that what was coming was a message I was meant to
hear that Louisa had been too shy bring up on her own. The reason for our
visit was about to be revealed.

Louisa: Há! No!

Javelina: I see, my sister, you are full of something. I see you are full of
something.

Louisa: I do have something, but can I speak about this work that we are
moving forward, to help orphans?

Javelina: Sister, so you know orphans here close?

Louisa: It is I, right here at home I have them.

Javelina: How many children"

Louisa: Three.

Javelina: Are they yours?

Louisa: No, they are my sister's, but they stay with me.

Javelina: Is your sister alive?

Louisa: My sister is alive; she stays in her home. Oh, things today . . . men
these days . . .

Javelina: [The children] are from another father.

Louisa: Yes. The father of these children died, and [the new partner] does not
want to live with these children.

Javelina: What would happen if they did not have family? But there are lots of
these cases.

Louisa: Yes, they exist. Even on my part, by the way. For this reason I decided
to live alone because it would be too much to lose my children. It is worth
living with my children and suffering together.

Javelina: Imagine if they did not have family?

Louisa: They would be alone, like these [children] that stay in the streets.

Javelina: It is sad. At your church is there much participation?

Louisa: Yes.

Javelina: But why are there so many more women than men?

Louisa: More women?

Javelina: Why are there more women?

Louisa: That's how it is in the world; there are more women than men.

Javelina: Do you think that's the reason?

Louisa: No, the question of motive, this case of having more women than men
is because of war. The war killed many men.

Javelina: Then do the women who are in church have husbands?

Louisa: Some, but the majority, no.

Javelina: But what brings the women to convert?

Louisa: It is to have help.

Javelina: What help?

Louisa: To have help from the church when you get sick or have misfortune.

Javelina: And so, it is a manner of getting family?

Louisa: These days, if you don't pray, you are left out.

When we left Louisa's house, I knew that besides helping me understand the role of churches in women's survival strategies, Javelina was showing me how much people who had assisted me in the past still hoped for material help from me, especially in the cost of raising the children born during my study who are now orphans due to AIDS and other sicknesses.

Jacinta: *A Case Study of Infertility*

During the years I knew Jacinta, I was able to follow several episodes of her quest to treat infertility under the care of a prophet from the Zion Christian Church. He was an older fellow who with his wife ran a bustling treatment center in their combined living and church compound in another bairro of Gondola. He was well known in Mucessua for his great success at curing infertility. Clay pots figured as potent symbols in his infertility treatments. In the sacred outdoor prayer and treatment space of his compound, I counted the burnished brown curves of nine clay pots buried by *mhanje* (infertile) women at the foot of a giant termite hill. The dirt was gray with the ashes of cooking fires located there before the termites began to build this natural phallic altar. At that site, under the guidance of the prophet, women like Jacinta underwent cleansing treatments involving strong laxatives, purgatives, emetics, and steam baths. Finally, each supplicant carved a hole and planted a lidded pot in the ground, leaving one section uncovered so that another supplicant would not unearth it accidentally, and so that it could be easily retrieved. This mosaic of pots protruded from the soil like a garden of miniature pregnant bellies shining in the sun, waiting to be uncovered, dug up, and carefully disposed of in the days before their signified's delivery, to ensure the onset of her labor and safe birth.

To begin her treatment, the prophet told Jacinta, she must have a consultation to find out what was wrong with her. Jacinta went to the prophet's consulting room dressed in her best clothes and prayed with him. Eventually, he began to *profetizar* (prophesize)—to use God's power through a holy vision to tell her what she has in her body. Jacinta was told she had a bad spirit in her body. To make the spirit come out, she was "*dado tatuagem*" (given tattoos)—small incisions made by a razor on her back. Blood from these incisions was put on money Jacinta had given to the prophet as an offering.

These bloodied bills were wrapped in Jacinta's clothes, which were thrown out in a special place known only to the prophet. After the evil spirit had been taken out of the body in this way, a cleansing of the body for conception could begin.

Jacinta's treatment involved five separate steps and a follow-up, with the prophet presiding over the process. For the first stage in the cleansing, Jacinta was given three forms of taero, a blessed tea made with black tea leaves, sacred waters, and other ingredients such as oil, butter, milk or salt. These mixtures may be taken orally as purgatives and emetics or anally as enemas, as well as added to baths, used in anointings, and sprinkled from containers in domiciles and on grounds that need purification. Jacinta's first taero, *chuacho*, was a solution of blessed water mixed with a large quantity of salt. She drank two to three liters of *chuacho* each morning for four days in a row. The strong cathartic action of the mixture provoked severe diarrhea, which lasted seven days. When the *chuacho* was finished, Jacinta was given *driza*, a *taero* made with a normal amount of salt. A potent diuretic, *driza* does not provoke diarrhea or vomiting but constant urination for three days. Following the *driza*, Jacinta was given *kugaba* over three days, an emetic taero with milk in it that provokes vomiting.

Her body having been cleansed from all orifices, Jacinta then underwent *kubvisa nyora* to remove nyora (dirty things with bad spirits, usually bits taken from a dead body, which have been secretly put into the body through magical writing, or secretly tattooed onto the victim by a witch or sorcerer, Sh., Tewe). In this ritual, Jacinta wrapped herself in a single capulana (a traditional woman's cloth wrap, Tewe). She sat in the hot sun with her shoulders exposed. The prophet painted another taero mixture of milk with other ingredients on her back. This mixture was left on her back to heat up for some hours, after which the prophet could see the *nyora* (writing, Tewe). Using his *bingala* (sacred staff, Sh., Tewe), he traced over the writing, lightly scraping her back. After this, he made superficial cuts with a razor where she had writing and removed impure objects from her body. She then had to take off the capulana wrap from her body and throw it away.

The next step in the treatment was a steam bath. Still naked, but covered with a blanket, Jacinta straddled heated rocks in a bed of coals burning on top of a low termite mound. For this *bafu* (steam bath, Sh.) *empiado* (standing up, Pt.), or *bafu ra kuima* (steam bath standing, Sh.), she poured a boiling hot taero onto the rocks as she straddled them. This, in Jacinta's understanding, was *"para o fumo entrar na confusão do sexo"* (for the steam to enter the [vagina] confusion of the sex).

After this steam bath, Jacinta was given another taero to drink while she rested outside the sacred taero preparation house, where no women could enter. The prophet finally gave her a recapped Fanta bottle filled with clear blessed water to drink at home each night before having intercourse with her husband until she conceived. When she did conceive three months later, the prophet changed the water prescription to a new preparation that Jacinta was told to use in her bath and also to drink. At eight months she was given another blessed water to drink and to massage herself with to prepare her for childbirth. Jacinta gave birth at the maternity ward to a robust boy she named Lucky, whom she loved with a passion. Lucky was as gorgeous and round as Jacinta, with his deep velvet glowing skin, burnished to a high gloss by Jacinta's constant kisses.

Full Cooking Pots

Clay pots appear, concretely and metaphorically, throughout all domains of women's activity, doing both secular and sacred work. The most essentially female of all home crafts, clay pots inhabit the center of women's domestic space, the cooking hearth, and carry and store the material staples of daily survival—food and water. Women's pots are as important in the concealed reproductive work of women as they are in women's more public social re-productive labor. When moved from the kitchen to the bedroom, the ubiqui-tous and thus inconspicuous clay pot is the symbol and repository of wom-en's reproductive secrets. The womb of an infertile woman is likened to a pot turned the wrong way inside her, or a pot whose cover is not tight enough, thus allowing the male seeds (sperm) to fall out of her without taking root.

The general Tewe term for treating someone for infertility is *ku-simikira*, from the verb *simika* (to plant, or to plant firmly as with a pole), whose verb root, *sima* (to transplant, or plant out from seedlings), also means to speak or converse. One curandeiro's cure for infertility involved gently uprooting a sweet potato, scooping the dirt from the hole left in the ground, and replant-ing the potato. The dirt removed from the hole is placed in a container of water and left overnight. The next morning, the water is poured off the dirt, which has settled to the bottom, and used to make cornmeal porridge. After the infertile woman eats the porridge from the pot in which it was cooked, some indigenous medicines are placed in the pot and the lid is placed firmly on it. Turned upside down, the pot is hidden under the infertile woman's bed or buried underneath a tree. When the woman becomes pregnant, she must uncover the secret pot in the last month of gestation in order to open her womb, or she will need a cesarean to deliver the child.

Two other methods indigenous healers use to help women who have diffi-culty carrying a pregnancy to term involve the symbolic and suggestive power of the pot. In one method, the healer prepares two kinds of medicine. One mixture is made into a paste, put into a clay pot, and covered. The other preparation is given to the pregnant woman to ingest. The jar is buried or hidden until it is time for the woman to give birth, when the healer presides over a ceremony for opening the lidded pot. In the second method, the pregnant woman collects a long reed into which she ties a knot. The knotted reed is treated with a medicinal preparation, then hidden in a pot beneath the woman's bed until she is about to give birth, at which time she takes the reed back to the healer to undergo another treatment and to undo the knot. Women in Mucessua have great respect for these methods, although they agreed that both involve the risk of permanent barrenness, should the healer die without the pot being uncovered, or the knot being undone. If this occurs, a treated woman will remain ritually "closed" forever, unable to give birth or even to conceive ever again.

If a woman should wish to intentionally "rest" from pregnancy, several forms of indigenous contraception were available that employed ritual means. These practices also frequently entailed the closing of the womb using a pot. One process is called *kumaidza nyoka* (from *kuruma*, to bite, sting, Sh.; or *rumatidza*, to join, link together, weld, Sh.; and *nyoka*, snake, uterus, soul, guardian of health, Sh., Tewe). A medicine made of dried, ground roots is mixed with the woman's last menstrual blood in a pot and covered. The pot is then hidden or buried in the ground until conception is desired. Kaler found four other "traditional" categories of home-based contraception engaged in by Shona women: practicing withdrawal (*kurasira panze*), drinking herbal preparations (*mishongwa yekunwa*), wearing herbs or beads on a string around the waist (*mishongwa yekupfeka*), and jumping over a certain type of tree or bush in order to "close the womb" (*kudarika bhenzi*) (Kaler 2000: 700). While female dependent, these methods were not necessarily female controlled, for "each method was embedded in a web of social relations and was dependent on someone, usually a female elder, to grant access and provide secrets that made the method work" (Kaler 2000: 701).

These contraceptive methods are likely not new to Shona communities. Beach (1980: 184) refers to a Portuguese writer in the 1780s who observed that "many Manyika women were taking medicines to avoid pregnancy." What was still in flux at the time of my research, however, was the power nexus of social relations within which negotiations and decisions regarding reproduction were being worked out.

Indigenous or "traditional" contraception, as women called these methods, was the only contraception reported by the women I worked with in Mucessua, and as Kaler found among Shona women in Zimbabwe, these practices were usually kept secret from husbands and *sogras* (mothers-in-law). Secrecy emerges as the strategy most often resorted to by women seeking to control their own reproductive labor. Indeed, control over fertility is one of the issues most marked by struggle. "For men, begetting children is inevitably mediated through a woman. Control over fertility, therefore, emerges over and over again as an area of conflict between husbands and wives"—and, I would add, in-laws. The swell in opportunities for women to engage in sex-work has exacerbated anxieties and struggles between genders and generations "over production and consumption of resources," including and especially reproductive resources and relations (Kaler 2000: 683).

When reproduction goes awry, the indispensable clay pot reappears, this time in an imperfect form. A large shard from a broken water jug is used to carry an aborted fetus or a stillborn infant to its grave. If delivered before nine months gestation, fetuses are considered incomplete pieces of a person and not fully human. These aborted or stillborn beings cannot be buried with adults or in the moist alluvial soils of river lowlands where children are customarily buried, and the mother cannot mourn this loss or she will take a long time to conceive again. An inappropriate display of grief on her part could even cause someone living in the same house to die. Neither should family or visitors mourn. No man or woman of fertile age except the mother should attend the burial ceremony. The tiny body must be carried away by postmenopausal women who no longer have procreative powers that could be ruined by such potentially defiling ceremonial acts. The grave is not carved with a hoe, for such distress must not be planted; it is interred in a grave carved out by the hands of women past childbearing age. These hands, the hands of pot makers, will also restore the broken mother by massaging her body in salt baths, and by picking, preparing, and administering healing herbs.

As the fetus is covered with earth, at the last moment the mother must bury her belt by its head, leaving one small piece above the ground. In the final gesture of the ceremony, she slowly pulls her belt from the grave as she turns and leaves, never looking back, unbinding herself from the loss. Only in this way, it is believed, will she be able to conceive in the future. She must hide the belt somewhere she will be able to retrieve it. If she forgets where she has hidden it, later when she goes to a prophet or curandeiro for treatment, she will not be able to secure (*segurar*, Pt.; *Kubata*, Sh.) another pregnancy.

Contagious Magic: Prescriptions and Prohibitions during Pregnancy

A broad description of pregnancy emerged from women's narratives regarding their current or most recent experiences. My own observations in Mucessua over the years confirmed that once pregnant, a woman's life changes little outwardly, and she is expected to continue her agricultural and domestic labor as before. Some husbands helped pregnant women with their work as heavy tasks become difficult, but women understood that such an indulgence was looked upon as a breach of codes of masculine behavior, and there was social pressure on men in Mucessua not to assist women in their work. Children were often asked to take up extra chores for which a pregnant woman had no energy. A woman without grown children, however, found this help harder than ever to mobilize. Javelina described the trend toward monetization of casual labor, social support, and trading of favors: "A woman can win people to work if you have something to give. In past times children worked for free if once in a while you had a little something to give. Now, neighbors are beginning to pay [children] money. Now I do, too, when I have it."

During pregnancy there are, however, behavioral prescriptions and food avoidances. Most of these pregnancy restrictions are symbolic and exemplify the principle of "contagious magic" (Sargent 1982: 207) inherent in much of Mozambican indigenous medicine. A woman who ate the prohibited foods would pass on undesirable physical or behavioral qualities to her developing child. For example, if a woman ate eel, her child would drool too much or slither on its belly instead of learning to crawl. Eating monkey meat would make her child naughty and overly active. Certain fish (*peixe cachão*, *peixe sapateiro*) would give a child ugly skin with scabs, and imbibing too much hot pepper would bring about irritated, red eyes and skin sores. Eggs and the liver of any animal would result in baldness in the infant. Eating eggs could also cause a newborn's fontanel not to move, which can kill the infant. Eating the meat of a small wild cat called *malumba* or *mulimba* locally, and *gato bravo* in Portuguese, would prevent a newborn from being able to cry. This was feared, for according to oral history, at some time in the past a child that did not cry at birth, or a child born attached to the placenta or inside the amniotic sac, was put in a piece of a broken pot and buried alive. Eating *rato bravo*, a large rodentlike mammal, was said to cause constipation in the newborn. Many women did not know of any prohibited foods, or had heard of them but did not believe in them. Nonetheless, eggs were the only item from the list of taboo foods mentioned that the pregnant women I interviewed ever spoke of consuming.

Other prohibitions suggest that specific actions and gestures of the mother could impact the behavior of the child or, more frequently, cause difficulties in childbirth. If a pregnant woman loitered in a doorway, her baby would come out and go back in during childbirth. Eating turtle or allowing a child to dawdle in the doorway of a pregnant woman's house could also cause obstructed labor. Tearing off a piece of meat or chicken instead of using a knife or yanking a banana from a stalk of bananas could cause the placenta, or a piece of the afterbirth, to be retained. Sleeping too much could make labor very slow and difficult. Pregnant women should also avoid wearing black, the color of mourning, to avert bringing upon themselves a reason to mourn. I remember smiling to myself as I wrote notes of these avoidances, and yet I soon found myself changing my mind about a black blouse or skirt

I had taken out to wear. By the end of my pregnancy, I was refraining from all these simple acts, just in case.

Most women agreed that by the seventh month, sexual intercourse should stop, as engaging in sex late in pregnancy could hurt the fetus by depressing its fontanel or making a dent in its head. They also feared that after the seventh—or some said the sixth or eighth—month, semen would dirty the fetus. The infant would be born covered in a thick, white substance, alerting anyone at the birth to a husband's abuse or the couple's joint impropriety. Becoming pregnant while still nursing (*kupundurira*, Sh.) was dangerous, for the nursing child becomes sick from breastmilk spoiled by its mother's having had intercourse during the period of postpartum sexual abstinence, an act that creates ceremonial heat in the mother's body. This period was ideally to last as long as the mother breast-feeds, reportedly from six months to two years among these women, but historically as long as four years.

Ntsuo: Preparation for Childbirth

In the seventh, eighth, or ninth month of gestation, women in Mucessua begin to prepare their bodies for childbirth. To avoid a painful, torn perineum, they begin drinking teas and applying herbal preparations as vaginal and perineal massages to prepare the *lugar* or *porta do parto* (place or door of birth, birth canal). Generally, a decoction or infusion is made from leaves, roots, or bark of particular plants and taken in prescribed doses. Women whose religious beliefs or affiliations prohibit them from using traditional medicine or roots of any kind can massage themselves with the juice from sweet potato leaves, the mucouslike liquid squeezed from boiled wild okra, or blessed waters from a pastor's wife or prophet. A woman under the care of a prophet during pregnancy is frequently given refillable containers of blessed water to consume at home in preparation for labor. This system guarantees the patient's close contact with the specialist as the delivery approaches. Church leaders and whole congregations also regularly perform prayers in the churches and during house calls specifically for a pregnant member's safe delivery.

The themes of secrecy and silence emerge again as the ideal female presentation at childbirth. The Tewe word for a woman who is about to deliver is *machinyerere*, meaning one who is silent, one who steals away. Crying out during labor is generally looked down upon and harshly discouraged. In a home birth, for example, a laboring woman who screams is sometimes hit or has a cloth put in her mouth so that she will reserve her energy for pushing. Women told me that at the maternity ward as well, the nurses would ignore a woman who cried out, forcing her to give birth alone.

Umai, Shona Mothercraft

Key contemporary ethnographic works exploring the symbolic and practical meaning of motherhood among Shona women in Zimbabwe make parallel claims about its centrality to Shona women's identities. Herbert Aschwanden, working in Masvingo Province (1982, 1984, 1989), Jane Mutambirwa in Central Mashonaland (1984), and more recently, Gurli Hansson in Maberengwa District (1996, 1998) suggest that it is not as wives, but as mothers that Shona women "attain a position" in their living compound, their husband's lineage, and their community (Mutambirwa 1984: 74). In the life cycle of Shona extended households, it is often only after the birth of her first child that a woman acquires her own kitchen separate from her mother-in-law's kitchen, and a man becomes the head of a household (*imba,* Sh.; *nyumba,* Tewe). "*Imba* marks the end of individual social development in Shona culture, [he or she] . . . has reached a stage of . . . maturity" (Mutambirwa 1984: 205–7). Motherhood gives women a new social and spiritual role, as they become the link between their ancestors and the next generation through the birth of male heirs.

To gain insight into these complex relational dimensions of motherhood in Mucessua, it is helpful to draw careful distinctions between the concepts of mother*hood,* mother*ing,* and being a *mother.* Andrea Cornwall, writing on infertility in southwestern Nigeria, has proposed a most useful framework for these terms:

> Mother*ing,* I suggest here, constitutes a cluster of social practices in which all women, irrespective of their fertility engage in at some stage in their lives. Mother*hood* is both an experiential state and a social status. In this context it is tied not only to having borne children, but having brought into the world children who survive into adulthood. . . . *Mother* is a relational identity, one that is used idiomatically to describe relations of dependency, care and guidance in other spheres, and one that can come to denote relationships between women and the children of others. (Cornwall 2002: 141)

The Shona word *umai* has been translated into English and defined in Hannan's *Standard Shona Dictionary* (1974) as "motherhood" or "mothercraft," a word interpreted by Hansson as the "art or skill to bring forth and look after one's child" (Hansson 1998: 47). Following Hansson, and as an extension of Cornwall's paradigm, I propose the term "mothercraft" to encapsulate the experiential, spiritual, and social status and economic dimensions of Shona motherhood and to signify the multiple forms of labor power that motherhood entails. Some scholars suggest that the experiential, economic, and status-related values of mothercraft constitute for women in Shona society acquiescence and unquestioning acceptance of uneven relations of reproduction (Hansson 1996, 1998). Aschwanden found, for example, that "although she is subordinate to men in other areas of life, she has no need for emancipation, for accepting . . . the role given to her by God and the ancestors, she becomes automatically the most important person in the lives of all Karanga; the mother. Therefore . . . to bring forth children . . . is her fulfillment" (Aschwanden 1982: 257–58).

Shona society is usually portrayed, on the one hand, as patrilineal and patrilocal (Mutambirwa 1984: 74), as is the case in Mukonyora 1999 (276):

> From the viewpoint of men as the official guardians of the land and lineage, women are unimportant in the pre-Christian religious heritage of the Shona peoples of Zimbabwe. Despite the roles they fulfilled in the ancestor belief system (e.g., as diviners and spirit mediums), women were and still are perceived as subordinates to men. This is reflected in literature produced by anthropologists who have drawn their conclusions on pre-Christianity among the Shona from observations made at rituals held in honor of the patrilineal ancestors. According to Bourdillon, for instance, there is a male focus in traditional Shona religion.

On the other hand, some Shona scholars propose that in practice, because they create and sustain the culture through bearing and raising children, Shona women achieve a "creative superiority" to men in both the cultural and spiritual realms, structures which have been described as "highly matriarchal" in their historical formation and current orientation (Aschwanden 1982: 257–58). Thus, below the official patriarchal and patrilineal orientation of Shona social organization, there runs a strong orientation toward matriarchy (Aschwanden 1982: 277). This "unofficial" matriarchy, with its "fluid and fugitive vitality" (White 1997: 328) is, in practice, so pervasive as to render the patriarchal system "extremely superficial," failing "to take the real situation into account" (Hansson 1998: 47).[3]

As the mother of grown children, a woman in Mucessua begins to reap some fruit from her reproductive labor. For the women I worked with, children were the single major source of companionship, as well as providers of personal domestic and agricultural labor. Children, especially those with some education, could undertake wage labor as well, for example, selling their mother's produce or baked goods in the market or bairro, while she continued with other tasks at home or in her grain plots or riverbed vegetable and fruit garden. For many reasons, then, women in Mucessua valued children. Besides bringing joy, pride, affection, and love to their families, children provided their mothers social security by linking them to their husband's lineage and repaying the debt of lobolo. Both boys and girls offered some economic security as laborers in the subsistence agriculture or urban labor economies, and girls also through their potential to marry and bring in payments of ma-sunggiro and lobolo.

However, mothercraft had a more "multivalent, negotiated and kalei-doscopic" character in practice, as timing, resources, and relational context all came to bear on the events of pregnancy and childbearing. Among the women I interviewed in Mucessua, only a handful recounted having sought or undergone an intentional abortion, which, under both colonial and inde-pendent Mozambique's legal code, was illegal and punishable by imprison-ment. From women's life histories, I learned that directly after Independence, girls and women who went to the hospital with injuries or other sequelae from clandestine abortions were often jailed immediately on being released from the hospital where they sought medical attention, or even taken, shackled, from their hospital beds.

In Mucessua, however, every indigenous healer I interviewed reported that the service most sought by women and on behalf of women was to *des-fazer*, undo or abort, pregnancy. None admitted knowing or assisting women who made this request, probably because of the potential criminal nature of such work. The Mozambican parliament is currently reviewing a bill to decriminalize abortion. However, the coexistence of reproductive sanctions and coercion on the part of the state, and the reported high demand for abortion on the part of women living in Mucessua, suggest that reproductive control among these women entailed, as Kaler found among Shona women in Zimbabwe, more dynamic and contested "everyday dramas of power and resistance" (Kaler 2000: 680; Kaler 2006). Mothercraft in Mucessua was cer-tainly about gender and intergenerational power struggles that led to subver-sion and secrecy surrounding motherhood (Kaler 2000: 679).

A Velha, Elder Women

In Mucessua's transforming social economy, in which the inflation of bride-wealth has made informal polygamy more common, older women's lives sometimes turn especially bitter. Many women complained that before the end of their fertile years, the toll taken by strenuous physical labor and long-term child bearing and rearing renders them unattractive to their husbands. In a final, cruel passage in a woman's life cycle, the wife becomes mother to her husband, as Dona Joana, age forty-five, explained: "To give birth fre-quently, you become old while he is still good (*bom*). He procures another woman. Now it is you who arranges the ring (*arnelle*, Pt.; *mhete*, love token exchanged as a symbol of agreement to an engagement, Tewe). You become his mother, finding a young girl (*menina*, girlfriend) for your husband."

Dona Joana and a few other women spoke openly and with pain of their shame regarding this loss of intimacy and substitution. However, they agreed that it was preferable to find a malleable young girl one could set up in one's own backyard and keep an eye on rather than lose one's husband, his affections, and resources completely to someone of his own choosing who might demand that he abandon one's household altogether. At any rate, they joked, if a younger woman has not enticed a husband to forego sexual intimacy with his wife already, menopause is likely to end it all together. The power of menstrual blood is potent, and contact with it is potentially dangerous, as described earlier. Senhor Matore, over fifty, a male elder in Mucessua explained that sexual intercourse "with a woman who stops menstruating can kill a man" because he becomes contaminated with the unclean blood trapped inside her that enters him during intercourse. "Others have medicamento [herbal and ritual means] to take the dirtiness [*sujidade*, filth] from the man. At any rate, the way of doing it [intercourse] every day won't do."

Postmenopausal women in Mucessua take on new social roles defined by the belief that their bodies, ostensibly no longer sexually active, are no longer *quente* (hot, ceremonially potent/powerful/polluted) (see also Kaler 2000: 696; Schmidt 1992: 23; Maxwell 1993: 374). For example, as we have seen, they can attend to other women who have miscarried, and only they can participate in the ritual burial of an aborted fetus, a process necessary to secure the future fertility of the woman who has miscarried. They are also able to attend to the burial of children without personal danger to their own fertility. Only women who are postmenopausal or who have not yet begun to menstruate can be involved in the hands-on preparation of the ceremonial beer brewed to propitiate the ancestor spirits. Thus, for two short periods in their life cycle, before and after their childbearing years, women achieve a fleeting state of balance and purity, as women of reproductive age who labor between these two points attempt to find safe passage.

As people's desires regarding reproduction are not always parallel even within a single household, and births are differentially valued based on the social and economic context in which they occur, reproductive futures are highly contested and bring significant power imbalances into play. Here again Mullings's notion of transformative action (1995) is useful, recasting the concept of agency in a way that explains women's everyday reproductive practices as frequently subversive and quite unfixed. As Ginsburg and Rapp have observed, transformative action defines agency "in a grounded way that does not require categorizing cultural practices as either dominant or alternative. [Rather] this concept helps us recognize the emergence of new social and cultural possibilities in the activities of daily life" (Ginsburg and Rapp 1995: 10).

Female gender socialization and the developmental cycle of the family in Mucessua are dynamic social processes within which women's reproductive lives are shaped and contested. As the mother of a baby boy, for example, Jacinta had begun to take pleasure in her position in her husband's compound.

However, when I left Mucessua, both Jacinta and her son, Lucky, wore amulets treated with strong herbs and prayers to ward off witchcraft and harmful spirits. Jacinta had been having recurrent dreams of a small casket, which her prophet informed her were caused by the rumors and gossiping of her co-wives. As the youngest co-wife and with only one child, Jacinta had many years to go before she could relax in her status as a mother of lineage men, that is, sons who belonged to her husband's lineage, who had a right to land as members of the patrilineage, and who were destined to carry on the lineage name.

CHAPTER 5

Controlling Women: Reproducing Risk

In Mucessua, people around me paid as much attention to the invisible and the unseen as they did to the visible, as they navigated a world vigorously inhabited by spirits and animated by rumors, gossip, prayers, rituals, and magic (West 2005). Another force at work in every aspect of Mozambican life is the not so invisible hand of the market. Under economic reform policies and structural adjustment austerity programs, social safety nets disappear with the wave of a wand, and at the same time, as if by magic, the country's GNP grows miraculously in the aftermath of wartime devastation. The devaluation of local currencies, reduction of state bureaucracies, privatization of state and parastatal industries, and prioritizing of debt repayment over social safety nets are policies all set into motion. Protections for the most vulnerable members of society—unwaged workers, especially women without adequate access to land along with their dependents—vanish into thin air or are cut through vital organs. The deregulation of markets associated with SAPs removes subsidies that include food for vulnerable populations, price controls, and direct taxes, meanwhile assaulting environment and labor protections. These tactics jeopardize the ability of economically precarious populations in general and women in particular to provide food, health, education, and other social supports for dependent household members (Demble 2002).

Signs of this surreal politics of abandonment were everywhere. In Vila Gondola along the Beira Corridor, just to the side of the road, people who were unhoused, unhinged, or simply in transit had converted a large covered bus stop into a sleeping shelter. Their sleeping bodies, wrapped in rags, grain sacks, or cardboard, are sometimes indistinguishable from the impromptu luggage and bundled trade goods of waiting travelers. People and things trade places, confusing what and who is for sale. Bales of people are piled in the back of a shaky pickup, and bouquets of live chickens tied together at the feet take up a full seat on a crowded bus.

Alongside and behind this shelter is the Gondola Central Bazaar, the largest market in the district. The mostly open-air bazaar is loud to both the ear and the nose. The odors of raw sewage, rotten produce, and festering meat vie for primacy, closely followed by the smells of fresh and dried fish and briny mounds of tiny dry salted shrimp, then the nose-stinging scent of long brown and blue loaves of homemade all-purpose soap.

After we had passed rows of vendors selling what seemed to be identical wares, Adelaide, whom I often accompanied to the market, stopped suddenly in front of an undistinguished stall and bought two cups of dried shrimp and a thumb's width of brown soap. Sticking her thumb toward the two newspaper-wrapped packets, she told me, "This will have to last a month," as she handed three bills, a thousand *meticais* each, to the vendor. "What I used to buy with this much money could get me through two months, at least." She had not yet made eye contact with the young vendor in his Joe's Garage bowling tournament jersey and ragged athletic shorts, but she raised her voice loud enough to include him. He, meanwhile, barely took his eyes off her.

"How do you choose which stall to buy from?" I asked as we walked on.

"I just paid half what I owe, but he knows I am good for it next week or so and doesn't yell, 'Thief!' about it, like some do. I'll buy fish on the other side where he won't see my *riqueza*." *Riqueza* in Portuguese refers to material riches or treasures, but also to richness of the senses and sensations, tastes, smells, pleasure, and physical attributes. Adelaide smiled furtively at me, tapping the spot between her breasts where she kept her money tied in her capulana, a mock seductive sway working its way into her next few steps, working it, knowing her body might have to serve later as her I.O.U.

Adelaide's constant juggling and patching together of scant resources and relationships is a common rhythm of life for all the women I worked with in Mucessua, acts necessitated by the "persistent injuries of uneven development" (Susser 2004: 612). Here, as elsewhere around the world, women's vulnerability to poverty is related to broader global processes. Over the last two decades, international development efforts have increasingly focused on the gender dynamics of these global economic disparities. Yet gender equity remains an elusive goal, and women get poorer (Gunewardena 2002). Mozambicans often joked ruefully that after Independence in 1975 and during the war of destabilization that followed, while foreigners despaired over the lack of goods in the stores, Mozambicans could buy almost anything they could afford on the informal market. Since the end of the war in 1992, the markets and stores are once again bursting with goods for consumers with dollars to spend, but most Mozambicans, people complain, "cannot afford to buy a damn thing!" Stalls in the Gondola bazaar sell just about everything, from basic household commodities like seeds, cooking oil, salt, matches, tea, batteries, nails, thread, and enamel cups, to luxuries—sugar, scented soap, macaroni, ultrapasteurized long-life cow's milk, baby formula and weaning cereals, batteries, instant coffee and margarine, sunglasses, Coke and Fanta in bottles, pens, razor blades, Hello Kitty backpacks, American Girl skin lotion, hair pomade, notepads, belts, plastic shoes, diaper pins, cigarettes, candy, cookies, yarn, marbles, tobacco, nail polish, and beer.

A central warehouse is almost exclusively occupied by fish sellers, along with purveyors of eggs, dried wild game, and the occasional cut of domestic livestock meat, less than fresh and swarming with flies. At the top of this pavilion, live chickens and, on occasion, live goats are for sale. In the field-burning seasons after harvest, one can buy field mice skewered on sticks and charred into black crunchy clumps, or as limp, furry clumps to char at home. From the country comes raw brown honey dark as engine oil and full of debris, homemade reed mats and baskets, metal pails, and on occasion, clay pots. Charcoal is sold from bulging sacks alongside bundles of wood for kindling, three-legged, cast-iron cook stoves imported from Zimbabwe, and choice recycled bicycle, car, and radio parts from the machine butchers.

Many pharmaceutical products were readily available in the Gondola bazaar without prescriptions; for the residents of Mucessua, self-medication with these products was often the fourth or fifth line of treatment, after waiting, praying, visiting a herbalist, consulting a spirit diviner, or all of these. It was rumored that drugs from government medical supply stocks were frequently diverted through various high-level channels into informal markets for public consumption. Some of these drugs found their way to the Gondola open market to be sold alongside drugs imported from Zimbabwe and South Africa. More than a dozen market stalls sold individual pills and capsules, from pain killers like aspirin and paracetamol to antibiotics, muscle relaxants, antidiarrheals, laxatives, quinine and chloroquin tablets, and occasionally mystery ampoules for injections. Vendors dispensed their wares for a spectrum of common illnesses, including whatever the customer was looking for or could be talked into.

Only one stall in the market sold pharmaceuticals exclusively. Besides the usual offerings, this well-stocked table held lindane pomade, tetracycline salve for conjunctivitis, multivitamins, iron supplements, gripe water, super-strength energy tonic, several antibiotics, antifungal cream, antiparasitic liquid, and throat lozenges. As Adelaide and I passed this stall, I casually asked the teenaged vendor if anything among his wares might "help" a pregnancy.

"To get rid of it?" asks the vendor, furtively.

"No, to protect it, to be well."

"Oh, no. Only to get rid of it, *desfazer*."

When I asked to see this medicine, he walked to another stall and quickly returned with a packet of oral contraceptive pills hidden in his palm. During the four years I lived in Mozambique, I heard of three separate instances where school-age girls connected to someone I knew had allegedly committed suicide with antimalarial pills. I suspected these apparent suicides might have been attempted abortions.

"Do I have to take them all at once?" I asked.

"No, like this, one after the other, but at one sitting." He scowled importantly, tracing with his finger the blue arrows printed on the foil back of the packet to show me how to take the pills. I thanked him and left without making a purchase.

Vendors of similar wares are grouped together in the bazaar grounds. Near the center of the market, several rows of covered stalls with faded cloths draped between them offer meals of meat or poultry stews with cornmeal porridge, roast chicken with oily fried potatoes or rice, bread with margarine, fried eggs, fragrant tea sticky with sugar, and sesame brittle in crisp, burnt chunks. Local fruits and vegetables of all kinds are for sale behind the tables of dried wares in baskets—beans, rice, sesame seeds, and raw peanuts. These vendors pay small stall rental fees to the local town council that is responsible for keeping the market clean. Local women, who come irregularly to the markets with their occasional surplus produce, often unable or unwilling to pay the fee to rent stalls, sit side by side on the ground in another designated area, their paltry wares in baskets or arranged on empty grain sacks. Each displays produce similar to that of the women on either side of her—bananas, oranges, tomatoes, onions, bound bunches of assorted greens, and the occasional pumpkin, pineapple, or sugarcane.

Beyond a transitional area dominated by sellers of bright capulana wraps and shoes, the entire eastern end of the market is devoted to stalls of used clothing. Arriving by the containerful in Mozambique from U.S. and European charitable organizations, these *calamidades* are given to local government and nongovernmental organizations to distribute, donate, sell, or consign to small entrepreneurs. The term "*calamidades*" sprang from the association people made between the Western hand-me-downs and relief aid distributions made by the Department for the Prevention and Combat of Natural Calamities—in Portuguese, *Calamidades*. *Calamidades* sellers without stalls lay their wares on old blankets.

At the front border of the market, along the edge of the Beira Corridor, mostly men sit passively beside large bundles of firewood, sugarcane, and sacks of corn and other produce for commercial sale waiting for wholesale buyers or transport to bigger markets. On the other side of the road, youths and children hawk fruits and homemade fried dough snacks, jumping from their perches on the stone wall of the crumbling Catholic church to accost potential customers from the buses and cars going west through Gondola toward Zimbabwe or east to Beira and the Indian Ocean.

On the northern border at the back of the market, a row of little bars regularly cough tipsy guests out of their doors and into the boisterous clamor. Under the gritty blare of pirated cassettes playing repetitive dance tunes from Mozambique, Zimbabwe, and sometimes Brazil, Cape Verde, South Africa, or Zaire, amplified to throbbing distortion, the bar customers' drunken lunging, muttering, and periodic brawls are quickly swallowed up in the smoky din of brisk business and loud hawking. Here is the best place to find Candies with a capital C—not *dolces* (sweets), but *meninas* (girls). Girls who frequent the bars go by the name of a brand of cheaply made plastic shoes, Candies, brought to the market from Zimbabwe and South Africa by truckers and traveling salesmen. Girls and women longed for these bright fashion statements and often got them as gifts and payment from men they met in these bars in exchange for friendly company, good times, or more.

In the face of material need, the line between sex work and other sexual relationships blurs; a primary benefit in either case is access to better material conditions. Although sex work was declared illegal and intensely persecuted by FRELIMO after Independence, the visibility of transactional sex has increased dramatically over the last decade. From full-time sex work in bars and hotels to casual exchanges of sexual favors for money, goods, school fees and passing grades, transportation, or meals (Chapman 1998; Chapman et al. 1999), the pervasiveness of sex work has generated widespread anxiety about the breakdown of families (Marlene, Chapman, and Cliff 2000). The spread of sexually transmitted infections and HIV/AIDS, the "immorality" of youth and their disregard for long-standing practices of intergenerational respect, and allegations of infidelity in households, especially on the part of women, tears families apart at the weak seam of tension over scarce resources (Pfeiffer 2003).

Perhaps related to this constellation of forces, a new theme emerged when people talked to me about the past: they painted a picture of an idealized though hardly idyllic time when everyone, especially youth and women, knew their place—nostalgic for the order and efficiency of the Portuguese colonial period or, increasingly over the years, for a rose-tinted version of socialism during the early years after Independence under the independent nation's first president, Samora Machel.

Mothers of adolescent girls often lamented that they were losing their daughters to this *nova vida*. To their dismay, the growing importance of money and decreased strength of extended kin networks for day-to-day survival was creating a new dynamic. Girls' greater need for and easier access to money and goods in exchange for sexual favors were leading them to resist long-standing institutions that monitor and control male and female sexuality, such as initiation rites, virginity examinations, and forced female confession of infidelity during childbirth (Chapman 2003). Within this economic push and pull lay the social space for women to redefine female sexual and social roles and expand female productive and reproductive repertoires in ways that presented new predicaments for the generation of girls coming of age. This potential for "strategic reversibility" of the situation wound in and out of our casual conversations and formal interviews (Foucault 1991: 5):

These days, when a mother says they have to be reviewed [checked for virginity], girls respond, "No, it is you who has to be reviewed." (Marida, age twenty-seven)

[The nova vida] is very negative because [girls] are becoming ruined. They see videos and learn many things that spoil them. They don't have respect! Long ago there were traditional dances [*chikweta*] that girls could not see. Now they see everything. (Woman in focus group)

Dona Banda, a Mucessua elder in her sixties, had spent much of her adult life doing virginity exams for families in marriage negotiations around Gondola. She had much to say about what she saw as a disastrous erosion of girls' social mores. During a visit to her house to show off my three-week-old daughter, she took a fussing Solea from my arms and soothed her with a strong, short rocking motion of her arms, and warned me about what I was in for: "Dona Raquel, the problem with girls today is that they are disobedient. While you are sleeping, they climb out the window to go to the houses of boys. They sleep around in whatever manner with lovers. Then when it comes time, you ask a girl's parents to know if she is a virgin to arrange a good marriage. But they want you to pay as if your son is the first lover, even if he is not!"

In Gondola, it is not commoditization itself that impinges most on reproductive practices but the intersection of commodification with female economic marginalization in an austerity economy that is reshaping the reproductive cycle. Monetizing the economy and gutting public-sector social safety nets have transformed kinship and gender relations and altered the reproductive cycle; the result has intensified reproductive pressures on women. The rise in the number of women and girls engaging in sex work and the expansion of a male market for their services is a troubling newer facet of the nova vida. The same is true for Zimbabwe, where what journalist Danai Mupotsa (2008) found "interesting is how women, women's bodies and sexuality have become increasingly commodified in the context of extreme economic inequality. In a country with an economy in crisis, women appear to be hardest hit by poverty, and transactional sex (by choice and otherwise) has emerged as one means of survival."

The commoditization of reproduction that is signaled by this explosion of sex work in Mozambique can be traced to the shift away from food, gifts, cattle, tools, and labor to money as payments for *masunggiro* (virgin seduction fees), *lobolo* (bridewealth payments), and *respeito*—the offerings of respect as a social debt made, for example, to midwives for birth assistance. This shift comes at a time when access to money is more important to women's survival than it has ever been.

The Girl in the Red Plastic Shoes

The bright red plastic shoes on Lilia's feet caught my eye first and worried me even before I took in her haggard face and protruding abdomen. The sixteen-year-old was Javelina's "niece," a petite, café au lait girl with an impish face, pimply adolescent skin, and a childish personality. Javelina is Lilia's madrinha—her godmother, the trusted older woman friend of the family whom her parents had asked to watch out for Lilia's training and initiation as a young woman. Someday she would be the agent to negotiate Lilia's engagement and marriage on her parents' behalf. I had met Lilia several times before at her home in another part of the bairro while out conducting interviews with Javelina. The pregnancy and strained features were a jarring contrast to her usual immature playfulness.

Lilia was uncharacteristically sullen, silent, and uncomfortably swollen by her advancing pregnant state. She breathed heavily as she mixed hot water from the blackened kettle on the cookstove and cool water from the clay water-storage jug in the corner of the cooking hut into a dented enamel pitcher to pour ceremoniously over my hands in preparation for the afternoon meal—thick cornmeal and a smoky stew of red beans. With this gesture of respect and welcome, she signaled me that she was acting as a daughter of the house and not another visitor. I wondered what was going on, but I had learned to wait for the story to introduce itself. When lunch was served and finished, Lilia cleared the plates and cups, moved away to rinse them in a plastic basin with a handful of water and a bit of sand, then went to rest in the shrinking shade under a breadfruit tree in the yard. Over tea and out of earshot of Lilia, Javelina filled me in.

After several months of no appetite and vomiting whatever she managed to eat, and after several trips to a healer and her church pastor's wife, of course it was uncovered that Lilia was pregnant. She refused to give up the name of the other responsible party. Making no accusation of violation or assault and naming no suitor to claim her and the baby put Lilia in a bad light, humiliated her parents, *and* deprived them of seduction fees or possible bridewealth payments. So her parents had chosen to throw her out to "wash their face" of the dishonor.

Lilia had at once confided to Javelina about her secret seventeen-year-old lover, Eusébio, and the dilemma they were in. "You can imagine," Javelina said, "a secondary school boy, he is unemployed and claims to have no money and no prospects of having any money for beginning engagement." Lilia's parents, of course, already knew this, and by publicly disowning Lilia hope to force the boy's family's hand a bit. Javelina was negotiating on their behalf with Eusébio and his family regarding their intentions with respect to Lilia. They were pulling together money for the seduction fees and engagement-starting bridewealth installment. "As Lilia's madrinha, of course, I have taken her in. So everyone is saving face while a financial agreement is finalized and a wedding arranged. Eusébio is avoiding a fat case at the bairro tribunal for unpaid damages [to Lilia's parents]," Javelina finished, shaking her head and sucking her teeth.

While everyone consulted had agreed that at least one source of Lilia's ongoing *problemas* were the symptoms of her pregnancy, Javelina had taken her to a prophet she trusted, just the same, to get her some protection from the various vulnerabilities she had incurred through her reckless actions—disapproval and withdrawal of support from her parents and potentially her ancestors over the unpaid seduction fees and bridewealth, and the possible jealousy of other girls in the bairro who might have had their eye on or been involved with Eusébio. As Lilia napped, evidence of her visit to the prophet peeked out where her shirt raised away from her *capulana* enough to reveal a thin protective braid of green, white, and red thread tied around her waist by the prophet to protect her and hold the pregnancy.

In Lilia's case, this prenatal care seeking was influenced by the understanding that reproductive threats are defined in relation not only to their potential to end in reproductive loss, but also to their association with actual or threatened ruptures in gender and kin power relations. Frequently, at the heart of social conflicts are struggles over avenues to material necessities and social mobility. The common aphorism Mucessuans offered in explanation of social conflict, and especially suspected sorcery, is that people do not like to see others do better than they are doing. Envy of others' material goods or economic opportunities is most frequently cited as the main reason for sorcery in the bairro. In the local economic context of inflation and deregulation, basic and status-associated luxury goods are available—from Nokia phones and Nike shoes to Peugeot scooters, Toyota Land Cruisers, and big new homes—but few can buy them.

What makes economic and social inequalities so keenly felt is that these conditions collide with the distorted international aid economy in which a few individuals in the community score jobs that pay salaries disproportionate to government salaries and even pay in foreign currency. Women's anxieties about pregnancy, and the way reproductive threats during pregnancy are categorized and addressed at the individual and collective levels, reflect these broader configurations of their vulnerability to economic and social instability and constant "insidious social comparisons." They need money to survive, but experiencing material gain is fraught with danger, as "getting more" makes one enviable and thus a target of others' resentment and, in some cases, violence. Sorcery, as a discourse, not only addressed the constant fear people harbored of falling into the growing gap between haves and have-nots, but also attempted to name the unlikely and unnatural circumstances under which someone otherwise like them suddenly became someone who had *more*.

After tea and our hushed conversation, Javelina and I went to sit by Lilia in the yard. Seated on another worn reed mat close enough for Lilia to over-hear us, Javelina explained to me how envy enters the body:

Say I am in my house, and I want to buy something nice. Next-door is someone who cannot buy that thing. If that person knows *feitishismo*, they will use it to get it, or to get me.

Rumor is what breeds feitiço. One day you are going to meet someone who knows a *feitiçeiro*. [Say] you gossip or brag. That rumor will get hold of someone who is going to do something by means of those rumors. It will happen without the person knowing whom because rumors travel far. But the prophet you go to in order to resolve the problem is going to know, because feitiço is always done in the name of the person who called it.

How did all this come about? Problems of war, communal villages—where there was one, now there are twenty. Each one has his thoughts. And you don't know who [the *feitiçeiros*] are anymore.

Coming from Javelina to Lilia and to me, this circuitous pronouncement was a serious warning. For my benefit, Javelina was hinting at the ambiva-lence she experienced regarding my presence in her life. I had hired her and paid her almost as much in dollars for one day's work as her husband made in a month. She was aware of the increasing envy my regular presence at her home was drawing to her, and she had begun mentioning frequently how worried she was about her health and that of her son, Abel. Even sitting with me in the yard might constitute bragging. To Lilia, she was hinting at the girl's literally growing vulnerability and cautioning her not to *zingar* (any form of showing off).

The double-edged nature of pregnancy as valuable and vulnerable is a most important clue to understanding why it is a well-kept family secret. But the secretiveness does not refer only to the hiding of pregnancy from those outside the family unit. It also suggests the intimate dangers that emerge out of the very familial relatedness that permits access to knowledge of intimate conditions and constitutes a burden attached to kin relations. In this envi-ronment of social disruption and competition for scarce resources, women reported feeling greater pressure to bear children that survive and more fear of harmful sorcery attacks from kin, neighbors, and spirits.

The reproductive cycle in Mucessua has been saturated with potent pros-pects, both perilous and tempting, as I proposed in Chapter 1. In this case, the allure *and* the threat lie in the possibility of making any *body* into a com-modity by transacting reproduction in an inappropriate manner, a manner not culturally sanctioned. A girl who gets pregnant out of wedlock with masunggiro, seduction fees, paid is a potential mother and wife. A girl who gets pregnant without masunggiro paid is considered a prostitute. A girl who shames her family can expect the withdrawal of parental and even ancestral protection, leaving her and the unborn generation she carries vulnerable to witchcraft and sorcery. By the end of the afternoon, I noted that Lilia had removed her red shoes, wrapped them in a piece of towel and placed them under her head as a pillow.

Cashing In on Reproduction

Reevaluating Virginity: Adolescent Sexuality and Seduction Fees

Local social dynamics reinforce women's perceptions that reproductive threats derive primarily from the breakdown of social and kin relationships. As women's sexual and reproductive labor assumes monetary value, female bodies become highly contested sites of friction (Agadjanian 1998a). I was repeatedly told that virginity (*utsvene*, Sh.) is an important aspect of a Shona girl's social identity, and that great value is placed on a girl's being able to demonstrate she is a virgin (*mandhuwe*, Tewe) at the time marriage arrangements are being made and bridewealth amounts negotiated. Whether this has always been the case, as some Shona ethnographers have claimed (Bourdillon 1991; Gelfand 1992[1973], 1979), the current high valuation of virginity in Mucessua is expressed in the intensity with which it is protected by social custom and the social and monetary price attached to the act of having sexual intercourse with a virgin, of figuratively "beheading" a girl (*decabeçar*). Until recently, girls entering puberty were routinely submitted to an examination of their hymen, a process called *kuchidza* in Tewe (*chidza*, a girl of marriageable age) or *kuringira* in Shona (to look up), when a prepubescent girl might be brought along for comparison; the Portuguese translation, *revistar a miuda*, means to "review a girl." Dona Banda, over sixty years old, described reviewing girls in Mucessua, a role she held in the area for more than twenty years. The metaphors of suitcases, baskets, cars, and vessels of water recur throughout women's coming-of-age narratives to refer to women's sexual and reproductive bodies:

> It was my work. When it was good news they gave me respeito (respect, status, social importance; also material and increasingly monetary compensation), particularly before a wedding. Now I do it once in a while. It makes a difference how much is paid in bridewealth. If the bride is a virgin, you pay more. You check to see if you have to pay for a full suitcase [a virgin]. You can still take an empty suitcase, but you pay less.

An "empty suitcase" refers to a girl who has had sexual intercourse and signifies the loss of virginity. When this loss occurs within accepted social parameters, specific rituals marking the change of a girl's status from virgin to nonvirgin and the initiation of engagement accompany the event. Called "seduction fees" in English translation of Shona customary law, the practice of paying masunggiro (Tewe) attempts to protect rights to a girl's reproductive capacity and assure sexual loyalty. A man must pay a woman's family if he is her first sexual partner (Stewart et al. 1990). In Mucessua, masunggiro is customarily paid to the mother, who has a right to "eat" masunggiro because it was she who felt the labor pains and the pain of birth and carried the child on her back, sometimes even having her back wet with the child's urine. In the past, masunggiro was an offering of two goats or a head or two of cattle the son-in-law made to his wife's parents at her first pregnancy. Today masunggiro is paid in cash and store-bought luxury goods after a couple initiates sexual relations.

After masunggiro is paid, a second payment or series of payments is made—lobolo, or bridewealth. Bridewealth payments traditionally extended throughout a marriage and included multiple disbursements of labor, cattle, gifts, and metal tools that passed through lineages from sister to brother and reflected an ongoing relationship of indebtedness between the bride-giving and bride-receiving families. Bridewealth must be returned if the marriage ends in divorce, especially in the case of infertility. In practice, the payers of masunggiro and lobolo are often different men. The bride's family is intent on not losing either payment, and the groom's family does not want to be unfairly overcharged. The payment of masunggiro protects both parties' interests and places some external constraints on young people's sexual relationships. What agency girls have in this arrangement is difficult to find, while the potential violence, symbolic and otherwise, is not.

The payment of masunggiro and lobolo formalizes both patriarchal rights in children and male prerogatives to quench sexual desire, also reflected in the linguistic treatment of the woman's body as a vehicle of transportation or a container in which to carry men's belongings—children who will be members of his patrilineage (see Brandström 1990; and Udvardy 1995 on gendered metaphors for HIV). Using this imagery, Dona Banda emphasized the continued importance of virginity for girls:

Since Independence [1975] we were told you could no longer *revistar* [physically examine] children. [Before that time], if you found a girl was *descabeçada* [beheaded, not a virgin], the only solution was to beat her, to kill her, or to force marriage. If the girl was *descabeçada*, it was said, "*Mala bonita, mais vasia*" [a suitcase that's pretty, but empty]. If she was "*mala cheia*" [full suitcase, a virgin], the family of the girl wanted lobolo and masunggiro. The two families were called to *revistar* the girl and agree.

When they see that the basket is empty, an old woman from the side of the girl will bring a half-cup of water on a plate. She takes a leaf, opening a hole in it in half down the middle, and puts the cup of water on top. She goes to deliver this to the boy's *padrinhos* (groom's guardians and intermediaries). [The outcome] depends on the taste of the boy. If he has courage, he marries without *masunggiro*. If he doesn't want the girl, he says to take away the *sokwata* [used car, Tewe]. There will be problems in his hearth. If he has to spend two or three days at a tribunal, he will say, "You are *uma mulhere da má vida* [a woman of the bad life—of the street, the night—a loose woman]. You went to where your other husbands are." There will be no trust. When the girl is full [*cheia*, a virgin], the leaf is pierced with a straw and a full cup of water placed on top. Today, control depends on the family. How many times a girl is *revistada* depends on the girl, to control her.

While checking girls' hymens as a practice may be decreasing, the pressure on girls not to give away first sex for free is mounting, as is the potential for masunggiro to bring money into family coffers, especially mother's pockets. Sandra's parents received money, drinks, and a cooked chicken from her lover's father as payment for masunggiro. As nineteen-year-old Sandra observed:

> Today it is not easy to be raised a girl, *todos momentos revistada* [at all moments reviewed (examined)]. [Girls] can't play in whatever way. There is control of their behavior to obligate the payment of masunggiro to the mother. It is the father who also controls this money. Masunggiro is only given to the mother as an offering. When it is not paid to the mother, the mother can have rancor and have the courage to treat her daughter with *medicamentos* [medicines, powerful herbal preparations used in sorcery from curandeiros] and arrange problems in her home [*lar*, hearth]. It is the great grandparents, ancestors who accompany all this. Not to pay [masunggiro] is considered a great sin. My father-in-law decided to pay to avoid problems later.

A girl's overall value as a wife is not necessarily diminished by the fact that she is not a virgin. However, a suitor's family cannot be held responsible for the payment of masunggiro of a girl who is not a virgin, an empty suitcase, at the time of her marriage. Thus, the payment expected from the groom's family is lower—the bride's family can rightfully claim only the bridewealth.

Several changes in reproductive practices come together in this scenario. On one hand, fewer and fewer young men are able to come up with the money for both masunggiro and bridewealth; on the other hand, girls' families count on these payments as a source of capital accumulation. In the changing social economy, masunggiro is less a symbolic down payment expressing the groom's family's intent to join lineages and more an opportunity for the bride's family to gain cash and store-bought gifts, an equity loan. Dona Banda explained further:

A boy must pay the parents to be a girl's first lover, even if he doesn't want to stay with her. For this, the parents demand much money. One million meticais [U.S. $200] is normal now; it used to be 200 to 300 [U.S. $40–$60]. Afterwards the parents ask to know [if the suitor intends to stay with the girl]. This money is not returned. It is payment of the expenses that the parents paid when [the girl] was a child. There is other money that they demand as payment when parents hand over a daughter in marriage. "Here. Now she is under your wave" [*Agora ela esta em baixa da sua onda*]. If he pays the second time, already he is known as the son-in-law of the house—lobolo. The amount depends on the parents—long ago it was 5 contos, then 50 or 60. Now everything with PRE [Economic Restructuring Program—structural adjustment] is ruined. It depends. If you agree, you could make a discount. Others don't ask much because [the suitor] is already *filho da casa* [like a son of the house]. If he doesn't pay, the children belong to the wife's parents.

People were astute in their analysis of what the cost-shifting equation of structural adjustment (PRE, in Mozambique) manifested in their daily lives. A girl who loses her virginity without *tradição*, that is, without masunggiro, loses valuable income for her family. In this sense, the illicitness of the un-sanctioned sexual act lies more in the failure to pay up than in the failure to refrain from sexual relations. It is widely believed that not paying the proper fee to a girl's parents can result in death of the seducer or someone in the se-ducer's family, and many people in Mucessua have heard of deaths provoked in this way. Anger resulting from a perceived theft of virginity, in this case of both honor and income, leads to the employment of feitiço. Recent cases of unpaid masunggiro brought to the bairro-level tribunal were familiar and frequent topics of gossip and speculation among women in Mucessua.

One of several bairro-level Customary Justice Tribunal cases relating to seduction-fee payment in Mucessua in 1995 involved a divorced couple whose daughter was raised by her paternal grandfather. When this girl mar-ried, masunggiro was paid, not to the mother but to the father and grand-father, who ate the payment, that is, spent and used it up. The mother claimed that this violation of tradition later caused her daughter problems in pregnancy and the death of the daughter and her infant during a cesarean section operation in the provincial hospital. The divorced mother charged the ex-husband and father-in-law in the bairro tribunal for ignoring their ritual obligation to pay masunggiro to her and accused them of having caused the death of her daughter and granddaughter by omission of duty. She was awarded 300,000 meticais (U.S. $60). Such cases illustrate not only the seriousness of this offense, but also the shifting valuation of virginity in the community economy and the ongoing weight of customary laws in regu-lating social behavior.

The current regime of value cannot be grasped in all its complexity without considering that the same bairro Justice Tribunal in Mucessua also heard a case against Dona Regina, a woman I interviewed for the study, for using witchcraft to make her son's girlfriend miscarry. The case was dismissed, but a cloud of suspicion followed Dona Regina long after. Women's potential value and persistent vulnerability as reproducers inflect and constitute one another through women's potential to be dangerous to themselves and others. The value/vulnerability binary pits women against each other as victims/aggressors. Reproductive threats are frequently perceived as stemming from conflicts in social relationships between women.

Transacting Marriage in Mucessua

Heavily overlaid by colonial interpretations and distortions, only a partial picture of regional marriage practices emerges from existing Shona ethnographic writing. The descriptions of a Shona village in the 1880s and 1890s by an anthropologist working in 1920 in the Chivero village near what is today Harare suggest that raiding and forced marriages continued to be ways of arranging unions. Women often resisted such arrangements, for "there were also many cases of young women running away from old husbands with a young lover, especially if they had been pledged when they were very young themselves," the anthropologist wrote. "The seduction of young women by young men—and the long negotiations about compensation that followed—also occurred and is reflected today in some Shona marriage rituals" (qtd. in Beach 1994: 52).

Records from the Chivero village suggest that although fertility rates were low, reproductive health was relatively good. Venereal diseases were mild and largely uncommon before the advent of migrant labor. Maternal mortality seems to have been infrequent, but infant mortality was high—a staggering 50 percent of live births. It is possible that infanticide played some role in these figures, for thirty years later, in 1920, judging from the fierceness with which a Manyika writer condemned the practice, it may have been a frequent occurrence in other Shona communities (Beach 1980: 184). Older women interviewed in Chivero in the 1920s maintained that in the past no woman wanted more than one very young child at a time because she could not run from the raiders with two (54). Their input suggests that women were certainly engaging available means of fertility control, and, as elsewhere around the globe, that this power was challenged and condemned when and where women's needs opposed male or state interests in increasing the population. Low rates of fertility may also have been the result of the uneven distribution of women in the community; a minority of wealthy men had several wives, while many men had no wife at all.

Colonial as well as more recent studies of Shona marriage describe a contract between two lineages established through a long and elaborate series of negotiations between two families (Bourdillon 1991: 36; Holleman 1952: 98). As Kaler observes: "Marriage in Shona communities has historically been a relation between two groups rather than between two individuals, between the lineage from which the woman comes and the lineage to which she goes" (Kaler 2000: 695–6).

More recently, choice of spouse is increasingly left to the individual partners concerned. Negotiations toward marriage still usually involve, largely through intermediaries, participation by the senior representatives of each family to finalize a marriage agreement. Following the private, often mediated, exchange of love tokens between a couple, an engagement becomes public when a third party approaches the girl's family on behalf of the suitor. The girl's father's acceptance of a gift as a token of intention to betroth (*ruvunzo*, Sh.) and the girl's show of her agreement to the engagement by her touching, wearing, or receiving part of the *ruvunzo* establishes affinal relationships (*kubatira*, to speak for after paying masunggiro, Tewe).

Following this engagement the two lineages are related as wife providers and wife receivers, a relationship that gives prestige to the former. From that time forward, the girl's father will be called *tezvara* (the father-in-law of the groom, Sh.), and the groom will be called *kuwasha* (son-in-law, Sh.). The new reciprocal relationship between the two families is expressed in the fact that any male in the bride's family is referred to by the kin term *tezvara* by any of the groom's kin, and any of the groom's male kin are reciprocally *vakuwasha* (sons-in-law, Sh.), all of whom should give *tezvara* the appropriate service and respect. Future marriages between these lineages that support these established affinal relations are considered most favorably (Bourdillon 1991: 37, 39).

At some time following the engagement, the go-between makes a second visit to the girl's family with a gift (*muromo*, to open the mouth, Sh.; to ask word of, Tewe) to induce the *tezvara* to tell the amount of bride-price he wants for his daughter. Bridewealth—lobolo, lobola, or *rovora* in both Zimbabwe and Mozambique—involved two separate payments. The first, *rutsambo* (Sh.) was customarily a utility item such as a hoe, a bracelet, or in some cases a goat. This payment is associated with sexual rights in the woman and is diminished or waived if the woman has borne children prior to the marriage (Bourdillon 1991: 41). In Mucessua, masunggiro was the only payment mentioned that was paid before lobolo, and it is also associated with sexual rights in a woman. However, as mentioned earlier, masunggiro payment is determined by proof of a girl's virginity.

A marriage transaction by lobolo involves many subsequent ritual interactions and exchanges of gifts (*zwipeto*, Sh.) between the two families (Holleman 1952: 128–47). Once a sufficient amount of the lobolo has been paid, the *tezvara* will hand over the bride to her husband's family. In a customary wedding in Mucessua, the young girls participating in this celebration might teasingly sing to the bride:

> *Wasara ndiwe*
> *Sara woi sara*
> *Wasara takuda kuenda.*

> You stay here
> You stay, you stay
> You stay here, we are already going.

When she arrives at her in-law's compound, the bride should show her intention to serve the husband's family well by sweeping their courtyard in beautiful designs before they arise in the morning. Joyce, eighteen years old, described her first day at her in-laws' compound in Mucessua, where she arrived early in the morning from the neighboring district of Sussundenga to sweep with her mother and madrinha: "If the in-laws are kind they may hide money in the hills of dust for the new bride to find. I must boil water for the baths of all my in-laws, and I should repaint all the dwellings with fresh mud."

Among the women I worked with closely in Mucessua, one-fifth described their civil status as single. The rest described themselves as married, but none of the women I worked with had participated in either civil or church ceremonies. Most commonly these marriages were in progress, that is, the man involved was at some point along the continuum of fulfilling his marriage payments or service, and the woman was at some point in the continuum of bearing children for her husband's lineage. Of the twenty-one women with whom I discussed lobolo and masunggiro payments, lobolo had been paid in thirteen cases. In two of these cases the payments had been returned due to infertility, and the union dissolved. Both women had since borne children to other men who intended to pay lobolo sometime in the future. One of these was Javelina, who has borne two children in her second marriage. She explained: "Since I had not conceived in my first marriage, my second husband and I were not counting on our having two sons together. I did not want to end up with a debt to my father if my husband paid out lobolo for me, and then wanted it back if I didn't conceive. Now we are going to do it one day."

"Civil status" described a number of different scenarios because of the processual nature of marriage in this part of Mozambique and the lack of official church or state records for most marriages. In most cases, a woman who described herself as married meant that somewhere there was a partner or a partner's family proxy who had paid or intended to pay lobolo for her. Of the eighty-three women I worked with, fifty-seven (68.7 percent) described their status as married (*casado*), and nine (10.8 percent) identified themselves as married in polygamous arrangements. There is good reason to believe that many more women than the nine were aware that they informally shared their husband's time, income, and sexual attention with women in other households. However, according to Javelina, shame and anger about such arrangements may have prevented many women from discussing them in our interviews.

Carla, at age thirty, was one of the women comfortable enough to describe the problems in her informal polygamous marriage (*barika*, polygamous union, Sh.), in which she is the around-the-corner woman. Though not married by church, civil, or customary process, she considered herself married to her husband: "In the beginning it was good. There was understanding with my husband. But now the first wife is saying to him to separate [from me]. Visits from my husband are weak now. In church they are also saying [for him] to leave me and stay with the first wife, but my husband does not want this. The first [wife] went to complain in church, and the high-ups are now insisting he leave. He is fulfilling this."

Carla bitterly explained the contradictory church rules and local community expectations that she felt trapped between: "Polygamy is not accepted in many churches. But in Mozambique when menstruation stops you cannot have sexual relations. For this [reason], most men look for younger women to have sex and more children. Many who join with a single woman with children does not want the children. These [children] are sent to live with the woman's parents. They grow up marginalized."

Since the primary contractual aspect of the marriage transaction is to ensure the reproduction of the male lineage, and this is the reason bridewealth is paid, "a woman only then equalizes the *rovoro* (bridewealth, Sh.) given for her when she actually produces offspring for the lineage which has given *rovoro* for her" (Holleman 1952: 148). Thus, only after many years, when the marriage has been "fruitful" in the birth of a number of children, are the obligations of the two families mutually fulfilled (Bourdillon 1991: 43). As Bourdillon observed in neighboring Zimbabwe, in Mucessua many marriages were in progress, meaning that few marriage transactions were complete in the sense that attention had been paid to all the details that may attend such transactions. The criterion for a marriage to be legally valid in terms of Shona customary law is whether "the performance as a whole reflects the expectations and intentions of the parties to contract a valid marriage" (Holleman 1952: 140).

The payment of lobolo, as noted earlier, extended over a long period, sometimes a lifetime, for the mutual benefit of both parties: "The groom would be unwilling to make the full payment, even were he able, until he was satisfied that his wife would fulfill all her obligations, and in particular that she would bear a number of children in a lasting marriage. The bride's family too have a vested interest in prolonging the payments since they can demand favors in the form of service and gifts as long as the son-in-law remains in debt to them; there is a Shona proverb which says "A son-in-law is like a fruit tree: one never finishes eating from it" (Bourdillon 1991: 43).

There are several other forms of marriage that are equally part of Shona custom (Holleman 1952: 109–28). In elopement marriages the couple pre-empt some of the lengthy formalities of traditional proposal marriage and eliminate control of family heads by announcing the consummation of marriage after the fact, forcing families to the negotiating table. Other marriages are prearranged between family heads without the consent of one or either partner, often when both members of the couple are still children. In such child marriages a bride may occasionally be promised to the lineage of her father's friend or associate even before her birth. When such an arrangement is made as security against a loan in time of need, the marriage is called a credit marriage. Sandra, nineteen years old, articulated her understanding of arranged marriage in this way: "They sell children because of paying respect, or because of hunger or tradition. It is how a man conquers (*conquistar*, seduces) while the wife is still in the belly. When born, the girl is already his. Nobody else can enter. It was already made, the marriage."

In one such arranged child marriage, Anita's parents gave her to her husband's family when she was about ten to be raised in their home. She was scared, Anita remembers, and went back and forth between her husband's and her natal home. Soon after her first menstruation, she had to consummate her marriage to a husband ten years her senior. No one had explained anything to Anita about what happened during sexual intercourse, and the experience was painful and frightening.

Arranged or credit marriages are not made only for children. At eighteen, Joana was forced to marry a man who had outbid the man she loved by buying her parents more gifts than her lover was able to. She could not refuse the marriage because her parents "ate" the payments made by her suitor and had nothing to return when she refused his proposal. Her parents' actions bound her to fulfill their obligations to her husband's family under customary law. At twenty-two, she remembers:

> I was seventeen living at home. He was eighteen. He arrived with his *padrinho* to get to know me. I refused to marry. My parents were afraid, with me almost eighteen years. They received his money without saying and ate it. It was arranged between his *padrinho*, my husband, and my parents. I was out. It was a secret. He paid my expenses and their expenses. Twenty thousand [meticais] for masunggiro. I fled to my aunt's house. She said, "You're married to a soldier! He is going to come here shooting!" My parents

sent the son-in-law to threaten me. He came with a pistol. I felt so bad. I loved another [who worked for the security force]. He brought chicken, eggs, and my parents also ate them, but my parents gave me to the other one. They forced me.

A fourth type of marriage is a service marriage, whereby a man without his own or family resources to pay the bride-price can work off payments through labor for his bride's family. Service marriages have become less common in Zimbabwe, where most men are engaged in wage labor. While the service marriage is dying out, new forms of marriage are springing up. Christians are opting to have church weddings, with as many European marriage customs and festivities as they can afford. Marriages may also be registered in government civil services. When the cake is cut and the time comes for signing the civil papers, the traditional song to the bride now goes:

Hoitara ndiwe, tara hoitara
Uone kuenda
Takuda kuenda.

You have to sign alone, sign, sign alone
For you to go tomorrow to respond yourself
We are already going.

The significance of this wedding chant, I was told, is that the modern bride signs herself into marriage alone when she signs the marriage license, a contract only between bride and groom, in contrast to traditional marriages that feature agreements between extended families from two lineages. From then on, she must respond for herself without the support of her kinswomen. The young, unmarried girls get to go home, still free.

By the 1960s and 1970s, the "idealized version of Shona marriage" no longer existed, if it had ever existed in any ideal form (Kaler 2000). Young men's ability to amass wealth by working in waged employment in the colonial economy had already weakened the material bases for the androcratic and gerontocratic norms that justified the control by males and seniors over women's and juniors' lives (Thompson 2000). The possibility for young men to be financially independent from their male elders, together with other forces—including the increase in de facto female-headed households, and the youth orientation of the liberation struggle and the participation in it by young men and women—contributed to the extended family's gradually weaker control of reproduction and a severing of the "bonds of obligation between the generations and the genders" (Kaler 2000: 698).

The High Cost of Lobolo: Women Pay the Price

With the shift of bridewealth payments from tools, livestock, or labor—re-distributed and valuable in different ways to many parties over a long period of time—to money, payments represent a father or son's personal property more than a lineage investment in future reproduction. Where formerly a lineage son would receive the bridewealth for his marriage from that received by his father from a sister's marriage, young men increasingly act as independent agents in their own marriage negotiations, thus eliminating the collective balancing element of exchanges of wealth between lineages (Thompson 2000; Bourdillon 1991: 46; Meekers 1993).

At the same time, the often extremely high lobolo payments demanded in Gondola proved an effective means for a father to reject an unsuitable suitor. Such a fate is lamented in a 1994 hit song from Zimbabwe by the popular singer Johnny Chibadura. In "Ndiri Kuchakao o Kama," the protagonist asks his true love's father for permission to marry her and is told he must bring five thousand dollars and thirty head of cattle (*zura zvi chanu zi madora na ngombe makumi matatu*, Sh.). The young man asks the father, "Why not just forbid the marriage outright?" In Mucessua, I was told that the number of marriages in which bridewealth is paid was declining because young men and their families were less frequently able to amass enough money.

On the other side of the coin, the high prices asked for lobolo were also an incentive for families to accept a suitor's offer or even to force a daughter's marriage (Modola 2007).[1] This dynamic has given rise to a range of "sexually violent relationships—from families accepting bribes to withdraw charges for sexual assault, to young girls (and their families) accepting money and gifts for relations with older men" (Mupotsa 2008). In her article documenting the costs of the commoditization of reproduction on women's lives in Zimbabwe, Danai Mupotsa (2008) uses the term "sexually violent relationships" inclusively to shine a critical light on a range of negotiations regarding sex and reproduction and the power hierarchies that condition them, explaining: "What I hope becomes clear is the expanse of this spectrum: I am speaking here of a variety of experiences and the negotiations of agency that are involved in them. I call it sexual violence to underline the question of power related to them."

Under FRELIMO, the economic basis of lobolo was clearly articulated and the negative social implications for both men and women widely condemned. In contrast, the incoming government in independent Zimbabwe made no move to officially eliminate bridewealth, an omission Tanya Lyons claims showed, "the unwillingness of the nationalist movement to radically change the social and economic position of women" (2003: 199). FRELIMO sought to end the practice through governmental policy, political education campaigns, community mobilization by OMM (Organization of Mozambican Women), and even by threatening to withhold government positions from polygamists and individuals who engaged in bridewealth payments (Urdang 1983: 27). The OMM second conference report from 1976 explains FRELIMO's analysis of polygamy: "In our patriarchal society, the man is the owner of all material goods produced within the family. Polygamy is a system whereby the man possesses a number of wives. As head and proprietor of the family, he acquires more wives to augment the labour force at his service" (ibid.).

Nonetheless, the idea and importance of lobolo lives on in Mucessua.

"So, what is different about the current bridewealth system today as compared to the times of your parents and grandparents?" I asked each woman I followed through pregnancy. From naive to caustic, women tended to agree that the system itself was the same, only worse because the prices were inflated:

I think [lobolo] is good when you give birth and there is not a problem in your hearth. (Anita, age 30-plus)

My father was a [migrant laborer, *viagante*]. But he kept coming back to my mother. [They] had eight children. We [eight children] paid [our mother's] lobolo in the name of my father to stay free, to not be ordered by my grandfather who bore my mother. (Adelia, age 35-plus)

It is the purchase of your children. (Ana, age 27; Domingas, age 24; Quina, age 15; Carlotta, age 29; Ana, age 22)

It is to guarantee the children for the husband. (Christina, age 30)

When he pays lobolo, the children are going to pertain to him. (Ana, age 22)

Lobolo refers to the purchase of both wife and children. (Victoria, age 29)

It is to serve your husband. (Amelia, age 24)

This payment is for the security of your marriage. (Rosinha, age 39)

It is payment of your children and just the same your son must take out lobolo. This has signified that it is your wife. (Matilde, age 42)

It is for the security of your hearth and your children. (Helena, age 28)

Payment for children and security for your marriage. (Cecelia, age 30)

I don't know. (Anastacia, age 22)

It is normal since it is a tradition. The second payment [lobolo paid after masunggiro] is normal. Others think they are purchased and they are not going to have any voice because they were bought. There needs to be understanding between husband and wife for it to work. (Trezinha, age 32)

Lobolo is to pay to not be ordered at home. To pay for these children to be taken by their father. In the case you divorce, you [the woman] don't take even one child. You are a toolbox [*caixa de ferramentas*]. A woman *lobolado* [with bride-price paid] doesn't have a right to nothing, but to fulfill all that her husband wants. When the ceremonies are done, the first and second payments [masunggiro and lobolo] paid, the parents hand you over eternally, not to separate until death. (Sandra, age 19)

Lobolo means that the woman cannot speak. Only when the man no longer needs her. (Marida, age 27)

Every woman in Mucessua whom I asked to describe the institution of lobolo argued that although they felt personally burdened by it, they would insist on receiving lobolo for their daughters. Lobolo was one of the few socially sanctioned ways women envisioned themselves getting money they would control. As one woman in a focus group mused: "We pray for one boy to take the father's name, and then a whole train of girls following behind for lobolo." As senior women with the capacity to control, and thus benefit from, the reproductive labor of daughters or daughters-in-law, they remained invested in the perpetuation of these practices, which represent a viable (albeit limited) route to socially sanctioned female material accumulation. Women defended their insistence on lobolo for their daughters in spite of their awareness that the practice heightened reproductive pressures on women and, in many cases, their own suffering.

As Acholonu has pointed out, it should be no surprise that "in many cases women are part and parcel, if not the power behind, the scattered instances of male domination" (Acholonu 1995: 28). The question to ask, however, is, What stake do women have in "practices once attributed to 'false consciousness'"? (Kandiyoti 1998). Reading Mozambican women's stake in bride-wealth as class interest in controlling labor power helps make sense of this instance, if our understanding is that class intersects with gendered positions in family and labor hierarchies. Richard Mabala's term "genderation" helps to locate and capture this power nexus, where women and youth—and young women in particular—can get trapped (2006).

Rosinha, a thirty-nine-year-old woman who spoke up confidently in a focus group discussion among women of childbearing age, struck a chord among the others: "It depends on the husband. No sooner than lobolo is paid, then no more words, only blows." The other women in the group all laughed, but uneasily. Domestic violence against women was certainly an issue in many of the households in the case study and for many other Mozambican women I knew. However, the problem was complicated by an attitude frequently expressed by women that a man will beat a woman only if he still cares enough about her to bother to do so. Thus, some women transposed violence into a sign of continued passion and, ironically, security for the woman in the relationship.

There was also general consensus that when lobolo payments have been made, it ensures that children will belong to their father's lineage in the case of a separation or divorce. Carmen, age thirty-six, expressed this view of women as borrowed reproducers for their husband's lineage matter-of-factly: "If you rent a car and put your baggage in it, does the baggage belong to the car? No. It belongs to the person who paid to rent the car. We women are cars. The baggage belongs to the dono [master, boss, Mr.]."

Of course, lobolo was not the only reason women wanted children. Women wanted children in their own right for joy, for pride, for companionship, or for help in the future. Many women wanted numerous children because they suffered so much from their children dying. A group of churchwomen in one focus group described their experience of vulnerability and the inevitability of infant mortality in terms of religious doctrine. Losing at least one child was every woman's destiny, they believed; God takes a child from each woman as a test of her faith. As one of them explained: "Diseases of God are an imposto [tax] from God. When you don't lose one, you are just waiting to lose one. No one gives birth to kill. That is why we need a comboio [train] of children."

Men's attitudes and gendered reproductive aspirations and obligations also play a part in shaping the pressure on women to reproduce, and in women's feelings of vulnerability. An all-male group of elders from around Gondola expressed a range of perspectives on bridewealth in relation to childbearing patterns and rights in children. Underlying each man's attempt to downplay the importance of lobolo, or his insistence that it is acceptable if a woman does not produce children after lobolo is paid, lies an element of entitlement that a man has a right to many children and that paying lobolo transfers rights in offspring to him.

We Africans like to have many children. Whites say, "Enough already!" Children are never enough for anyone. God could take all ten. Mwana ana kuanda no kuanda kwao [He who has children needs nothing to be great,

Tewe; *não tem nada dele estar muito*, Port.]. Ten . . . twenty . . . thirty children is nothing. (elder Senhor Matore, age fifty-plus)

I paid lobolo. If God gives me children, even if I separate from my wife, I don't stay thinking about this money I paid for her, because the children are mine because I paid lobolo. (Nyusai Raul Muchikwame, age sixty-plus)

Lobolo does not refer to the child. After I had the luck to have children, I forgot the money to think about my children. [Lobolo] just means that the children are not ordered by the wife's lineage. (Louis Nzugu Jakachira, age fifty-plus)

When I didn't have a child, there is always my wife. I didn't marry to have children. If I don't have children, it is God who wants it. It is for this [infertility] that they insist on a second wife. (John Chipanela, age fifty-plus)

A key aspect of the strong double standard for male and female infertility is that male infertility is not often acknowledged or divulged in public. Given this context, John Chipanela's comments stand out from those made by the other men for his acceptance of his marriage to his first wife, which did not result in children. He was the only man in the group who described the meaning of his marriage as being primarily about the company of his wife, and although he and his wife had no children, he did not take a second wife. A man's social and economic security is to some extent guaranteed by having offspring, whose productive and reproductive labor is ideally under the control of their father or their father's parents through the payment of bride-wealth. As Kaler found among Shona-identified men in Zimbabwe, there was a range of more and less economically based responses to the meaning of bridewealth and the value of children, including what Kaler called "a sort of cultural essentialism" (Kaler 2000: 688).

Having many children was also seen as part of being "African" in contradistinction to "white," a race sometimes represented, as in Senhor Matore's comment, as seeking to limit African fertility and family size. The institutions of polygamy and socially sanctioned concubinage protect men from the threat of infertility and reproductive loss in ways that do not protect women. In this environment, women reported feeling pressure to decrease postpartum sexual abstinence from the traditional period of up to two years to as little as three months. The goal is both to keep men from seeking new sexual partners and to quickly give birth to children who survive in order to repay the lobolo, which cannot be returned if the marriage proves unsatisfactory because it has been eaten.

This related common thread ran through women's accounts of their experiences of bridewealth: the enormous daily pressure to conceive that they felt because of lobolo. The multiple issues involved in this dynamic were laid out for me in each of the group discussions I had with women and in many individual life stories. Women believed it was their duty to bear children for their husband and his family, who had paid lobolo to her family. Through bearing children, especially male children, a woman earned the right to eat under her husband's roof, to defecate within his compound. This dynamic is apparent in the story Javelina told of her first marriage:

> I had my first lover when I was eighteen. I went to the town of Dondo to live with him in his family. They were Sena. Three years passed without conceiving. I saw things were getting worse. [Some members of his family began to taunt,] "Give food to someone who does not bear [children]? Hah!" Others beat me. Every lunch, every dinner. You could never forget it. I grew really thin. I finally begged to leave Dondo. This Senhor [the husband] arrived at my parents' home and handed [me] over: "Take your daughter." He had paid masunggiro of 1,500 meticais and lobolo of 4,500 meticais. My father gave back the lobolo because his daughter did not produce. "Arranjou-me sokwata [used car, a lemon, Ndau] que não nasce!" [You arranged for me something used that looks good, but doesn't birth (work)]. This same thing is happening now to my niece, Lidia. She has sought treatment for infertility in the hospital and traditional medicine.

If lobolo has been paid and a woman does not bear children, she can be divorced but remain responsible for paying back the lobolo exchanged for her. This requirement can keep women trapped in miserable relationships in which they are treated poorly, unable to leave because of their lobolo debt. Stephanie Urdang (1983: 22) found in her research on women's status after Independence that the desire to pay off lobolo in cases of unhappy marriages drove some women to seek waged labor. In Mucessua, where female employment opportunities were rare, women shouldered the lobolo debt by giving birth to "enough" children. How many children were enough? The answer over and over was, as many as you can have, or until you can no longer give birth. When men and women in Mucessua described wanting as many children as possible, they were not referring to an arbitrary ideal number, but to their experience that there can never be too many children born who survive (Bledsoe 1998). Bridewealth payments anticipate the commitment on the part of the married woman to bear and raise as many lineage members as she can, and represent a debt on the part of the bride-giving family until children are raised.

Not only has the going rate of lobolo payments been inflated in the current austerity program economy, but also it is paid in large sums of cash quickly spent or *comedo* (eaten) by in-laws. Remember Joana, who at seventeen was forced to marry a man who outbid the man she loved by paying cash and buying her parents more gifts from the shops than her lover was able to buy. Speaking angrily about the forced marriage from the perspective of age twenty-two, she explained what had sealed her fate:

> It happens often. Parents eat the lobolo without consent from their daughter. These marriages often go wrong because they are love that has been forced. Obligatory love! Later when you suffer, it must be in the name of the parents. "See what you forced on me?" Many women abandon these marriages—flee. In such a case, if the lobolo has been paid, the parents must reimburse the husband. If they do not have the amount, the man may persevere and follow the woman until she ends up in jail. If she is with another man, he must repay [the lobolo]. Since FRELIMO entered, the situation is not better. It's worse. The charge has gone up so much higher than they were.

She could not refuse the marriage because her parents ate the payments made by her suitor and had nothing to return when she refused his proposal. Her parents' actions bound her to fulfill their obligations to her suitor's family, which are protected by customary law in Mucessua's Justice Tribunal.

Sorcery and the Commoditization of Birth Assistance

Like seduction fees and bridewealth payments, where a few trusted women elders were the keepers of authoritative knowledge (Jordan 1997; Davis-Floyd and Sargent 2004) and family secrets in childbirth, midwifery practices are also the target of challenges and changes as they become increasingly monetized. Customarily, in this area of Gondola, a female family member— often the mother, co-wife, or sister-in-law—assisted women in childbirth (Metraud 1993). Mothers-in-law were, and are still, avoided as midwives, ostensibly for incest-related reasons; it is considered a serious impropriety to see one's daughter-in-law naked, because she has had sexual intimacy with one's son. Women said that midwifery in the past was a highly respected health specialist role in the area, and women reputed to be excellent midwives had special skills in delivering babies, assisting with some obstetric complications like breach presentation, and sorting out social complications that could occur during childbirth or as the result of a birth with questionable legitimacy.

The ceremonial power associated with assisting a birth is so strong that women or the rare men who perform births are at risk of losing their eyesight unless they protect themselves with traditional medicines, as noted earlier. As a respected community specialist, the birth assistant is accorded the affectionate kin title of *mbuya mwana* in Tewe, *vovo* in Portuguese—grandmother to the child—and paid respeito (respect) with an offering of cloth, corn flour, wine, and, increasingly, money. Like the relationship between a son-in-law and his wife's family, the social relationship between a midwife and the baby whose delivery she assists is a lifelong connection, symbolized by a series of displays of respeito paid to the midwife at milestones in the child's development, for example, when the child first sits alone, walks, and speaks.

Women reported that seeking assistance from someone outside the family had become more common as families increasingly feared a family member might be to blame for a reproductive loss. This outsider is called less as a birth specialist or assistant than as a birth witness. Childbirth has become an opportunity for material gain through this bond of social and material debt. Some women felt that even family members expected to be paid money these days. For example, when asked where she preferred to give birth, Marida, age twenty-seven, responded: "The maternity is much better. There is no confusion of mbuya mwana, mbuya mwana [midwife this, midwife that]. When you give birth at home, you are not going to endure. You have to give stew, money, capulana. If it is family who assists, you have to give something to family, too."

For these related reasons—fear of ongoing indebtedness and of family members being responsible for reproductive mishaps—over the last decade women have become increasingly afraid of home births. Signaling another shift in birthing practices, in the nova vida many women in Mucessua are opting to give birth in the government maternity clinic to avoid paying a midwife.[2]

The competition for access to women in childbirth as potential opportunities for economic gain constitutes another level of women's reproductive vulnerability. When this work becomes lucrative, compensated with money, the potential for competition and corruption to enter the relationship increases, and the motives for assisting in the birth process become suspect. Any potential midwife might vie for the opportunity to profit from a birth or intentionally create a need for her presence by precipitating a crisis through magical or spiritual means. This possibility haunts a process already fraught with potential danger for mother and infant.

Pregnant women fear aggressive strangers, persistent neighbors, even jealous relatives who could be competing for the role of birth assistant for the cash and gifts involved, and who might resort to witchcraft or sorcery to achieve this end. A person who uses witchcraft or sorcery to provoke a problem during childbirth, such as obstructed labor or retention of the placenta, must be summoned to the bedside of the woman in childbirth to undo the feitiço. Failure to call the interfering individual could result in the serious injury or death of the mother, the infant, or both. An example of this trend came from Jorda, who at age forty-two had been pregnant five times, twice failed to go to term, and had three children, offered the following story:

Long ago we never thought of going to the hospital to give birth. An assistant had the right to a capulana, a belt, a plate, five liters of wine, soap, flour. When it happens within the family, do you think all this is going to happen? A person from outside, to succeed in having all of this will even do witchcraft. Now, it is said if something bad happens when you are alone with your mother, they say it is because you didn't invite someone who could know how to treat it. And so now you have to invite someone else. If you have ten children, you have ten assistants.

Now many people are going to the Maternity, because if you do not call the person in the zone who wants to serve as your midwife, and you don't call, you are not going to give birth until people call the prophet or curandeiro to say the name of this *velha* [old woman]. As soon as she arrives, you give [birth]. For this reason many people are going to the hospital. What angers the person is if you call someone else, or even more when you go to the hospital. Everyone loses. After you give birth, you have to gather up everything you have in your home, money, food, capulana, and give it.

When I was pregnant, a prophet told me that a woman short and dark skinned wanted to assist me. I went to that prophet to find out why I was always sick and in pain. The prophet said that someone was waiting to assist my birth, and if I didn't call her on the day, I was also going to really suffer. And so I went when it was dark to the hospital to give birth to avoid this person. That woman was scared and surprised when she saw me already with my baby born.

Javelina's sister-in-law, Marida, was not so lucky. Marida, age twenty-seven, had been pregnant six times and carried four pregnancies to term; she had four children. From the beginning of her pregnancy, she suspected that her elderly neighbor was closely watching her pregnancy progress, waiting to take part in the birth. On the day she went into labor, Marida had been doing her work in her courtyard but had finally gone inside to avoid her neighbor's inquisitive stares.

I felt this neighbor [was saying], "You are suffering with [labor] pains. Now you have to say [my name]." When I was seated inside my house the day itself, the old woman stayed seated to wait in her house to come assist. I stayed inside and then called to my husband to wash my shoes for going to the Maternity, but I felt the baby already coming out. I delivered alone. When my husband entered, he saw the baby already out lying near the corner. But the *jasuri* [afterbirth, Tewe] was still inside. I told [my husband] to bring my sister-in-law.

First Javelina arrived and saw the baby out already and did massage for fifteen minutes for the rest to come out. After a while, she saw that it still did not come. It is tradition here that when someone wants to assist and you do not call her, [the birth] is always delayed. To treat the handiwork of sorcery that a woman has done to you, you must call her.

In the end we called this old woman to help deliver the placenta. She said she saw I hadn't come out of my house so she knew it was my time. When she arrived, she prayed. She did massage and blessed water with a little salt in it. This was Javelina's idea, who had suffered the same problem. I drank the water that the old woman blessed. She began to do massage and soon pains started. She stayed at it until [the placenta] came out. She had the idea to cut the cord with a millet cane. Javelina refused and said this creates problems of tetanus and went to bring a new razor blade from her home. Javelina cut it. The neighbor showed her how. Now I have to organize a capulana, soap because she touched the child, money, and flour. It is for this that people do this [sorcery], for these goods.

Pregnant women's fear of others using witchcraft or sorcery to cause problems in childbirth so they can serve as midwife is so pervasive in the community that any friction between a pregnant woman and her neighbors is interpreted as a potential reproductive threat, and measures are taken to avoid harm. When Juliana argued with her neighbor, she suspected at once that the woman was trying to find a way to assist her birth. Juliana is twenty-five, has been pregnant three times, and has three children.

When I was six months pregnant, I got treatment at the prophet [Zion Apostle]. You see, there are those who want to assist [the birth]. I was arguing with my neighbor, and we exchanged words that were not pretty. She was really mad, so later her husband came to beat my husband. Even after that she was full of rancor, [saying to me], "I want to see you on the day of your birth." That is what I heard from the prophet. [My husband and I] went to learn if I had something in my body put there by sorcery. It appeared in the [prophet's] vision that I had argued.

Ironically, prophets who diagnose this problem in their patients are often asked to assist in births jeopardized by intervention of witchcraft or sorcery. A debt of respect that a woman might wish to avoid in the first place is thus created between the woman and her prophet. Payments to prophets, however, are almost always described as gifts and never as payments. This free reproductive health care explains in part the growing popularity of churches among poor women with little access to monetary resources. The following conversation between Javelina and her niece, Lidia, took place at Lidia's house in September 2008 when Javelina and I visited women in Mucessua from the original prenatal care study.

Javelina: At the time we were doing our prenatal care study, many times mothers talked about *mfukwa* spirits. Now, these days does there still exist many who do *mfukwa* very much?

Lidia: This thing about *mfukwa* still exists, but since there are many prophets now, when I see that I have been grabbed [by a bad spirit], I run to get treated.

Javelina: Now, where do people go most to be treated for bad spirits—to prophets, curandeiros, or to the churches.

Lidia: More go to prophets.

Javelina: They go to prophets?

Lidia: Yes, to prophets.

Javelina: That is to say that in other churches, prophets exist?

Lidia: In other churches it's different because Assemblies [Pentecostal] don't have prophets. Xigubu [Zion] has prophets, but they have less than we Apostles.

Javelina: What church are you in?

Lidia: I go to the Apostles.

Javelina: What's the name of the church?

Lidia: Kukiera dos Apostólos that came out of Magodi em Mandigo.

Javelina: Aham, Mugodi Church?

Lidia: Mugodi Church is the one I am in.

Javelina: Does it have prophecy?

Lidia: It has prophecy. We are congregated there by Father Jessi.

Javelina: Aham, it's Father Jessi's church?

Lidia: Yes!

Javelina: OK, so he does prophecy?

Lidia: He does prophecy.

Javelina: Does he treat with taero?

Lidia: He makes taero.

Javelina: OK! Does he use taero for all illnesses?

Lidia: He only uses taero. He doesn't do that where you cut remedies [into the skin].

Javelina: For people with bad spirits in their body does he take them out?

Lidia: He takes them [out].

Javelina: They don't come back anymore once he has taken them out?

Lidia: (laughing) When you get treated, [the spirit] really goes. Or if it comes back, it is the kind I can grab myself.

Javelina: Aha!

Lidia: Even when it is sent by those old women [witches], it goes.

Javelina: Now, these days are there many people [treated by prophets] who don't pray, or do people pray?

Lidia: These days there are only believers.

Javelina: Are there many?

Lidia: Those that really don't pray are few.

Javelina: Even people drinking, sinning, are praying? Many people go to church?

Lidia: There are many believers.

Javelina: You're saying that there are few curandeiros in the Vila, in the bairro?

Lidia: Here in the bairro, none. Only there on the far margins, but real curandeiros, none.

Javelina: Don't exist? Only prophets?

Lidia: Only prophets.

Javelina: Do they help other people that come from other churches?

Lidia: If you leave the other church and join this one.

Javelina: But they help for nothing or do you have to pay?

Lidia: It depends on the church where you came from, if there is no interference. Because the churches that came out of this one, no problem, you're not charged money. But when you come from another church, like Assembly, Zion Church, then they charge money.

Javelina: They charge ... But does your church allow going to the hospital?

Lidia: Ah, they go.

Javelina: You go? They don't prohibit it?

Lidia: You go, yes, to the hospital.

Javelina: Now, when you get sick, what is the first thing you do? Before you go to the hospital, but you see the person is gravely [sick]. What would your idea be?

Lidia: When it is only illness or for other things, right away you go to the hospital to be treated. They allow it.

Javelina: You're allowed?

Lidia: You're allowed.

Javelina: Even if the person is pregnant?

Lidia: Even if the person is pregnant, they don't prohibit it.

Javelina: That doesn't exist where a pregnant person can't go stay at the hospital, they must be treated here [in church]?

Lidia: Not at all.

Javelina: Why do they let a person go the hospital?

Lidia: Because here they succeed taking out other things [spirits]. Now, for a birth you might not get it right. Someone could need an operation. To give birth, here there is no one capable of doing it, and that's when you start thinking about going to the hospital.

When you take out the spirit, there at the hospital you are received. And there is where they know whether you need water, if you need more blood.

Javelina: In past years when we had our conversations, there were things mothers talked about, that often people did not go to give birth there [at the hospital] because there were children there [young nurses] and for this reason mothers refused to go and be seen nude by these children. Does this still happen?

Lidia: Not at all. These days this doesn't exist because they help you, because these children [young nurses who are not yet mothers themselves] are trained for a year, so women going there are well assisted during birth. By then they don't feel shame because they are already feeling [labor] pains!

Javelina: Aha! That doesn't exist anymore.

Lidia: Not anymore. You give birth well assisted during the delivery.

Javelina: OK, you say that things have changed. Mothers no longer say they are being assisted by children?

Lidia: No, it doesn't exist. It is all modern. In that time, it was like that because women were oppressed. Now we have opened our eyes. There is no oppression. We give birth in hospitals, the mothers are giving birth [at the hospital].

Javelina: Why in that time did people say if you wanted to give birth there [at the hospital], you had to bring money? Is that still happening?

Lidia: No, this thing about money.

Javelina: People say that you must have a little something tied in the knot of your capulana.

Lidia: This thing about something in the knot of you capulana is something other women do. It's up to each one who goes to the hospital to pay their respect, but myself, of all the children I bore, I did not pay.

Javelina: Uhuh.

Lidia: I already stopped giving birth, and I didn't even pay 50 contos [small coin].

Javelina: How many children did you give birth to in the hospital?

Lidia: (counting) I gave birth in the hospital to two girls, and a boy . . . five, six . . . eight, nine children.

Javelina: Not one you gave birth to at home?

Lidia: Ah! All were born in the hospital.

Javelina: You didn't even give birth to one child at home?

Lidia: I, not one of my children was born at home. I gave birth at the hospital only.

Javelina: When a person gives birth at home, what do they do there at home for respect?

Lidia: After you give birth at home and are assisted by a person, it is necessary to take flour, a bar of soap, when you have it, a chicken, and a capulana to go give to the midwife of the child.

Javelina: Uhum, OK.

Lidia: Go give this to the midwife of the child.

Javelina: Go to her house to give it to her?

Lidia: To her house.

Javelina: On the day she is going to assist you, you go to her house, aren't you going to give her something?

Lidia: On the day she is going to assist you, it is necessary to buy a bar of soap to wash the dirtiness. You have to buy a bar of soap to wash with.

Javelina: Aham!

Lidia: When you are done with this, then you can go out of the house after completing a few months, you go pound corn and go with the child to the midwife's home. Now, these days, this doesn't exist anymore.

Javelina: Now when you go to the house of the child's midwife, what would the midwife do?

Lidia: When you give this to the midwife she says, "Thank you, my granddaughter," and receives that flour. These days this thing about child's midwives doesn't exist. Only in the hospital.

Javelina: But in the past, if you didn't do this, what would happen?

Lidia: Nothing happened, but the granny who assisted the birth would murmur, "I assisted the birth and even touched your filth, your blood. I didn't even get respect, flour, soap." She goes on murmuring and then the child becomes unwell.

Javelina: The child gets sick?

Lidia: It gets sick, that child.

Javelina: Uhum!

Lidia: Now, these days this doesn't exist. When you feel real labor pains, you run to go to the hospital. No one will be murmuring because no one worked [assisting your home birth].

Javelina: Aham! OK, now all that is left to do is go to the hospital?

Lidia: The hospital is better. [*laughing*] It's better to go to the hospital.

Javelina: But in the past when people gave birth at home, was it good or was there some law you had to give birth at home?

Lidia: A long time ago there was a law that you couldn't go to the hospital. They said that when you went to the hospital to give birth to a child, they would kill it. You had to give birth here [at home] when you were a daughter-in-law. You had to give birth here at home for you first child.

Javelina: Why did they do that? Why did the first child have to be born at home? For what, actually?

Lidia: Some say that when you give birth either at home or at the hospital for your first child and then the child weans itself, that means you prostituted yourself or something. Now they want to hear themselves in the moment you give birth, so you have to be at home. It was very hard to give birth outside of the home.

Javelina: Nowadays do they still try to discover who prostituted?

Lidia: Some confess, and from there, they take *mfuta* [a seed from a castor-oil bush] and give it to you to swallow to see if you can deliver because you mixed *mutupo* [sperm, totems, expression of taboo].

Javelina: So when you take this *mfuta*?
Lidia: When you take *mfuta*, you birth fine.
Javelina: Aham! So it is a remedy to find out who prostituted?
Lidia: You mixed [sperm], and so for this people don't give birth at home
    because whether they prostituted or not, they go to the hospital.
Javelina: To the hospital?
Lidia: To the hospital.
Javelina: When you get there, you don't have to confess?
Lidia: You don't have to confess. This doesn't exist anymore.
Javelina: Aham! That's right.
Lidia: Uhum.

Home birth is also disparaged by younger Mucessuans who, striving to succeed on the new terms of the money-driven, urban economy, increasingly desire to distance themselves from practices associated with their rural roots. For example, more than thirty years ago, Lucia learned from her mother how to deliver her own children. Lucia has had twelve pregnancies in her fifty-odd years and recounted how she had given birth each time alone. She has nine living children after losing three infants to fever. Her six grown daughters, however, want nothing to do with their mother's birthing traditions. The knowledge that Lucia is not passing on to her daughters is the accumulated experience of generations that resided in her own mother's practice as a midwife and curandeira.

Lucia: From the first until the last, I always gave birth alone. I only went [to the clinic] for the weighing of the child afterwards. I never had a single [prenatal] consultation since my first pregnancy. My deceased mother knew medicine that she gave to all her daughters to succeed in having a normal birth when we were in another country or where there was no family, so you could give birth alone. There are two types of medicine my mother gave me. One treatment makes the child grow well—*akura bom* (*kura*, to grow, Sh.; *bom*, well, Port.). When you are two months [pregnant], you already begin to drink this root that is put in cold water and drink once a month. I don't know the name of it, but it is hard to come across. The second medicine is *nsukumo* [Sena] or *ntsuo* [Tewe]. This medicine is for the child to come out so fast, without delay, that it causes pain. Even when the child is *mfutete* [Tewe; *contrario*, feet-first presentation, Port.] or *pelvica* [breech presentation] they come out just the same.
Rachel: Have you given this medicine to your own daughters?
Lucia: No, because it is not easy. You see, you cannot mix this medicine with pills from the hospital. When you mix them, you destroy the child in your belly. No, [my daughters] are already following the nova vida.

As Crandon-Malamud has proposed, "Local constructions of health and illness are fluid, borrowing from different systems of thought. The apparently conflicting 'bodies of knowledge' represented in the different medical systems can be drawn upon simultaneously and without contradiction" (1991: 24). Yet, in the antagonism and danger Lucia detects between her own inherited and time-tested reproductive health practices and those of the biomedical hospital, she recognizes that the nova vida and its shifting economic and social opportunities harbor significant hazards for those least able to fully take up those opportunities.

Like Taussig's (1980) Bolivian tin miners and Colombian sugarcane cutters who could see the contradictions of capitalism from their vantage point on the periphery of the world capitalist economy, women in Mucessua sense that the nova vida is, among other things, an expanding range of options that are most precarious, even hostile, to those caught on the margins of economic and social participation. They are *bricoleurs*, patching together an improvised mix of what services and certainties they can lay hands on, frequently unable to follow any course of action fully. It is clear to people in Mucessua that to make good in this particular market, one must buy or sell something that should not be bought or sold, use strong magic, or make deals with a demon. However, not all mixes are good for you, and the systems you are trying to access are in some fundamental ways competing with each other.

In 2009, sitting with tea in Javelina's house, Marida described her experience of this competition to me another way: "Rachel, you can't have one foot in each camp. If you are going to use roots, use roots. But these roots are what call bad spirits to you. Because the way one knows which roots to use is by being guided by spirits. One person could take roots and not be cured because they do not know how to use them. Someone else knows through spirits which roots to use and how to use them. If you go to a curandeiro with a problem, they are always going to find something. You have to give them this, this, and this, and then do what they tell you. If you don't comply with this, you get worse, and they are going to say, 'See, you didn't do as I told you!'

"If you want to get out of all that [endless diagnoses, accusations, payments], you stay in the church and use only prayer. With my daughter, the day she told me her [labor] pains were already increasing, I prayed with her. Then we went along to the maternity [clinic], and even there we prayed. 'God, we hand over our daughter to these nurses to be in their care. May her fate be your decision. In your name we pray that everything should happen as is pleasing in your sight.' And then, thanks be to God, when we arrived during visitation, we found her well and her baby with no problems. When you use roots, stay with roots. When you pray, stay with the church.

"Let me give you an example. If you work, you cannot have two bosses. If you are a guard and you have to be at work at seven, you can't also be at another place at seven at the same time. You can't have two masters."

"I see," I said. "But sometimes women know their problems are caused by *mau espirito*. What do they do then?"

"It is not that nurses treat you any better now. They are still young, still yell at you, still leave you alone to labor, no food, blankets, or hot water. But if you have problems of *mau espirito*, it is not the fault of the nurses. It is you who must resolve the problem yourself."

The small group had grown slowly throughout the late afternoon to six women and a smooth, sleepy, sweet-smelling two-day-old baby. During our discussion the young mother frequently nursed, cuddled, and burped her baby, passing him around the group for others to rock, tickle, and kiss. Everyone nodded when Rosinha spontaneously started preaching:

> Since the time of the war until now, I see that prayer is what is securing our lives, because when we sit and we want to measure who prays and who does not pray, those that pray are many. Because to follow worldly things, because when you go provoking worldly [traditional, spirit-related, curandeiro], he is going to lie to you. This could separate you from your family. For this [reason], people are praying. For this, the churches are already many. Also, you feel freer since that time until now. People are now praying. Even in my house, even as suffering arrives, but not to the point where we can turn away. I only stay firm in a single thing, which is God, who is the single Creator. He says, "It is I who take away, and I who gives."

Recent shifts in childbirth practices do not signal trust in the biomedical sector to handle the event of birth. Women's birth narratives were full of complaints about the Gondola District maternity clinic, in particular the inexperience and inattention of the younger nurses, and the lack of material necessities such as blankets, hot water, mattresses, and food. Rumors circulating about the dangers to pregnant women of being transferred from rural maternity centers to the provincial hospital exposed laypeople's perceptions that a parallel process of monetization and corruption was occurring at all levels of the formal health sector. Such rumors abounded in Mucessua and in the capital city, as well. One widely circulating rumor was that the provincial hospital had a "foreign contract" and was receiving money for each corpse they could produce. Thus, health workers were feared to be intentionally letting people die, or actually helping them along. I was told that in 1993, a strike of maternity nurses had led to the deaths of many women in the maternity ward but could find no other evidence of such a strike.

Great distrust was also expressed in relation to the increasing medicalization of birth made possible by the technology available at the provincial hospital. This anxiety was articulated, for example, in the fearful rumor circulating about the maternity ward operating room at the provincial hospital, where cesarean sections were performed for emergency high-risk births—

from the dreaded operating room, the saying went, no one leaves (*Da sala d'operação ninguem sai*). For women sent to the operating room, death was imminent; if not there on the operating table, within two weeks the woman would bleed to death. Most laypeople I spoke with in Manica Province asserted that the hospitals are generally where people go to die.

Even to an outside observer, the provincial maternity ward seemed to live up to its bad reputation. I knew or knew someone related to seven women who died in the hospital of childbirth-related causes in the spring of 1995. Eleven maternal mortalities were recorded in one month that spring under circumstances that catalyzed a national Ministry of Health inspection of the provincial maternity ward conditions, and resulted in the removal of one foreign doctor from the staff. Despite real problems of poor facilities and insufficient staff and resources, the situation at the provincial hospital was shaped by its role as the only facility in the province with tertiary-level services. It was the final stop for the most serious cases transferred from the districts.

Senhor João Manuel, the Gondola District health director during my first year in Manica Province, was trained as a second-level nurse and agent of community medicine. As the district health director, he was often called to the Gondola maternity clinic to attend women who had obstetric complications. He was the only person in the District Health Department with the official power to authorize an ambulance transferal to the provincial capital, half an hour away. In his experience, the biggest problem in maternity care in Gondola District was the referral service. Most of the emergency obstetric cases seen at the district level arose during attempted home births and arrived at the district health center or maternity ward when they were already extremely grave. Even with referral authorization to transfer a patient to the provincial capital hospital, there was no telephone at the maternity clinic, and the health center phone rarely functioned. Assuming that the need for transport could be communicated to the proper facility, the ambulance, which served the health transport needs of an entire district of 50,000, was rarely available.

The causes of maternal deaths were not officially recorded at the district level. However, according to Manuel, the most frequently seen obstetric complications were obstructed labor due to cephalo-pelvic disproportion and abnormal presentation of the baby, and ruptured uterus due to the use of indigenous labor-inducing medicines or the custom of sitting on pregnant women in cases of prolonged labor. Atonia of the uterus and fetal distress were also common, as women were frequently instructed by home-birth assistants to push before complete dilation. Maternal hemorrhaging due to incomplete delivery of the afterbirth was also a frequent occurrence. By the time such cases reached the provincial hospital from the rural areas of the districts, they were often past the point where intervention would help, and the hospitals, especially the provincial surgical rooms, were indeed places where many women died.

Even in the face of what many believed to be a risk of imminent death for pregnant women transferred to the provincial hospital, many perceived the social risks of feitiço and economic debts incurred through home-birth assistance as the higher cost. These perceptions of reproductive threats have transformed local strategies for managing risk during pregnancy and birth. At the beginning of pregnancy, women purposely delayed entering the formal biomedical system for prenatal care in an attempt to reduce reproductive vulnerability, which they believe stems from public knowledge of their pregnant condition.

By initiating antenatal consultations late in their pregnancies, women circumvented national norms and relegated formal biomedical services to a partial role in guarding or guaranteeing community continuity through children. Ironically, at childbirth, women may reject home-birth assistance and utilize hospital maternity facilities to avoid witchcraft and sorcery threats. In this way they also escaped senior females' interference with their reproductive aspirations and deflected claims on precious monetary resources in payment for birth assistance. These patterns of women's use of biomedical services reflect women's strategic decisions to protect their pregnancies from social, spiritual, and economic threats that are rampant in the nova vida; these decisions do *not* indicate a lack of knowledge of the value of these services.

The intense social preparation of girls for their future roles as reproducers, the significant cultural resources mobilized to keep procreation under the control of male and senior female-dominated patrilineal kinship structures, and the limited routes to female social and economic autonomy define the contours of reproductive vulnerability for women in Mucessua. The reproductive practices of masunggiro and lobolo are long-standing institutions that control sexuality and reproductive labor that have been altered by monetization but remain resilient in the current socioeconomic context. Many women, especially those forced into sex work by poverty, are redefining female sexual identities and challenging rules of reproduction regarding the appropriate transacting of reproductive and sexual labor and the control of its profits. Like young men, young women act as individual agents and resist being mediated and managed in the ways that were expected of their mothers and grandmothers. *Cada um para cada um.* Each one for each one.

I was still worried for Lilia, though, even with Eusébio now in the picture to claim her pregnancy and baby as his responsibility, and to legitimize her pregnant state through the payment of respect to her parents. Her problems were far from over. Her candy red shoes glowed like a neon symbol for HIV/AIDS risk and other pressures and predicaments of the nova vida.

CHAPTER 6

Seeking Safe Passage:
Pregnancy Risk and Prenatal Care

"Ah, Dona Raquel. Since we last met, I have suffered so terribly." Two weeks after giving birth, exquisite, cherub-faced Amelia was puffy in the cheeks, dark under the eyes, and thinner than I had ever seen her. Her health had been poor on and off near the end of her pregnancy, but she had given birth to a healthy baby boy, James, named after my husband. She proudly held her two-week-old son, in an intricately detailed blue sweater, pants, booties and hat, and soft baby blanket she had knit on a new knitting machine, just like the one she had made for my daughter. In a setting where male names carry on lineages and families are lifelines, this honor of "naming after" was also a line she had thrown out for help. It was a subtle gesture by someone with a weak social network, and therefore, I learned, with a baby at risk of not surviving, to reel in a bit closer foreigners who might not be in her social network for very long. Amelia had needed the lifeline, but it had been too little, too late.

I had known Amelia before I started the prenatal care study. She was one of the only two women who participated in the research project who had a wage-paying job. At thirty-two, she was a young widow and the mother of two girls, and she was also caring for her two younger sisters. She managed all this at the moment by working as a domestic, cleaning and serving tea and water in the office of a small international health organization operating in Gondola, for which she earned about $120 a month, one and a half times the government's official minimum salary. Now she was also knitting and selling acrylic baby sweater sets. The only difference between Amelia and her Mucessua neighbors who had little formal education, no employment history, and few marketable skills was Amelia's courage and tenacity: when the NGO arrived in the district, she walked to their office every day for weeks asking for a job, until a spot opened up when a woman took maternity leave. She had filled in and quickly won over the entire staff with her dry humor and assiduousness.

I had not recruited Amelia into the prenatal care study—she had enlisted me. She had heard about the project and approached me conspiratorially,

I assumed to participate in the research. When I first interviewed Amelia, soon after she had discovered she was pregnant, she requested to speak to me alone. With a combination of desperation and aloof determination, she asked me if I knew someone at the hospital, one of the foreign doctors maybe, who could arrange an abortion for her. She was not wavering or asking for advice. She needed me to *arranjar* and *colocar*, to arrange things and hook her up to my network. Abortions are illegal in Mozambique except to save a mother's life, as noted earlier; however, some doctors were known to "help" women. I encouraged her to set up a prenatal care appointment at the provincial hospital and heard nothing more from her for over a month.

When Amelia and I met two months later, she was lithe and energetic. I was not sure if she was still pregnant. "I'm still in this study of yours," she grinned when we sat down with tea in the kitchen of the small office where she worked. "You'll still have to bring me some gifts, after all." She had not been able to arrange an abortion and had decided to make the best of things. A new relationship with one of the kindest fellows who worked as a driver at the same organization was going well. She felt supported, adored; she was beaming.

Over the next months I had seen Amelia only briefly now and then as I went about my interviews with other women in Mucessua. She had a way of disappearing and showing up when she wanted to be found, and I knew she was busy with a new relationship, impending pregnancy, and her jobs. Now we were sitting down together to catch up. Amelia had been pregnant six times before this unwanted pregnancy; four of her children had died; she now had three living children, two daughters and baby James.

Since our last interview and the birth of her son, things had been going from bad to worse for her. Amelia settled delicate James, with his full head of curls and serious dark eyes, to nurse before she started in on her postpartum update. She was shaken and preoccupied over a fight with a neighbor.

"It was during my second month of pregnancy. My neighbor said that I would see someone die. 'In your house you will see death, or you will see how it is going to be, your pregnancy! Or not give birth.'"

This was a serious threat, a kind of curse. "Wait! What?" I said. "Start at the beginning!"

"This *confusão* was provoked over a cookstove!" Amelia continued. "A boy stole the stove from [my neighbor] and hid it close to *my* house. When my neighbor woke up to cook, she didn't find the stove and accused my sisters of having lifted it. The girls denied this. She insulted my sisters, saying they had hidden it. They exchanged words until five o'clock.

"When I got home at five thirty, my neighbor arrived and entered my kitchen. She searched there without permission. I asked to know what she wanted, but she just insulted me and left, so I closed the door and later went to the market. The boy returned the stove when he heard the woman was causing *confusão* in my house, but the neighbor said nothing. Oh, I got feeling so bad! She had disgraced me about something I had not done. She sullied me in the bairro. She didn't ask forgiveness, so I cut my trust [with her]. My neighbor walked around talking with my other neighbors, gossiping. I just left it at that.

"After one week, I became sick. I went to the hospital and did analysis [blood test]. It accused malaria." Here, Amelia employs "accuse," the Portuguese for clinical diagnosis (from *accusar*). Indigenous practitioners also use the term to diagnose the ultimate cause of sickness by identifying and "accusing" the witch, sorcerer, or client of either who has sent bad luck, *azar*, or a bad spirit, *espirito mau*, to cause misery.

"I was given a prescription for chloroquin—three pills, three times a day, since I was"— here Amelia made a gesture of a protruding pregnant stomach—"aspirin, oral [rehydration] mixture, and *sal ferosa* [iron supplement]. But the malaria continued. I vomited at all hours. So I went again to the hospital and checked in overnight. I took intravenous quinine, got an injection and some small green pills. I became even worse.

"Then I got another idea [about the cause of the illness]. I had already gone to the hospital, so I went to a prophet. When I arrived there they attended to me. [The prophet] began to pray over me. He did some treatments. When he prayed over me, he never missed mentioning [the neighbor's] name! He asked for milk, a candle, a chicken, three drops of *agua cassimba* in a cup—the first water on the morning grasses. [It cost] twenty contos [+U.S. $2]! He took the chicken and cut it, took the blood and put it in water. First, I took a bath in this water. Then the milk was put in water and boiled. I took a bath in it. He melted the candle in water. I took another bath. The drops of dew he put with blessed water, which I took to drink at home. In the prophet's house I felt my body free after the treatment. As soon as I arrived at home I felt bad all over again—dizzy, fever."

"How long had you been sick by this point?" I asked. I marveled at the creative steps of the triple-layer bath that began by using blood to attract and draw out the malevolent spirit to make its wishes known, milk to purify and nourish Amelia and the unborn, and wax to seal this treatment in and leave a protective shield. The sacred water, prepared with drops of dew, vital to starting fresh, was to continue the purification process at home. Sufferers were frequently asked to gather water from a specific source that mimicked the action the body needed to heal: water that flowed smoothly or churned roughly bringing up silt from the bottom, water that sat stagnant, rose as mist, or collected in the fork of a tree or a hollowed rock. Using various procedures and preparations, these four processes were central, recurring therapeutic practices in Mucessua: drawing out the spirit or individual involved in the sickness for consultation; diagnosis; cleansing/curing/strengthening; and protecting/closing. These modalities often formed the basis for a wide range of improvised and idiosyncratic therapies in both indigenous and church-related healing practices.

"This was the third week. Then I heard from a person who gave me directions to a curandeiro. [The curandeiro] did a consultation. A spirit came out of his body. [The spirit] began to speak of all that had happened—the stove, the promises to kill someone. He said I couldn't go home. First, he gave me medicine to take to treat the diarrhea, fevers, vomiting, body pains. It was powder . . . a flour, to take. He cut [my body] with a razor and put more medicine [on the shallow incisions]. Then he bet with me that he would cure me. He could cure me, but he needed to go treat my house [*kuvara*, to clear (of sky); *mucha*, village, house, Tewe]. The neighbor had put medicine there."

"[At the house] the spirit came out again and asked for a hoe. My husband, my mother, and the curandeiro's assistant went outside, and my husband dug into the ground. They found medicine tied up with black string and coins from Zimbabwe put there to make me suffer. [The curandeiro] took it out and treated the house. He closed the house and pathways. When we finished closing everything he asked for two hundred *contos* (thousand meticais notes) for treatment *and* enough to pay for his bus fare to and from Pungue [where he had come from] on the top of it! Yes, all this was after having been treated in the hospital. Because whenever I came back home, I became worse. I did take the iron supplements until the end of the month of the birth."

Amelia coughed throughout our interview, and little James was fitful at her breast. He died before he reached one year, and Amelia dragged herself to work for months after she could no longer do anything once she got there but sit in the kitchen, cough, and doze. She died a year later, a slow and wasting death in which she became unrecognizable under her sheets; within a year, her new partner, the driver Ernesto, who had worshipped her, also died. Amelia's first husband had died before people spoke about HIV/AIDS very much. When Amelia and Ernesto died, testing was rare and drugs for HIV/AIDS treatment were available only in expensive private clinics. Only in the last five years has antiretroviral treatment become available to anyone but the extremely wealthy, and it is still not universally accessible.

Amelia's story illustrates the way tensions in the bairro between neighbors are played out as reproductive threats. Her prenatal health-seeking trajectory may be unusual in that she earned more income than any of the other women in the study. With her wages, she was taking good care of her children and sisters. She had also begun to relax her hair at a hair salon and use skin-lightening lotions from Zimbabwe that were very popular. There was even enough money to buy the knitting machine, with which she was churning out acrylic baby sweater, bootie, and blanket sets to sell to whomever she could. She had begun to stand out.

Amelia's income and her control over it also allowed her to take her search for safe passage through her pregnancy farther than her cash-poor neighbors could have in such a short time. For peasantariat women without consistent incomes, gathering that kind of money meant convening extended family, often traveling to ancestral lands and relatives in other regions, taking on new home industries and projects, and selling whatever they could part with, sometimes even pride. However, this movement among health options was common among the other women in Mucessua I worked with. Amelia sought biomedical care for the "incidental" occurrence of malaria early in her pregnancy. Then the symptoms grew worse, continued longer than expected, and did not respond to biomedical treatment. Suspecting the use of sorcery by her hostile neighbor, she sought appropriate informal-sector experts to diagnose, cure, and protect her, her unborn child, and her home from *espirito mau*.

The diagnosis of Amelia's illness also changed as her relationship to her neighbors changed. The words of a curse that resulted from conflict over a woman's key resource, a cooking stove, followed by the resistance of Amelia's symptoms to multiple levels of treatments, steered her health-seeking trajectory away from the clinic. She was propelled to seek ever-costlier therapies further and further from the realm of biomedical care as her bodily suffering increased.

The broader context of Amelia's bodily suffering has many levels. Beyond her body and home there is the conflict-filled community, in which dynamics of distrust, jealousy, and theft characterize daily interactions between neighbors. I never saw the stove, and I do not know what happened with its leaving and returning to Amelia's neighbor, and in between these, its hanging out behind Amelia's house. But I do know that the curse and the gossiping that followed the incident made Amelia ill, and that through the use of poisonous language, the neighbor opened the way to being called to Amelia's birth and thus to being paid respect, as mentioned earlier. Amelia was well aware she made more money than those around her, enough to provoke jealousy, so she was convinced that when the opportunity arrived to bring her down a notch by maligning her as a thief, or to find a way to be present at her delivery should something go wrong, the neighbor had made a move.

At the district level, the health system could not diagnose interpersonal discord and had neither the creative nor the technological capacity to go beyond the resistant malaria diagnosis to treat the ongoing and worsening symptoms Amelia experienced. She might have needed an HIV test, as well as access to antiretroviral treatment for herself, nevirapine, an effective drug used to prevent mother-to-child transmission of HIV, and pediatric AIDS treatment for small James—all services available in Manica Province only in the last few years. In terms of causes at the national and international levels, people in Mucessua were crowded and poor as a direct result of war-related violence funded by four countries interested in the destabilization of the region in general and socialist Mozambique in particular: Portugal, Rhodesia, South Africa, and the United States of America. The high cost of food, the absence of medical infrastructure, the fees for schools and medical services—all were related to the economic restructuring that permitted Mozambique to keep up with financing its debt to Western banks. With so many tiers of danger involved, a pregnant woman needed every layer of protection she could get.

"No One Gives Birth to Kill": Maternal Morbidity and Loss in Mucessua

Despite all the risks to pregnant women, there was no doubt that women were delaying or avoiding prenatal care in the clinical setting. Data showed this at the national and provincial levels, and among the women I followed through pregnancy, a majority, 85.5 percent (71), reported that they did not initiate prenatal consultations during the first trimester. Most initiated prenatal care between the fifth and seventh month when pregnancy is hard to hide and many women report fetal movement, but late, for example to prevent fetal damage from syphilis. The mean time for initiation was sixth months' gestation (Table 1).

To understand why women living within 3 kilometers of free services at the maternity clinic delayed prenatal consultations, I needed to discover what motivated women to seek prenatal care at all. What were women's experiences of reproductive loss and vulnerability, and what problems did women experience and perceive as threats to their well-being, to their pregnancy, and to maternal and fetal health during pregnancy?

I use the term "reproductive loss" to refer to miscarriage, perinatal deaths (stillbirth to seven days postpartum), and infant deaths (one week to one year postpartum). I include deaths of infants up to the age of one in this category because women in Mucessua believed that the death of a nursing or weaning-age child had a negative impact on the mother's future fertility, and so was a serious threat to conception, pregnancy, and reproduction (Chapman 1998). The number of previous pregnancies for the women I followed in Mucessua ranged from none to eleven, with an average of four total pregnancies. Almost a quarter of the women in the group were pregnant for the first time. Of the sixty-four women with a previous pregnancy, 67 percent (forty-three) reported at least one pregnancy ending in reproductive loss (see Table 2). Reproductive losses may have been underreported due to the stigma placed on women who have repeated reproductive losses and thus are suspected of being witches or spirit's wives.[1] Taking that consideration into account, women in Mucessua were extremely vulnerable to reproductive

Table 1. Initiation of Prenatal Care in Maternity Clinic, by Trimester, 1995

When Prenatal Care Was Initiated	Number of Women (%)
First trimester	6 (7.2)
Second trimester	43 (51.8)
Third trimester	23 (27.7)
Not initiated	5 (6.0)
No information	6 (7.2)
Total	83 (100)

Table 2. Reported Lifetime Reproductive Losses, 1995

Number of Women N=83 (%)	Reproductive Losses
21 (25.3)*	0
26 (31.3)	1
9 (10.8)	2
3 (3.6)	3
2 (2.4)	4
2 (2.4)	5
1 (1.2)	6

*Of the twenty-one women reporting no reproductive losses, nineteen (22.9 percent) reported that they were pregnant for the first time.

morbidity and loss throughout their reproductive years. They had reason to fear losing their pregnancy or infant during its first year of life.

The reported reproductive losses of the women in the group I followed were primarily infant deaths, as is apparent in Table 3, which also indicates the outcomes of their pregnancies. Because induced abortion is illegal, it was difficult to obtain information regarding its practice; women were reluctant to discuss it. For those who can afford abortion and know how to navigate the system, quasi-legal induced abortion services are available on request in a number of hospitals in the country (Agadjanian 1998; Mugabe 1998; Machungo 1997). Nonetheless, clandestine abortions performed by curettage or with the use of herbal and other nonpatent abortifacients remain common (Agadjanian 1998).[2]

"You remember the pretty secondary school girl who worked at the pharmacy?" Javelina asked me one day as we walked through Mucessua to the house of our next interviewee. As my own pregnancy progressed, I moved more and more slowly along the sandy paths. "Well, I heard she committed suicide. With chloroquine, I heard." Over the years I worked in Gondola, stories circulated about three young teenage girls who had allegedly committed suicide over lovers, usually older or secret. In each case, I did not doubt the shame or desperation that could lead to such an act, but I had also learned of the lay perception that bitter medicines taken in high doses, chloroquine in particular, could induce miscarriage. Perhaps no one would ever know the intentions of these girls. However, in Mucessua, as I have noted, the indigenous healers and all other informal providers I interviewed reported that the most frequent requests they received were to "undo" pregnancies and to cure infertility. Though none of the bairro healers admitted to performing abortions, five women in my group reported having had an induced abortion in the past. Because of the severe criminalization of abortion at the time, I did not press to know, and did not learn, where and how the abortions had occurred. Although no one disclosed that induced abortion was an outcome of any pregnancy I was following, the women very possibly reported induced abortions as miscarriages. Of the eighty-three case study pregnancies, eleven (13.2 percent) resulted in reproductive losses, including miscarriages (Table 3). It was lucky that the number was not higher and that, in the folk epidemiology of the bairro, the losses were not associated with contact with me.

Pregnancy Illness Episodes

As Javelina and I followed the 83 women through their pregnancies, we recorded all episodes of sickness they experienced during pregnancy and charted each action (or inaction) taken in response. I defined sickness as any unwanted change in a woman's state of being and probed by asking, "Since discovering you are pregnant . . ." or "Since our last interview, what problems, pains or sickness have you suffered?" Each incident counted as a pregnancy illness episode—any health problem or perceived threat to health that occurred during pregnancy. The women reported a total of 380 illness episodes during pregnancy (see Table 4). Most reported physiological states and symptoms, but they also spoke of feelings, premonitions, dreams, altercations, and emotions, especially fear. Types of illness episodes ranged from problems of the reproductive system and genitals to headaches and fevers;

Table 3. Pregnancy Outcomes, 1995

Pregnancy Outcome	Past Pregnancies (%)	Case Study Pregnancies (%)
Successful birth	267 (80.4)	71 (85.5)
Induced abortion	5 (1.5)	0
Miscarriage	6 (1.8)	3 (3.6)
Stillbirth	7 (2.1)	4 (4.8)
Perinatal death	8 (2.4)	1 (1.2)
Infant death	39 (11.7)	3 (3.6)
Maternal death	0	0
No information	0	1 (1.2)
Total	**332 (100)**	**83 (100)**

stomach, chest, lung, and heart problems; lack of blood; pains in bones and teeth; and fear of witchcraft or sorcery.

I also talked with every woman about each treatment she had sought during her pregnancy. I recorded ignoring an episode, waiting, or doing nothing—enduring—as a noteworthy response to an illness episode, for such responses tell us something about the ways people suffer and deal with suffering. The women reported 409 treatment-seeking episodes, and I estimated an additional 87 visits to the maternity clinic from maternal antitetanus vaccination records, making a total of 496 health-seeking episodes (see Table 4). Women did not seek treatment for 43 (11.3 percent) of the total reported illness episodes. In these cases women reported enduring illness episodes until they experienced relief from symptoms without intervention or until symptoms changed on their own.

Etiology of Illness Episodes and Reproductive Threats

Understanding what women thought was the cause, or etiology, of each problem, illness, or negative state gave key clues to where they would seek diagnosis and treatment, and what specialists they would deem appropriate. When asked to identify the cause of each reported pregnancy illness

Table 4. Characteristics and Frequency of Pregnancy Illness Episodes, 1995

Characteristics	Frequency (%)
Reproductive system and genitals*	120 (31.6)
Head and/or fever	76 (20.0)
Fear of personalistic threats**	60 (15.8)
Stomach/abdomen	37 (9.7)
Blood-related (Anemia)	32 (8.4)
Bones and extremities	17 (4.5
All-over bodily symptoms	15 (3.9)
Chest and lungs	10 (2.6)
Heart	10 (2.6)
No information	3 (0.8)
Total	**380 (100)**

* Any symptoms of the reproductive system, including genitals
** Fear of witchcraft or spirit threats to reproduction

episode, women's responses fell into two broad domains—naturalistic causes and personalistic causes (see Table 5). Drawing on Foster's classic typology of causality beliefs, I use the term "naturalistic" to refer to illness caused by natural forces or conditions such as germs, heat and cold, contaminated food or water, or an upset in the balance of the basic body elements. I use the term "personalistic" to refer to illness causality assigned to "an active, purposeful intervention of an agent, who may be a human (a witch or sorcerer), non-human (a ghost, an ancestor, an evil spirit) or supernatural (a deity or other very powerful being)" (Foster 1998: 112).

Two prominent naturalistic illness subcategories became evident as the women narrated their pregnancy histories and trajectories. One included illnesses the women considered unrelated or coincidental to pregnancy. They regarded malaria, colds, and some forms of tuberculosis, for example, as naturally occurring "illnesses of the world" or "illnesses of God" (*doenças do mundo, doenças do Deus*), sometimes also called "God-given" or "God-sent" illnesses (*doenças dado por Deus, doenças mandados por Deus*). Such illness episodes were reportedly caused by agents of the "natural" world, such as mosquitoes causing malaria, contaminated food or water resulting in diarrhea, or contact with an infectious person.

Table 5. Pregnancy Illness Episodes by Reported Cause, 1995

Etiology	Number of Episodes (%)
Naturalistic Causes	
Illness world/God	70 (18.4)
Symptom of pregnancy	124 (32.6)
Preparation for childbirth	75 (19.7)
Health improving (vitamin supplements)	12 (3.2)
Personalistic Causes	
Pregnancy protecting (protection from witchcraft or *mal espirito*)	51 (13.4)
Treatment for symptoms of witchcraft or *mal espirito*	38 (10.0)
No information	10
Total	**380 (100)**

The second subcategory included naturalistic illness episodes that women referred to as "symptoms of pregnancy" (*sintomas da gravidez*)—health problems caused by pregnancy itself resulting in discomfort or severe symptoms. The women considered these routine, though often debilitating, physical manifestations of the normal process of pregnancy, for example, toothaches, sore legs, back pain, or varicose veins.

Personalistic illness episodes included many of what women considered the most serious reproductive problems, from difficulty conceiving to hemorrhaging, threatened miscarriage, constant illness, lactating during pregnancy, previous reproductive loss of any kind, and all birth complications. These problems were most frequently diagnosed as the result of witchcraft or sorcery, *uroya* in ChiTewe or *feitiço* in Portuguese, or by intervention of *espirito mau* (bad spirit).

Significantly, of all the reported illness episodes for which pregnant women sought treatment, they reported almost one in four (23.4 percent) as caused by witchcraft, sorcery, or *espirito mau* (see Table 5). Under certain conditions, a diagnosis shifted from naturalistic etiology—God or symptoms of pregnancy—to personalistic harm caused by a human or spirit foe. This occurred when one or more of the following conditions applied: (1) the problem is undetectable or dismissed untreated in one sector, especially biomedical, despite acute sensation of symptoms by the sufferer; (2) following diagnosis, the problem does not respond to indicated treatment within the expected time; (3) symptoms are unusually acute; (4) the condition persists over an unusually long time; or (5) the problem occurs simultaneously with an unusual combination of other symptoms. These were exactly the shifting circumstances that Amelia faced during her pregnancy, as we have seen, and her health-seeking strategy changed accordingly. Table 6 indicates the range of illness episodes women in the case study reported during pregnancy and shows the potential shifting etiological categorization of some episodes depending on context and course of the affliction.

What women told me, and what I saw and learned, suggests that, contrary to the assertion that no parallel prenatal care system exists in Manica Province (Lafort 1994), a lively informal sector of popular healing options offering prenatal and other reproductive care does exist, as I had suspected. Perceptions of the source or cause of reproductive threats influenced women's health seeking during pregnancy in several ways, as they utilized different providers and services in this medically plural setting (see Table 7). Illness episodes considered naturally occurring and coincidental to pregnancy were most frequently self-treated with pharmaceuticals or at the district health center. For symptoms of pregnancy, women sought treatment from many sources but primarily from the one private pharmacy and open-market drug sellers, the district medical center, and churches. Illness episodes diagnosed as caused by a human or spirit agent directing harm at the pregnant woman were almost always treated outside the biomedical sector by church prophets, church pastors, and curandeiros (Table 7).

"They Don't Know the Pains": Barriers to Biomedical Prenatal Care Seeking

Within the universe of illness episodes pregnant women described, and the causes women identified for each episode, four forces emerged as the most influential on women's pregnancy management strategies and prenatal patterns of resort: (1) a woman's reproductive history; (2) a woman's workload; (3) health care provider–client relationships; and (4) fear of personalistic reproductive threats.

Reproductive History

Women's individual histories of reproductive health problems, especially in their most recent past and current pregnancies, influenced women's decisions about whether, when, and where to initiate prenatal care. For a small number of the women, problems in past or current pregnancies were reported as the primary catalyst for initiating clinical prenatal consultations. In current pregnancies, they referred to the problems reported as illnesses "of the world"

Table 6. Complaints during Pregnancy by Etiology

| | Etiology | | |
| | Naturalistic | | Personalistic |
Pregnancy Complaint	Illness of World/ God	Symptoms of Pregnancy	Witchcraft or Evil Spirits
Fever	X		XX
Malaria	X		XX
Headache	X	X	XX
Diarrhea/stomach cramps	X		XX
Genital itching/STD	X		XX
Tuberculosis	X		XX
Colds	X		XX
Heart problem	X		XX
Weight loss	X		XX
Anemia/lack of blood	X		XX
Dizziness		X	XX
Nausea		X	XX
Bloated stomach		X	XX
Pontadas (pain under ribs)		X	XX
Vomiting		X	XX
Lack of appetite		X	XX
Cramps		X	XX
Weakness		X	XX
Body heating up		X	XX
Laziness		X	XX
Sore feet/legs		X	
Backache		X	
Labor pains in back and abdomen		X	
Varicose veins		X	
Aching joints		X	
Nosebleed		X	
Toothache		X	

continued on next page

Table 6. *Continued*

Pregnancy Complaint	Etiology		
	Naturalistic		Personalistic
	Illness of World/God	Symptoms of Pregnancy	Witchcraft or Evil Spirits
Amenorrhea (unexpected cessation of menstruation)			X
Infertility	X		XX
Bleeding			X
Abdominal cramping/ threatened miscarriage			X
Miscarriage			X
Stillbirth			X
Hemorrhage			X
Early lactation			X
Painful, itchy breasts			X
Misunderstanding at home			XX
Malpresentation at birth			X
Bad luck			X
Cold body			X
Constant illness			X
Previous death of many children			X
Bleeding umbilicus			X
Whole body pricked by sun			X
Infant or child death			X
Maternal death			X

X = Common diagnosis
XX = Secondary diagnosis under the following mitigating circumstances: untreated in another sector; unresponsive to treatment; acute symptoms; long duration of condition; unusual combination with other symptoms

Table 7. Treatments and Providers Sought, by Reported Cause of Pregnancy Illness, 1995

Treatment or Treatment Provider	No Information	Naturalistic Causes			Personalistic Causes		Number of Times Sought (%)
		World/ God	Birth Prep.	Pregnancy Symptom	Pregnancy Protecting	Witchcraft	
No treatment	7	1	16	17	0	2	43 (11.0)
Pharmaceutical*	2	33	39	0	8	0	82 (22.0)
Herbal*	0	0	5	49	0	2	56 (15.0)
District health center	0	20	34	0	3	2	59 (15.5)
Church	0	5	23	2	0	30	60 (15.8)
Curandeiro	0	1	2	0	0	12	15 (4.0)
Prophet	1	0	1	3	0	34	39 (10.0)
Prayer*	0	0	0	4	1	7	12 (3.0)
Mission clinic	0	3	3	0	0	0	6 (2.0)
Traveling nurse	0	5	1	0	0	0	6 (2.0)
Maternity Clinic	0	0	2	0	0	0	2 (0.5)
Total	**10**	**68**	**126**	**75**	**12**	**89**	**380 (100)**
(%)	(2.6)	(17.9)	(33)	(20)	(3)	(23)	(100)

* Self-treated

or "of God," both related and coincidental to pregnancy. These illnesses included sexually transmitted infections, malaria, and nonceremonially provoked tuberculosis—tuberculosis diagnosed in the informal sector as caused by contact with ritual "heat" (for example, caused by attending a funeral) that has been left untreated. Women resorted to clinical care when the problem did not respond to self-treatment and was perceived as falling within the purview of biomedicine. Women without problems or histories of reproductive problems more frequently reported being influenced in their decision of when and if to initiate prenatal care in the formal sector by work, time, and resource constraints and fear of spirit or human harm.

Women's Work, Time, and Resource Constraints

Few women named time, distance, or financial barriers as their primary reason for delaying consultations in the formal biomedical sector. However, watching and accompanying women in their daily activities over the years, I saw evidence that time and resource conflicts resulting from the journey to and from the medical center (a one- to five-kilometer walk each way) influenced health seeking for many more women than the eight who brought it up. As we have seen, women in Mucessua are primarily responsible for meeting the basic needs of their households, and their extremely labor-intensive agricultural and domestic tasks do not change or decrease significantly during pregnancy. It was a general expectation that pregnant women, even in labor, should continue working, cooking, or cleaning without complaint right up until the moment they stop to give birth.

Adding to the burden, while a prenatal exam in the Gondola maternity clinic took between five and ten minutes, the wait to be seen ranged from one to three hours (Lafort 1994: 10). When a woman had to wait in several lines for a child to be weighed, examined, or vaccinated, that time increased. It is a twenty-minute to one-hour walk one way to the medical center from the different quarters of Bairro Mucessua. Most women described their visits to the clinic as taking half the day. Health workers with low salaries and poor working conditions sometimes charged fees for officially free services, thus adding economic burden to time conflict. Pregnant women who did not feel that they were suffering from urgent health problems often could not afford to use their time or energy to stand or sit in line for a routine prenatal checkup.

Provider-Client Relationships

Several aspects of their experience with prenatal care at the government-run maternity facility also influenced women's use of clinical prenatal services in the first trimester. In four cases, maternity clinic staff directly undermined national norms for prenatal care that encourage its initiation in the first trimester by turning women away and telling them to come back when they had something to "see" or "measure." Two of these returned in the second trimester and one in the third; one did not return. Jacinta was among them; at twenty-nine, she had been pregnant twice and lost one child: "I saw them also send away the woman in front of me who came in at two months to come back with four months. The second time I went at five months. [The nurses] grabbed my belly very forcefully. Finally they agreed [I was pregnant]. They had told me to leave and come back when one could note the pregnancy [*quando gravidez se nota*]."

Jacinta's experience was not unusual. Many women in the study expressed the common concern that if they went when the pregnancy was too small, they would be sent away or ridiculed. The practice of actively discouraging women from coming into the clinic early in pregnancy might be related to the Gondola prenatal clinic's most common methods for assessing gestational age: measuring uterine height and palpating the uterus externally.

The attitudes and practices of maternity clinic health personnel also influenced women's attending the prenatal clinic in other ways. Five women reported going to antenatal consultations only or primarily to obtain the prenatal evaluation form and antitetanus vaccination (VAT) record card as proof of attendance.[3] These women saw limited if any value in attending the clinic. None of these five went to the clinic in the first trimester. Nonetheless, they worried that if they did not have the prenatal form or vaccination card, it would be assumed that they had not attended the antenatal clinic, and they might be turned away when they presented to give birth.

Many other women expressed the same concern, that the maternity nurses would interpret their not having a prenatal form and VAT card as their failing to attend the clinic and either treat them less well or deny them admission at the time of childbirth. While a majority of women planned to give birth at home, they all would depend on the clinic if an obstetric emergency occurred. The nurses were evidently using this unauthorized negative reinforcement mechanism to pressure women to come into the clinic for antenatal care. Anecdotal evidence suggests that the practice was common.

Most women knew or had heard of someone who had been refused admission for these very reasons. Lucia, who was turned away from the Gondola District maternity clinic for failing to appear at the clinic for prenatal care, gave birth to a son alone by the side of the road as she tried to return to her home. Retaining the placenta inside her and bleeding heavily, and with her infant's umbilical cord still attached to the placenta, she had made her way back to the maternity ward, where she was then admitted and treated.

Javelina and Dona Joanna, the district secretary of the Mozambican Wom-
en's Organization, had together helped another woman in labor who had
been turned away from the maternity ward by accompanying her back to
the clinic and insisting on her admittance. Trezinha and Victoria recounted
that in previous pregnancies they had been turned away because they had
not brought their antenatal vaccine and consultation card as proof they had
attended the maternity clinic before birth.

Other obstacles that impeded women's use of the maternity clinic in
the first trimester were their lack of information and their misconceptions
regarding the preventive aspects of formal antenatal services—antitetanus vaccinations (VATs), treatment of anemia with iron supplements, and
syphilis screening. Most women reported they had received VATs; however,
confusion over the difference between VATs and Depo-Provera contraceptive injections was evident in the community. In the early 1990s when the
Gondola maternity clinic had introduced the use of Depo-Provera in the
family-planning clinics, a rumor had circulated in the area that pregnant
women were being injected with something that would make them infertile.
As a result, so many women refused to get the VAT at that time or stopped
going to the prenatal clinic that the district health personnel had mounted
a door-to-door public health education campaign to dispel the misinformation and sway public opinion, the district health director, João Manuel, told
me in April 1994. Nevertheless, ambivalence toward all vaccinations at the
maternity clinic remained. In each of the group discussions we conducted
with women in Mucessua, questions came up about the possible dangers
of the VAT and the fear that "the injection" contraceptive (Depo-Provera)
might leave them unable to conceive when they did desire another child.
Many women were unable to find their prenatal vaccination cards at the
time of my interview with them to allow me to confirm their having received
vaccinations.

A short time before I began the study, the maternity clinic stopped dis-
pensing a free month's supply of iron supplements to all pregnant women
attending prenatal consultations, a change that also negatively influenced
women's early initiation of prenatal care. Women unanimously perceived iron
supplements to be "good" for pregnancy and helpful to the development of
their baby. Several women specifically credited iron supplements with reliev-
ing dizziness and fatigue and restoring diminished appetite. Yet, according to
the nurses at the maternity clinic, a shortage of medical supplies meant they
could dispense iron supplements only to pregnant women with clinical or lab
diagnoses of anemia. Many women felt that without the free supplements,
the prenatal clinic had lost its most beneficial service, greatly reducing, in
their opinion, the value of going to the clinic at all. Twelve of the women
took iron and multivitamin supplements, seven of whom purchased them in

the private pharmacy or open market. The remaining five had received free iron supplements or prescriptions for supplements at the antenatal clinic to treat anemia.

Women in Mucessua knew or understood nothing of the preventive nature of the prenatal syphilis-screening program offered through the maternity clinic. During the period of research, contrary to national norms requiring all pregnant women to be screened for syphilis, the maternity center regularly referred only women with clinical diagnoses of sexually transmitted infections to the laboratory for syphilis screening. The reason for this policy was a provincewide shortage in reagents for the test (Lafort 1994). Of 40 women referred to the laboratory, 39 had undergone the test; of these, seven had tested positive and undergone treatment with penicillin, 1 reported testing positive and not undergoing treatment, and 31 reported negative test results. However, only 2 women of the 83 understood that the blood test given to some pregnant women could detect an illness that might affect the fetus. I did not find a single woman in Mucessua who knew that the test screened for syphilis infection. Not a single laywoman whom I spoke with throughout Mucessua knew what the purpose of the blood test was in relation to pregnancy, or remembered having had the purpose of the test explained to her. Fifteen women reported having been charged an unauthorized lab fee at the time of screening or to receive their results—one woman reported forgoing the test because she did not have the cash demanded at the laboratory. Ancha bought half the prescribed dose of penicillin, because she could not afford the whole prescription.

Official Ministry of Health policy was and continues to be that all antenatal clinic services are free to all women, and required medicines are subsidized for those who cannot pay. However, evidence shows an increasing demand for under-the-table fees for lab tests (Lafort 1994) and for hospital childbirth assistance (Hanlon 1996). This increase has elsewhere been attributed to the inadequacy of government wages under inflation (Hanlon 1996). The anger and frustration I experienced hearing from women about these unauthorized fees was tempered only by learning that an average health worker's salary was not enough for a family to eat meat or chicken each month, as one chicken cost the equivalent of one-tenth of a mid-level health worker's monthly salary.

Women's Perceptions of Biomedical Prenatal Services

Women considered the formal biomedical sector to offer the best treatment for very few categories of potential reproductive risk. They believed the maternity clinic was the best option for care only for problems during childbirth that required surgery, such as obstructed labor or postpartum hemorrhaging, or for some other medical technology, such as contraceptives. They considered biomedical services somewhat effective in treating infertility and sexually transmitted infections (STIs), although they more often rated prophets and curandeiros better at treating infertility, and curandeiros better at treating STIs.

Several women expressed the belief that any sick person should go to the hospital first, perhaps the response they thought I wanted, as this was a much-emphasized public health message. A majority expressed a more nuanced approach to negotiating health seeking during pregnancy, for example, Sara, age thirty-two, who had been pregnant three times, had lost one child, and had two surviving children: "When some women conceive they always have pain. This kind of pain could provoke a miscarriage. They must find the person who knows how to treat this [pain]. A curandeiro or pastor could treat this, but it depends on the woman. There are some cramps that are from your body, and there are [illnesses provoked by] *mau espirito*. Only a prophet or curandeiro can say which is which. In the hospital they don't know how to differentiate. But neither the hospital nor the curandeiro can cure without God's help." Women reported only curandeiros, church pastors, and prophets to be effective in addressing spirit-provoked reproductive threats of sorcery and *mau espirito*.

Among the entire group of eighty-three women and the 496 reported treatment episodes, only 2 episodes that women diagnosed as having personalistic causality were treated in the biomedical sector. One was Anita's episode of "pain in the abdomen"; the other was Yvonne's weight loss in the last month of gestation. Both Anita and Yvonne had gone first to the maternity clinic to diagnose the problem, but neither was given treatment. Anita then sought treatment from a curandeiro, and Yvonne at a church. With the exception of these two cases, women's patterns of resort were consistent with the general consensus among participants that problems caused by spirit intervention need to be treated outside the clinic. It is the commonly held view that an aggressive spirit has to be removed from the sufferer's body before treatment or even diagnosis in any sector will be effective. In the eighty-seven remaining spiritual or human threat-related pregnancy illness episodes, the women sought intervention from popular healing options.

The women most often mentioned *medicina tradicional* (traditional medicine)—the general Portuguese term for all methods employed by curandeiros—as the best treatment option for pregnancy and childbirth complications with personalistic causes (see Table 7). In practice, however, more prophets and churches than curandeiros treated these kinds of pregnancy illness episodes. This contradiction between traditional ideals and the women's patterns of treatment choice represents an important change in preference among women, especially the shift away from curandeiros toward churches and faith healers reflected, for example, in Sara's observations about the efficacy of "traditional" versus faith healing:

> The sickness where milk comes out of the breasts before birth [is best treated] by traditional medicine. In traditional medicine, [the curandeiros] know it well, because at times [this sickness] is provoked by our ancestors. First they have to take out the *mau espirito*, and after give roots to take. But, prayer and fasting are also forms that are utilized in the treatment of milk coming out before birth. The treatment really depends on the sufferer and which side [church member or not] one is linked. If it is the church [one is linked to], it is better to be treated in church.

Some women who were church members never mentioned curandeiros at all as a source of treatment for problems related to reproduction or pregnancy. Seeking help from curandeiros who work with ancestral spirit mediation and use traditional medicines is against most churches' doctrines. Anecdotal evidence suggests, however, that despite church rules, women with serious reproductive problems do not exclude any treatment option they can access. In fact, members of churches often seek help outside their churches. For example, Javelina left her father's strict church congregation to pursue treatment for infertility. Her father, a bishop in Johane Malange, an African Independent Church that originated in Zimbabwe, prohibited members from seeking any medical treatment. First she sought treatment in the biomedical sector and later with a Zionist prophet, even though the use of all medical interventions outside the church's healing therapies are forbidden by the teachings of the Zimbabwean prophet Johane Malange.

The reverse also occurs. People unaffiliated with any church who become afflicted with a serious reproductive problem will join the congregation of a prophet whose specialty it is to treat that particular affliction. When eighteen-year-old Paula, who did not belong to any church, began feeling abdominal pains in her first month of pregnancy, with the help of her mother she sought treatment immediately from a curandeiro. The 70 *conto* (U.S. $7) treatment helped "a little." When the pains continued in her third month, at the insistence of her boyfriend she went to the maternity clinic. The nurses sent her to the laboratory to be screened for syphilis. The test came back negative, so she was not given any treatment. When the pains continued through her eighth month, Paula went to a well-known prophet from the Zion City Church, who gave her blessed well water to drink every day until she gave birth. The pains subsided only after she delivered a healthy baby girl. Curiously, women most often described churches as the best treatment option for symptoms of pregnancy discomfort such as headache and toothache. In women's health-seeking trajectories, however, use of pharmaceuticals was the most frequent recourse for relief from symptoms of pregnancy, followed by going to the district health center (Table 7).

Prenatal Care Strategies and Pregnancy Management

Seeking Safe Passage: Fluidity of Movement and Layering of Treatment

Women's use of formal- and informal-sector health care options in succession or simultaneously creates layers of protection and treatment from different sources. Ancha's search for a cure for syphilis is a good illustration of this fluid movement among options in reproductive health seeking. At five months' gestation, Ancha suffered from intense vaginal itching and pain when she urinated. Following a routine clinic consultation, the nurses at the district maternity clinic sent her for a blood screening to confirm a clinical diagnosis of a sexually transmitted infection. She tested positive for syphilis and was given a prescription for twelve antibiotic tablets that cost 12,000 meticais (+U.S. $1.20—half a week's salary at minimum government wages). After paying 5,000 meticais under the table to get her results at the laboratory, Ancha had only 7,000 meticais left, so she received only half her prescription for penicillin tablets at the pharmacy. The six white pills did not reduce her pain and itching.

The next month, Ancha proceeded to a curandeiro, who gave her an infusion of roots for another 5,000 meticais. The itching diminished but did not stop completely. She continued taking the infusion for three months, but also bought six mystery injections from a traveling nurse from Zimbabwe, who charged 30,000 meticais. This nurse administered the injections to Ancha and her husband once a week over three weeks. The injections seemed to finally overcome the itching. Still, to make sure it would not return, Ancha went in her seventh month to a Zion Christian Church prophet, who gave her a blessing and sacred water to drink and bathe in. The treatment was free, but Ancha left the prophet 5,000 meticais as an offering (*chipo*, Sh.). At twenty-seven, Ancha had been pregnant eight times, had experienced three reproductive losses, and was the mother of five children. She believed that all the treatments had played a part in her ultimate healing:

> They all treat [sexually transmitted diseases], but it depends on the luck
> of where you go to be cured. Three treatments are the limit, though—the
> Father, Son, and the Holy Spirit! The hospital is really better because at the
> hospital they do analysis. So first I finished the hospital's pills. But everything
> helped. The curandeiro cleaned inside me for the baby not to get infected, but
> he didn't cure the illness. It was only diminished. The injections attacked the
> bridge of the illness [*tsine ye nhenda*, Tewe], where the illness is fixed inside

you. Like a tree, [the illness] already had deep roots. The prophet's treatment was to cleanse my body and to not have more bad luck.

For women in Mucessua, prenatal care is a process of layering protection against the various reproductive threats they perceive around them. The combined tactics of layering prenatal care from different sources and of adhering to a local relational and behavioral code for pregnant women involving secrecy and late disclosure of pregnancy are elements of what I came to call *safe passage*—a survival strategy from preconception through childbirth, and from menstruation to menopause.

Early Prenatal Care Seeking from Alternative Sources

Contrary to the story the institutional data were telling, many women sought prenatal health care during the first trimester, but not at the maternity clinic (see Table 8).

In their first trimester, more women sought prenatal health care from alternative sources than attended the maternity clinic. While 86.7 percent (72) of the 83 women reported seeking treatment from alternative health options, only about 7.2 percent (6) went to the maternity clinic, and 19.3 percent (16) to the district health center. In the second and third trimesters, visits to the maternity clinic increase significantly, but these visits occurred after the gestation time the national Safe Motherhood Initiative had promoted for beginning prenatal consultations. Most significantly, while women continued to experience an increasing number of illness episodes during pregnancy, they did not report seeking treatment at the maternity clinic. Instead, their patronage of spiritual healing specialist and use of herbal treatments increased in the second and third trimesters, as women addressed threats to pregnancy they believed lay outside the expertise of the biomedical sector and prepared themselves at home for childbirth.

Increased Use of Alternative Sources of Prenatal Care across Trimesters

Following the patterns of fluid movement and layering of treatments and seeking early prenatal care outside the formal sector, a third general pattern of women's movement between and among therapeutic options in Mucessua became evident: as pregnancy progressed, women increasingly sought nonclinic prenatal treatment for spiritual and social threats to reproduction. In the third trimester, alternative care use overtakes the biomedical prenatal care use that dominated in the second trimester. Three factors might help explain this pattern. First, in the third trimester, many women begin preparing for birth using local plant preparations and other substances for ingestion

Table 8. Treatments and Providers Sought, by Trimester, 1995

Treatment or Treatment Provider	Trimester		
	First	Second	Third
No treatment	6 (7.2)*	8 (9.6)	8 (9.6)
Pharmaceutical**	31 (37.3)	25 (30.1)	23 (27.7)
Herbal**	3 (3.6)	4 (4.8)	49 (59.0)
District health center	16 (19.3)	25 (30.1)	21 (25.3)
Church	21 (25.3)	23 (27.7)	27 (32.5)
Curandeiro	5 (6.0)	5 (6.0)	5 (6.0)
Prophet	7 (8.4)	13 (15.7)	17 (20.5)
Prayer**	4 (4.8)	4 (4.8)	8 (9.6)
Mission clinic	1 (1.2)	3 (3.6)	1 (1.2)
Traveling nurse	0	2 (2.4)	3 (3.6)
Maternity clinic	6 (7.2)	58 (69.8)	56 (67.4)

*Percentages appear in parentheses.
**Self-treated
Note: N=83. A woman might have selected more than one type of treatment or treatment provider in a trimester or selected one option more than once.

and for massage of the birth canal and perineum. Second, the diagnosis of chronic and severe problems during pregnancy shifted from originating in the world or God to being provoked by spirits or sorcery. Third, women saw all illnesses late in pregnancy as more serious reproductive threats. The "bigger"—closer to term—the pregnancy, the more vulnerable the mother and unborn child were to harm. By the third trimester, nearly the entire group of women were using extraclinical prenatal health care. These three trends are illustrated in Table 8.

The Folk Epidemiology of Social Threat

In contrast to the multiple layers of social meaning expressed in women's responses to reproductive threats, formal biomedical services reflect a narrow concern for the control of women's fertility using a medical definition of pregnancy and obstetric risk factors. Women in Mucessua view these services as inadequate to respond to certain salient reproductive threats and pregnancy health needs. Delaying consultations in the maternity clinic until late in pregnancy is frequently a conscious and, from these worried mothers' perspective, a conscientious prenatal care strategy, just as delaying care in the maternity clinic early in pregnancy is a preventive and protective health activity.

Importantly, women's pregnancy management strategies reflect priorities consistent with the goals of national maternal health norms and WHO Safe Motherhood Initiative policies in three significant ways:

1. Women in Mucessua identify themselves to be at high risk for pregnancy and obstetric complications.
2. To protect themselves, women seek preventive and curative prenatal care throughout gestation that is intended to diminish reproductive risks and detect and avert complications.
3. In cases of pregnancy and obstetric complication, women consult specialists deemed appropriate to treat both the cause and the accompanying symptoms of the complication.

Women purposely delayed entering the biomedical system in an attempt to reduce reproductive risks that they perceived stemmed from public knowledge of their pregnant condition. By initiating clinic-based prenatal consultations late in their pregnancies, they circumvented national norms and relegated formal biomedical services to a marginal role in safeguarding or guaranteeing community continuity through children.

Early in pregnancy, nonmedically trained popular providers of reproductive health care such as prophets, pastors, and occasionally traditional healers are privileged over biomedically trained health providers in the formal sector. Women have more trust in these informal healers as sources of authoritative reproductive knowledge and therapeutic processes that address meaningful aspects of women's experiences—social tension, jealousy, isolation, economic instability, and the reproductive vulnerability that these conditions engender. In the context of economic insecurity exacerbated by congested living conditions, an account of how women seek protection from pregnancy threats they believe are related to their social and economic vulnerability helps explain their patterns of delaying and underutilizing formal prenatal care services.

Following the patterns of women's experiences of pregnancy and prenatal health seeking also challenges the characterization of high-risk women in developing countries as unmotivated or noncompliant victims. On the contrary, under conditions of frequent reproductive morbidity and loss, little access to cash, immense domestic and agricultural work burdens, and limited routes to female social and economic self-determination, many women demonstrated significant initiative in mobilizing the resources they deemed necessary to influence their own reproductive labor and decrease the odds of poor pregnancy outcomes.

The existence of a wide universe of women's options for prenatal health care outside the biomedical sector does not make them beneficial or more capable of treating pregnancy and obstetric complications. Rather, the biomedical system could more effectively promote prenatal service use by integrating local idioms of protection into its health messages. Activities of the maternity clinic—antitetanus vaccinations; vitamin supplementation; blood screening; and screening, prevention, and treatment for sexually transmitted infections, including HIV—are all compatible with women's desire to protect their unborn children from harm and need to be promoted as such. More importantly, however, health care givers in the formal sector must recognize the sensitive nature of pregnancy threats and reorganize the delivery of services to provide confidential prenatal care.

The implications of these findings for public health are vital, since women's beliefs seem to have a bearing on their delay in seeking prenatal health care from health facilities. For example, women's explanatory models were significant influences on their perceptions of reproductive health risks. These findings are consistent with those of several studies of reproductive health of women in third-world countries. For example, in Nigeria, Adetunji found that Yoruba women preferred "traditional" over "modern" prenatal care because "the traditional prenatal care included ideas of physical as well as metaphysical sources of illness and tried to combat both, whereas the modern care focuses only on the physical" (1996: 1566).

Ethnomedical beliefs alone, however, are not sufficient to explain patterns of women's behavior in seeking prenatal health care. Asowa-Omorodion (1997: 1823) identifies the influence of local health beliefs on pregnancy and childbirth management in Nigeria:

> The Esan people often see most health problems arising from one's sins. Illnesses are believed to be caused by unnatural events (Omorodion 1993). Hence complications in pregnancy are often assumed to be the result of the woman's sins, such as having committed extra-marital affairs, or bewitching their spouses. The researcher believes that because of these interpretations of illness, the men are often lukewarm over providing financial assistance or allowing the woman to seek the best treatment even preferring the woman to die for her sins. The women tend to accept complications in pregnancy and after delivery as punishments for their sins.

Asowa-Omorodion goes on, however, to elaborate the link between ethnomedical beliefs and women's gender-related economic dependence on men. The Nigerian women "lack access to the means of production, and they certainly cannot control it despite the fact that they provide most farm labor" (ibid.). Jirojwong's (1996) study of Thai women and pregnancy also finds that women's perceptions of susceptibility to and severity of illnesses during pregnancy contribute to their underutilization of biomedical prenatal services and support the use of alternative prenatal care providers. Jirojwong concludes, however, that economic and social pressures, including poor treatment by biomedical personnel, also account for delayed and inadequate prenatal care in the biomedical sector.

On the other end of the spectrum, studies of reproductive health management strategies need to pay attention to ethnomedical beliefs. For example, Schmid et al. (2001) document the need for emergency transport to improve obstetric outcomes for women experiencing complications in home deliveries in rural Tanzania. Facilitating access to emergency obstetric care for poor women in developing countries is a critical problem that must be addressed. However, if the patterns and underlying reasons for home delivery and delayed transferal of women with obstetric emergencies go unexamined, we may overlook key economic and social negotiations that precede and contribute to the progression of an obstetric emergency. The reasons for delay need to be scrutinized (Asowa-Omorodion 1997), as well as the broader context of rural Tanzanian women's interrelated economic, social, spiritual and physical vulnerability. In other words, analysis should not stop at the level of explanatory models but should go on to link culturally shared beliefs to the political economic context of the social actors. Neglecting these additional data leaves out crucial aspects of social relations of production and reproduction that inform women's reproductive health beliefs and pregnancy health-seeking behavior.

An analytical model that takes into account individual experiences, socioeconomic conditions, and the structure and practices of the health system in historical perspective allows greater insight into the formation of explanatory models and their influence on health strategies. It also begins to reveal the mechanisms by which both risk perceptions and health strategies might change over time (Atkinson and Farias 1994). More importantly, such an approach can begin to expose the fundamental causes of health burdens and their unequal distribution within and across communities in ways that can help redirect much-needed health interventions, as well as social and economic justice policies.

CHAPTER 7

Segredos da Casa

No one dies of natural causes in Mozambique. People may have heard of someone who lived the right life and died peacefully in old age, but nobody actually knows this person. For a person to have an accident or to become sick and then to die, there has to have been some breach of protection, and people work hard at finding it. Following a death, there are always stories and uncertainties, rumors and suspicions, and people worry these thoughts around and around in hushed conversations.

If someone dies from driving at night down a road they drive down every day and crashing into a truck with no lights that has broken down in the middle of the road, it is not an accident; it is only the final event in a series of ill-fated events. If that same truck hit a cow and killed it, also damaging the truck, both the owner of the cow and the driver of the truck begin to comb back through an inventory of their relations and interactions looking for clues. People immediately trace back over every possible sign or signal or step that could have led to the moment of misfortune, the knowledge of which could help improve the future course of events by some corrective action.

The appearance of an owl is always a warning, and usually a sign of impending ill fortune in Mozambique, often of death or serious sickness. When an owl entered a bank in the town of Chimoio where we lived, it was a terrible omen. As the story goes, someone was sent in to kill the owl. When the man who killed the owl died a few days later, the news circulated all around the town, accompanied by trepidation, awe, and grim understanding. The owl was a portent of that very man's own approaching death. This story made sense to everyone, though no one would tell me why anyone would agree to kill the owl in the first place unless it was his job, as in this case; the owl killer was the bank's custodian. I was not sure what to think two weeks later, when a foul smell in the tap water in our house led to the discovery of a dead owl in the water tank on our roof. I did not know whether to be relieved that the owl had died or afraid that a dead owl was a doubly serious warning. People hedged their answers when I asked how to interpret the owl incident. Everyone agreed that *estrangeiros,* or foreigners, were exempt from the dangers of witchcraft and sorcery unless they were sleeping with or married to a Mozambican, in which case they were susceptible. My being a person of African descent put me in a betwixt and between category, so people advised that it was best to play things safe, scour the water tank and my conscience, take care of my family, and watch my back.

I had learned of women's particular fears of being harmed by sorcery during pregnancy in my first individual in-depth interview session. Clara, a young pregnant woman, had agreed to be interviewed where she lived, at her mother's compound very close to Javelina's house. However, when we arrived—Javelina, Jorda, who was helping us mobilize women in Mucessua for the focus groups, and I—Clara's mother greeted us rather coldly, a woman who just days before had been jovial and welcoming when I had met her with Javelina. We three guests sat on the family's three chairs. The mother sat near us on a mat, and Clara sat at a distance on another mat. Throughout the interview Clara kept her gaze on the ground, while her mother gave minimal or no answers to the questions.

After this disastrous experience, I asked Javelina what she thought was going on. She matter-of-factly explained that the girl had miscarried less than a year ago, and that Dona Jorda, who had come with us, had been accused before a bairro tribunal of helping the mother of the baby's alleged father use sorcery to cause the miscarriage. Significantly, Clara was one of the five women who reported she sought no clinical prenatal care and delivered at home. Her child was also one of the three infants born during the prenatal care study who died within the first year of life, and one of the three babies who had been given my name. Coming from someone who had just met me, the honor of naming a child after me was a sign of shallow social support, signifying deep social and material jeopardy for the child.

Embodied perceptions of reproductive vulnerability and social tensions are linked, as we have seen throughout these chapters. Women attribute the most serious pregnancy and obstetric complications to personalistic reproductive threats of witchcraft and sorcery; this in turn shapes women's responses to reproductive threats. In this chapter I explore how the threats directed at women's reproductive bodies and responses to those threats are negotiated through horizontal and vertical female envy, as well as through socially constructed female identities of witches (*ngozi*), spinster ghosts (*zinyaumba*), and wives of spirits (*mkadzi wa mfukwa*). Pollution and purity beliefs and the commoditization of childbirth also play key roles.

Celia: Horizontal and Vertical Female Envy

The main reasons for witchcraft in the bairro come down to jealousy and envy. Envy in particular is expressed in ways that women experience as dangerous to their reproductive health—horizontally in relation to living relatives, neighbors, and co-workers or sexual rivals, and vertically in relation to ancestral spirits (Swantz 1979: 170) and future or unborn kin. These categories of reproductive threat tend to overlap. Yet the havoc is always brought close to home by the belief that these threats could not be operationalized without the expert working of witches, "shadows of fleeting, improvised [wo]men" (Lacan, cited in Geschiere 1997: 232). Witches and sorcerers, in turn, could not breach the sanctity and balance of the body and spirit of another without the aid of jealous kin or vengeful ancestor spirits trading in lineage names. At the heart of the hearth-hold—"the mother-child units between which men move and in which the heterosexual relationship is one among many others" (Ekejiuba 1995)—reproductive threats are frequently perceived as stemming from conflicts in social relationships between women.

Celia secretly accused a spiteful maternal aunt, her mother's oldest sister and a kin role socially prescribed to be nurturing and protective, of using witchcraft to cause problems in her second pregnancy. In her eighth month, Celia complained of severe pains in the bottom of her abdomen. She had been to the maternity clinic, but the nurses had not offered any treatment for her pain, only told her to come back the next month to give birth. Counseled by her husband, she had gone to a prophet. The prophet brought forth a spirit from Celia's body which, speaking through possession of Celia's mother, began to identify tensions between family members who had gathered for the ceremony. During the summoned spirit's tirade, one aunt became especially agitated and expressed a wish to die. Celia believed that this aunt had sent the spirit to harm her: "My mother's sister sent this spirit. She has a crazy daughter and a crazy son. She has hate. The spirit told me that it doesn't want me to give birth. This aunt is bad. She is also a curandeira. This sister of my mother had an eldest daughter. Her mother sent a spirit to make her go crazy [kupenga, Sh., Tewe]. She stayed crazy. Up to today she is still in her mother's house."

At this point, I asked for more explanation about the daughter's misfortune, and Celia went on: "[The aunt's daughter] had married a soldier and moved into his house. But when [my aunt] drank, she arrived at the house and insulted her son-in-law. She said [to her daughter], 'You are showing off. You didn't pay me my lobolo money. You already have a husband, but you don't want to see me, don't want to give me any money to buy capulana, stew. As it is with my mother and father, I also want [lobolo].'"

These insults and curses were what drove the daughter crazy forever. As Celia explained: "After this, the husband said, 'Now that you made your daughter go crazy, I no longer need her,' and sent her home."

Celia believes that her aunt's bitterness at having been deprived of her own daughter's lobolo, along with her envy of Celia's good fortune, led her aunt to use powers she possessed as a curandeira to ruin Celia's reproductive health. This aunt was angry not only at failing to receive bride-price for her own daughter—an example of a vertical breach in payment of respect between different generations in the same family—but also because Celia's reproductive health would bring wealth to Celia's mother's household through the payment of masunggiro, or virgin seduction fee, and bride-price, an example of horizontal female envy between sisters. Celia felt she was the vulnerable target the aunt used to rage against her own irresponsible daughter and her more fortunate sister, Celia's mother. While Celia's story portrays the aunt as the aggressor, the accusation of the aunt is embedded in a broader criticism of weak kin support, for it is Celia's own mother and her maternal ancestors whose protective roles are called into question.

Celia's father-in-law has paid masunggiro to her parents, but her young husband had not yet earned enough to pay lobolo. Because of this unpaid sum, Celia, who was nineteen, worried about her ability to protect her first son's health from witchcraft: "[My husband] is going to arrange [lobolo]. But, at times [my son] Jaimecito is not well at night. At night his body heats up, and he cries. As soon as morning arrives, it stops. Curandeiros are accustomed to keeping the lights burning until morning. I don't know if it will come again at night. I'm usually afraid."

Florencia: Mother-in-Law as Reproductive Threat

Reproductive threats often stem from other struggles for power within the domestic sphere. Daughters-in-law frequently view their *sogras* (mothers-in-law) as envious and see them as a potential source of reproductive threats from which daughters-in-law must seek protection. It is as a sogra that a woman in Mucessua achieves her greatest status, for as a senior female in an extended family she has a social right to make claims on the labor of her sons, unmarried daughters, and daughters-in-law. A sogra often supersedes her son's influence over his wife and vies discreetly or openly with a new wife for control of her married son's income and labor. Until her children are productive members of the family, a wife represents a drain on the sogra's resources. Much as Wolf found in China (Wolf 1972), in Mucessua, the daughter-in-law's building of a uterine family to counteract her isolation and establish security for her old age may interfere with her mother-in-law's consolidating power through building her own uterine line. As Lamphere contends: "Strategies which females use to manipulate and influence males who control power include strong and subtler methods such as gossip and playing one person off against another" (Lamphere 1974: 123).

Because of the contentious nature of this relationship, wives often fear their sogra—especially new wives without male children through which to establish strategic power in their husband's lineage. This fear is projected as reproductive threats, and women often blame sogras in cases of sorcery-induced pregnancy, obstetric complication, and reproductive loss. Knowing that their sogra may suspect them of stealing her son's allegiance and resources generates a common feeling of vulnerability among young wives in relation to patrikin. Florencia, pregnant for the first time, for example, tells of sorcery sent by her sogra to increase her husband's favor toward a more docile second wife:

> During the seventh month of my pregnancy, I experienced severe cramps, vomiting, and diarrhea for a week. I went to the district health center, where they treated me for malaria, but my symptoms got worse, and I could not sleep. I decided with my husband to return to the same prophet who had treated me for feitiço during my first pregnancy. During the *consulta* using water gazing, the prophet asked me if I had in-laws in my house. "I live with my in-laws!" I told her. I told her that my husband had married that other woman, and now his parents preferred that he leave me and stay only with this new wife. The prophet agreed that indeed it was they who wanted to give me *problemas* and had gone to a sorcerer. Since I live in the same compound with them, I had to carry out my treatment very clandestinely.

Nonetheless, warned the prophet, the danger remained that Florencia's in-laws might learn of her actions to protect herself the next time they tried to send the spirit to harm her, and the spirit might refuse to go. For extra protection at multiple layers, the prophet gave her milk mixed with blessed water to put in a bottle and drink for three days whenever she was thirsty. She received another blessed water to secretly flick from her fingertips to purify her in-laws' home and courtyard from the sorcery. To protect against a miscarriage, Florencia received a cord of red, green, and white braided threads to wear around her belly and untie only when she was about to give birth.

Despite her efforts, Florencia's son was born with an umbilical infection locally called *urongorongo*—an illness caused by sorcery and fatal within seven days unless the infant is kept inside until its umbilical stump falls off and given treatment to close vulnerable openings in the body. This closing is accomplished by squeezing herbal paste onto the infant's umbilicus, mouth, and anus, and into the water used to bathe the baby and wash its clothes. Treatment also involves closing the vulnerable openings of the house and pathways to the house from strangers and anyone who is ritually "impure" or "hot" from intercourse, especially adultery, or from the "sacred danger" (Jolly 2002) associated with menstruation, a long journey, levirate rituals, or a funeral.[1] In her competition with a second wife for resources and legitimacy,

Florencia leveraged the diagnosis of *urongorongo* to curb her husband's sexual contact with the second wife, claiming it endangered their infant son.

In a patrilocal marriage, where a wife moves to live with her husband and his patrikin, a mother-in-law can also exercise considerable influence over her son's wife if she experiences trouble with childbirth. Infidelity on the part of the pregnant woman is widely believed to cause problems during childbirth, especially prolonged or blocked labor, and it is the right and duty of a mother-in-law to extract this information from her daughter-in-law. Armed with such a confession, the sogra can inform her son, often initiating a break in relations between the young couple or even catalyzing divorce proceedings, thus fortifying her own position of influence with her son. Senior women's power in this setting is linked to their ritual control over certain diagnoses in pregnancy and birthing that carry social meaning.

Recently, however, junior women have begun to defy these customary sanctions on their sexual freedom, protecting themselves by inventing new rituals that preclude the necessity of a public confession and undermine the power of senior women in their time-honored roles—the mother-in-law who witnesses labor, the midwife (*mbuya*, Tewe) who assists laboring women, or the indigenous healer (curandeira) who controls access to medicamentos to aid labor and protect adulterous women in childbirth—to use junior women's secrets against them. Josefa, age thirty-two, explained how women can resist this control as she described an invented private ritual of self-protection to avoid adultery confession:

> When a pregnant woman joins with another man, it is certain she will have an *operação* [Cesarean section] if she doesn't confess the name of her lover. The treatment for [birth complications caused by adultery] is with *mfuta*, a tree that gives *mfuta*. You take the fruit, part it, and take one seed. When you have the seed, you [hold] it in the hand with salt. Then, go with a *massador* [a heavy stick used to pound grains] to where you cook in your house—the three cooking stones. Put the seed in your mouth and swallow it whole. Dump the salt in the fire. Then bite the *massador* on the end that is held. Jump over the fire. Like that you can stay safe without confessing.[2]

This new ritual demonstrates the fluidity of long-standing practices as they are adapted to new and evolving conditions of social vulnerability. In another instance of privatizing formerly public reproductive health practices, when women are suspicious of their sogra and do not want her present at their delivery, they may go to the hospital instead of giving birth at home. Although women most often employ indigenous, informal-sector methods of healing and protection to deal with social threats, such cases demonstrate that they can also strategically employ biomedicine to reduce social vulnerability.

Julia: Vertical Envy and Spirit-Inherited Infertility

Because of the role played by matrilineal kin (vadzimu) in protecting and ensuring female reproductive health, a history of infertility and reproductive loss in a woman's family may be blamed on a jealous kinswoman who died childless. One specific sign of this situation is the culture-bound affliction called *zvinyaumba* (plural of prefix *nya*, guardian, user; and *-umba*, inability to bear children that survive, die soon after birth, Sh.). As was the case with Julia, a woman with *zvinyaumba* is believed to be haunted by the spirit of a childless female relative who returns to steal a living relative's child for herself. The condition manifests as early lactation during pregnancy and is considered fatal to the unborn child, who will die in utero or soon after birth. Julia told of her experience with *zvinyaumba*:

> After twelve years without conceiving, I gave birth to a baby girl who died halfway out of the *lugar do parto* [birth canal] while I was giving birth at home. This birth was in danger from the foot coming first instead of the head. Less than a year later, I was pregnant again. During the first four months I felt extremely tired and always sick and with pains. But after my experience *de não dar* [infertility] and the death of my daughter, my family suspected the intervention of evil spirits, so I went for treatment by this prophet rather than attending consultations at the maternity clinic.
>
> The prophet saw that a small, dark woman in the bairro was scheming to serve as my birth assistant, and to receive the customary cloth, food, wine and even cash paid as respeito to midwives. She warned me that if this woman was not called to assist the birth, I would see how much I would suffer even more on that day. The prophet gave me a mixture of blessed water and powdered milk called a taero to drink. I returned with that bottle to refill it every week over four months.

In her seventh month, Julia began to lactate. She was diagnosed a second time by the prophet who was already treating her as having *zvinyaumba*—an illness caused by the intervention of a deceased maternal great aunt who had died a barren spinster. The prophet led her through a ritual cure in which she had to make a doll of clay and carry it like a child on her back to a special river. There she waded naked into the river and released the doll from her wrap into the water calling, "*Zinhaumba*, here is your baby. *Zinhaumba*, take your baby." Julia then turned from the river without looking back, and leaving her clothes there, she returned to the church wrapped in a new cloth, where the prophet bathed her with a special mixture of blessed waters. A cord of white, green, and red thread was tied around her breasts to wear until she gave birth.

At this point in the story, Julia provides another example of strategically choosing biomedicine to deal with social threats: she reported that to be "safe," she intended to deliver at the hospital to avoid having to call the small, dark woman to assist the birth and thus avoid having to come up with cash and goods to pay her. However, Julia went into labor while praying at the home of the prophet and gave birth precipitously to her second son. The prophet tied a cord identical to the one around her breasts around the newborn's waist for protection. Though she was not expected to pay for the prayer treatment or birth assistance, Julia joined her prophet's church and continued bringing offerings of cash and food.

Marcelina: Wives of Spirits

The persistent link between kinship, economic tensions, witchcraft and reproductive vulnerability is most apparent in the institution of "spirits' wives"—*wakadzi wa mpfukwa* (women bound ceremonially as a wife to an avenging spirit or spirit of a dead relative, Sh., Tewe; *mkadzi we* (woman, wife of); and *-pfuka* (haunt, turn away from, leave in the lurch, abandon of amiable spirit); or *mulher d'espirito* (spirit's wife). A girl becomes a spirit's wife when her parents or other kin relatives with guardianship rights attempt to pay off debts of respect to a stranger, another lineage member or an ancestor who has been robbed or murdered by a family or lineage member by ritually marrying a daughter, niece, or granddaughter to the avenging spirit of the offended party. As Sarah, age nineteen, explained the process:

> You will need blood, because when a bad spirit is attached, it is done with blood. They do it like that, people who are sorcerers, attach a spirit to you with blood of a dead person who was murdered. [To bring out this spirit] you take the blood of a chicken and put it in a cloth. Carry it to the prophet's house. When it comes time for the sprit to come out, it is going to speak how it arrived. The family can all come, if the spirit demands this. They take out money for the spirit to speak. The whole family convenes to find out what the spirit wants. "We want to pay. How much do you want?"—if it wants money, a girl, or a goat, as contribution to [pay off] this debt.

Characteristic of spirits' wives was poor reproductive health. Any woman who experiences frequent miscarriage or stillbirth or whose infants and children do not survive is suspected of being a spirit's wife, as is a woman who has difficulty in delivery except when she gives birth within the confines of her father's compound. A spirit's wife and her offspring are threatened by spirit intervention if her social, especially sexual, behavior knowingly or unknowingly contradicts her status as a spirit's wife. Javelina, age thirty-eight, first explained the institution of spirits' wives to me.

Javelina: In the past people lived far apart. Maybe family living together, but still sons and daughters, once they marry they must leave home and build their own houses. If they stay, people begin to suspect them of bad spirits.
Rachel: What does it mean to "have" a bad spirit? Like an illness?
Javelina: This bad spirit comes from assassinating a person, maltreating a person. His spirit stays in your house. If this person is from far away, you have to arrange a girl for his family. But you, the girl, don't know. In this case the father must construct a house, and put a daughter, and give her the name of this person who died. The girl marries this spirit. "Here. This girl is your wife." She cannot marry now. If someone wants to marry this girl, they have to tell [the spirit]. If this girl bears children, the children belong to this spirit. The other [man] serves as a rooster only. He can't hit her. If he does, he could become sick or die, because she is the master's.

In the course of discussing other topics, the subject of spirits' wives surfaced as a central, recurring theme. Everyone in Mucessua knew of spirits' wives and had a story to tell about one, usually in their own family. For example, in a focus group with female adolescents in Mucessua, when I asked Lorinda, a sixteen-year-old girl without children, if she and other girls of her generation would prefer not to have bride-price (lobolo) paid for them these days, she responded vehemently:

No! Women who are not loboloed are *mulheres da casa* (women of the house, spirit wives). Where the mother came out not loboloed, the daughters also cannot be loboloed. A spirit's wife stays in the house of her parents, and her children stay to be spirits' wives. Many [spirit wives] have children with many men. Many [of them] note that men are scoundrels, but the family and the woman just say this to hide their secret. They live badly. Sometimes when they find a husband, he dies. Each child has his own father. Eh! But society accepts this.

Some women know of their status and live according to the restrictions placed on spirits' wives. While they do not marry, meaning lobolo is never paid for them, after appropriate ritual permission is requested of the spirit through their father or guardian, they can have partners. Spirits' wives are considered a kind of sex worker whose temporary partners pay respect for the right to sleep with them, a practice thinly veiled in the common euphemism for a spirit wife as a "woman in search of a husband."

Men who had slept with a spirit's wife described sensations of weakness and being drained of energy during intercourse, or a feeling they were making love with a man. Some had even heard the spirit speak through possession of the spirit wife. As Sr. João recalled: "In the middle of the night the spirit comes out of the girl screaming and screaming, 'You have the courage to be with my woman?'" Mateus told the story of a friend who lost most of his tongue when a spirit's wife who became possessed while they made love bit it clean off.

While the diagnosis of spirit wife is often given to women with reproductive problems who are seeking a healer's treatment, other women claim the identity for themselves. Dona Marcelina, who was over fifty, had been pregnant six times, and had lost three of her six children, spoke of herself and her deceased mother in these careful but revealing words:"I wasn't paid for with lobolo. Do I want it paid now? Who is going to eat this money with my parents dead? My mother didn't want [lobolo paid for her] when she was alive. She always birthed and lost, birthed and lost. She wasn't secure. My mother didn't want the debt."

Because of her poor reproductive health, Dona Marcelina's mother had accepted or actively taken on the diagnosis that she was a spirit's wife. She had refused to enter into a marriage contract in which she would be responsible for repaying lobolo should her husband divorce her if she was unable to produce offspring that survived. She did, however, live with a male partner and had five children. Following her mother's example, Dona Marcelina had also never married, that is, lobolo had never been paid for her. Like her mother, she attributed her own poor reproductive health history—six pregnancies, two infant deaths and one stillbirth—to having a spirit husband. She claimed that her eldest daughter's recent miscarriage was evidence that she had passed on to her daughters her fate as a spirit's wife.

This strategically fluid role of a spirit's wife takes on new meaning in an economy where sex work is increasingly one of the few viable means of survival for impoverished women without education or adequate access to land. Yet many women, especially those with one or both feet in the rural social economy, require a more socially acceptable identity than sex worker to maintain their social identity. Like the woman-invented ritual Josefa described to avoid confessing adultery during a difficult childbirth, claiming the spirit's wife identity provides a strong example of women improvising on a construction of selves, sexualities, and genders that is not rigid and strict, but a "system of possibilities" (Wekker 2006: 104) in ways that suit their economic and social needs.

Stories abound of women unaware of their status as spirits' wives. In these cases, their parents unwittingly accept bride-price payment for their marriage. With cash so precious, however, parents who have made a deal with a spirit sometimes knowingly accept bride-price from a suitor without telling their daughter her status. In both circumstances, it is believed that to stake his claim, the betrayed spirit will manifest his presence as sickness, if he is a good spirit, or death, if he is bad. Sometimes the "adulterous" wife is struck down. Sometimes it is the living male interloper or "rooster" who dies.

No real escape, however, is available from this gendered role as lineage scapegoat. Parents maintain control over the productive and reproductive labor of an otherwise marriageable grown daughter and perhaps, as some respondents hinted, profit from her sexual labor through gifts from suitors. Josefa asked me: "If you only take out the spirit, where will it go? A prophet could take it out to speak of what is happening with the girl. But a family can only take [the spirit] out and attach it to another daughter or granddaughter. Anyway, paying off one spirit doesn't always buy peace. A row of others [spirits] can line up behind when you show your money. So people here say, 'A son-in-law cannot confront the problems of his father-in-law.'"

Many women expressed the belief that the only treatment for spirit wives is to follow the prescriptions mandated by their status. They pay the price with their bodies through multiple partnerships that may actually put them at risk for compromised reproductive capacity through exposure to sexually transmitted infection or by passing the blood debt on to another generation of female relatives. Some women labeled spirit wives because of reproductive health problems have recently found a new solution: as part of a burgeoning social movement, they enter African Pentecostal and Zionist churches to seek relief from the financial burden of healer's costs and from the social stigma attached to being a spirit's wife (Pfeiffer 2002). So, while the "row of others" Josefa refers to are spirits, there is also a living row of others who line up when people seek desperately to understand and end misfortune. These are the prophets, pastors, and curandeiros who make their living diagnosing and treating people who suffer on any level, especially women with reproductive problems who find themselves or can conveniently be diagnosed as afflicted by spirits.

While the unprecedented commercialization of women's sexual and reproductive labor provides some young women with the means to contest ritual practices older relatives employ to control them and the fruits of their labors, this freedom does not come without associated reproductive dangers. Because of Mucessua's location at a pit stop for truckers along the AIDS Highway, as the Beira Corridor has been informally labeled, sex workers in Mucessua are increasingly in danger of exposure to sexually transmitted infections, including HIV.

Strategizing Reproduction

Several recent public health studies that seek to explain patterns of women's reproductive health seeking, especially variability in antenatal care utilization and low compliance with high-risk obstetric referrals, have considered the relation of risk perception to women's prenatal care use. These studies are limited by their focus on physiological risks, however. For example, Magadi et al. (2000) found that the frequency and timing of antenatal care in Kenya is similar to that in other African nations and associated with a range of socioeconomic and demographic variables. Variations in health-seeking practices between different births to the same woman, between different women in the same community, and between communities remain unexplained. The authors conclude that unspecified "traditional beliefs and cultural practices" common to the community might account for the variation and contribute to inadequate use of "modern" health services. This discourse reinstates the binary association of "tradition" with incompetent health service consumption, and "modernity" with biomedical service use compliance.

In another study, Myer and Harrison (2003) concluded that rural South African women's lack of information regarding potential physiological risks and the benefits of prenatal care accounted for their late initiation and low use of this care. However, the researchers ignore the potential influence of social threats on pregnancy management. Furthermore, women interviewed in the clinic setting may have declined to expose their health seeking from competing or "subjugated" alternative healing modalities (Root and Browner 2001; Davis-Floyd 2003) that compete monetarily or ideologically for "patients."

Women's representations of their own reproductive subjectivities suggest that their perceptions of reproductive threats correspond to gendered, corporeal experiences of social and economic marginalization. Women's narratives show that they process bodily experience and risk perceptions as social phenomena that influence their health-seeking behavior. In the face of their fears and frequent reproductive complications and loss, women make strategic use of both biomedicine and multiple forms of indigenous and newly emerging religious forms of healing; they seek protection from multiple sources of health care in a vibrant, medically plural system.

This system is shaped by and in turn shapes women's vulnerability to rural poverty and the gender-specific consequences of changes in Mozambique's rapidly transforming political economy. By political economy I refer to "the attempt to constantly place culture in time, to see a constant interplay between experience and meaning in a context in which both experience and meaning are shaped by inequality and domination [and the] attempt to understand the emergence of particular peoples at the conjunction of local and global histories, to place local populations in the larger currents of world history" (Roseberry 1990: 49; Lancaster and Di Leonardo 1997: 4).

Missing these connections among experience, meaning, and the history and contexts of inequality can significantly limit questions and findings regarding women's reproductive management repertoires. For example, Dujardin et al. (1995: 534) examined low compliance with obstetric risk referrals in Zaire and found that geographic accessibility and women's perception of their risk status in relation to biomedical norms were the factors most associated with compliance, although they suggested that qualitative research data were needed to help explain the role of "cultural perceptions of risk." The study minimizes the extent to which the social meanings of pregnancy and birth might be as important as biological outcomes; its authors conclude that perinatal loss is less traumatic or important to women in Zaire than it is to women in "industrialized countries." On the contrary, evidence from Mozambique and elsewhere in Africa suggests that perinatal death may direct women away from the clinic and toward informal-sector healing specialists (Adetunji 1992). From a social threat perspective, Zairian women's request for spirit healers to be present at births underscores the importance of social aspects of birth that are absent in the clinical sphere of interest and diagnostic expertise. It also becomes clearer from this perspective that ethnomedical beliefs alone are not sufficient to explain patterns of women's prenatal health-seeking behavior.

For many African women, a "trouble-free" childbirth may be as important as the birth of the live infant to demonstrate that a mother is sin free and has obeyed social-sexual mores (Asowa-Omorodion 1997). Indeed, a woman's achievement of this identity is crucial to the material and social survivorship of both mother and child. These dual priorities do not diminish the importance placed on live births but illuminate the conventions people use to manage the loss, grief, and disruption of social order that reproductive crises provoke.

It has been a productive shift to begin to consider how a range of women's experiences of reproductive threats both constrain and engender reproductive agendas—"a complex set of individual goals and priorities" that includes proverbial virtues, cosmological concerns, status aspirations, and medical concerns (Sargent 1982: 70). For example, in Mucessua, while economic marginalization intensifies the isolation of women and distrust during pregnancy and birth, dependence on male earnings keeps women under pressure to reproduce throughout their fertile years. Long-standing patterns of intrahousehold male dominance of monetary resources are supported by the control of women's sexual and domestic labor and the social constructions of women's mouths, vaginas/wombs, and homes as potential sources of reproductive threats and as targets of reproductive attack (Martin 1990). Horizontal and vertical female envy and the containment of women's reproductive bodies is also negotiated through the assigning, adopting, and defying of such stigmatized socially constructed female identities as witches (*uroya*), spirits' wives (*mukadzi wa mupfukwa*), and barren spinster ghosts (*zinyaumba*). Through these institutions, the control of women's reproductive bodies is both negotiated and contested, and women's reproductive vulnerability becomes manifest both bodily and socially (Marlins 2000).

As women navigate dangerous social and biological processes in their effort to demonstrate fertility and thus attain social womanhood, these conditions increase their perception that their reproductive capacity will be harmed and help explain the high rate of reproductive loss. In this setting, where limited resources restrict routes to female social and economic self-determination, "it is the moral value, not the truth value of risk claims that is crucial in shaping perceptions of risk and influencing health behavior" (Oaks and Harthorn 2003: 6).

The narrative of Mozambican women's reproductive agendas demonstrates how bodily experience of social threats not only shapes women's perception of maternal risk, but also informs their prenatal actions. These portraits also make it clear that anthropology, public health, and biomedicine need to expand the definition of risk to include not only embodied social risks, but also structural vulnerabilities that inform perceptions and limit choices. Examining how structural conditions generate and maintain the social suffering expressed through local risk discourses reveals systems of politics and power that institutionalize inequality at the local and broader levels, including systematic deficiencies in the health system (Barnes-Josiah, Myntt, and Augustin 1998).

Policy makers should not be blinded by constructions of economically and socially marginalized third-world communities as "traditional" and the blanket interpretation of "tradition" as static. Such discourse serves to "reinstate global imperial relations" in the domain of African health, reproduction and sexuality (Wekker 2006: 255). Far from being "traditional," these women's pregnancy beliefs and practices articulate contemporary expressions of distress and resilience in response to modern circumstances of social isolation and intensifying interpersonal and economic competition.

Safe Motherhood Initiatives to date have failed to account for these complexities of "abjection," to again use James Ferguson's term. Addressing the dissociation between biomedical constructs of risk and the idioms poor women use to construct individual and collective risk subjectivities requires the insights ethnography provides to map new sites for resource investments. Blaming tradition only mystifies the effects of this dissociation and obscures the "disparate, hybrid, messy on-the-ground phenomena" of reproductive health seeking on the margins. Plural health systems exist, and women are creatively using their options to minimize both social and biological risk. On-the-ground ethnography shows that maternal health initiatives must take this complexity and creativity into full and accommodative account to achieve viable improvements in reproductive care and outcomes. This insight will prove even more consequential as rising HIV/AIDS infection rates and the policy of universal AIDS screening during prenatal care in Mozambique delivers medical diagnoses that may confirm a new layer of vulnerability for already marginalized women and their families' social health and economic well-being.

CHAPTER 8

AIDS and the Politics of Protection

New Worries: Life along the AIDS Highway

Each time I have returned to Mucessua over the last ten years, it seems at first that very little has changed. There are still no paved roads or city plumbing, except in the older colonial houses along the Beira Corridor. The district's largest open-air market has moved west down the Corridor, but the *bazaar*, as it is called, and the individual market stands in the bairro look much as they have for the last fifteen years, with the same kinds of goods, though prices are a bit higher. But many changes, large and small, have crept steadily into Mucessua. On my most recent visit in September 2009, more cement houses were going up here and there, and the crumbling preschool with three walls where I held my first meeting with pregnant women has been replaced. The Gondola District Ministry of Education, impressed with the community women's initiative to improve the school structure over the years, has built an airy four-room primary school painted bright yellow and terracotta with shiny red waxed floors and new blackboards.

As I walk the dirt paths, I see that more people are raising small animals for sale or making bricks to sell or use to improve their homes. The district has extended electricity to some parts of the bairro, which has allowed many more households to pirate a line to their homes. Now, by night, along with the flicker of cookfires in the open air or winking through cooking-hut walls, single bulbs hanging in one or two rooms cast a cool glow in some houses and even a few of the market stalls. One of the broken bore-hole pumps has been repaired, so there are now three working public wells in Mucessua, one with a new spigot instead of a hand pump. More women are wearing shoes. People tell me more women are returning to school. For the first time since Independence, the Gondola district administrator is a woman, as is the prime minister.

However, the improvements are not widely or evenly spread. Rosinha and Marida agreed that change is something reserved for the lucky few. "[Life] is changing for those who are doing a little better already," Rosinha said. "We see some have cement houses, have electricity. Now, those of us who don't have, we are the same. That's how we are."

Marida agreed. "Um! Right now in the bairro, it is changing for others who have money. When you don't have money, it seems like nothing is changing. Now, for one that has money, it is changing for him. When you don't have money, nothing has changed. That's it."

The most relentless changes are the erosion of a familiar human landscape. After our greetings, friends begin our conversations by recounting each death they have experienced in the time between visits. The lists are longer now, and the patterns of loss are changing. Women have always lost infants and sometimes older children, but now more and more they name teenagers, fathers, brothers, and husbands as well.

In the circle of ten women who have come to meet with me at Dona Victoria's in September 2008, it was a time to take stock, mark the changes and mourn losses. Rather than starting with a FRELIMO party call-and-response cheer, community gatherings and meetings now more often begin with a hymn. After the women sing, Victoria starts a prayer, and then everyone joins in. There is a long period of collective oral prayer, each woman with eyes pressed tightly shut uttering a nonstop stream of thanks, praises, requests, more praises, and more thanks. Then the ten of us sit on the cool cement floor in Julia's new brick house. The front room has one table pushed to the wall and no chairs. In the corner of the room, a white chicken—powdered with the same fine layer of red dust that gets on everything—sits on a nest, two thin poles cut the same length and leaned against the wall as an open tent for protection while she sits on her eggs. I have brought rice flour cakes and butter from the bakery. The women have each contributed enough together to buy a palm-sized bag of coarse brown sugar, and Victoria has made tea. Marisa, Sara, and Sandra have brought precious store-bought ceramic cups and saucers from their homes so that Julia will have enough to add to her three to serve us all. As we sip our tea, a gray hen bobs cautiously into the room from farther inside the house and eats a few crumbs before leading her brood of six peeping chicks out the door into the sunlight.

I ask everyone what they think has changed most in the bairro since we started the prenatal care study in 1993, and over the last few years, especially. Around the circle, the women quietly chime in, each waiting her turn. Many reach back to touch on the end of the war, the time we met, and their pregnancy that I followed. Then they mark out time up to the present in lives born and lost, punctuated frequently by prayer and by the need for work.

Louisa: "After that child that you assisted, I gave birth to a baby boy who died. After that I had twins that lost their lives." Women have come to refer to me as the midwife to the cohort of children born to women who participated in the prenatal care research. "Then I had two more, so three children are left, but now the father of these died. These children that were born after your child have a different father. Your child now doesn't have a father and is suffering. There is no pick-up work nor do I have a trade or business. If I had some trade, that would be worth it. Now, without a trade or anything, I'm barely existing."

Adelia: "I see that things related to the church are developing. Since I gave birth to Magireta, I gave birth to Ervilha. I had two children with God's help. Now I am no longer able to give birth. I lost one male child. If there was work, those of us who can no longer go to cultivate our fields so far away, we would have work, and that would be a change!"

Ilda: "Change, perchance, has existed since 1991 up to today, that is to say, there are changes. For example, the child I had when you were assisting me was stillborn, but after four years I had two twins. I lost one, the other is alive and just turned ten, and another named Gelma, who is seven. Last year my father died . . . [a long silence while she blinks back tears] Another change that has occurred in the country and in Gondola, because in the time of the war, there was nothing, but we have seen that there is already a market opened, there is now something for people to do, only that it is not enough [work], because there are so many people and there is not enough with all these people. Now, we are asking if we could at least have something to give our children bread. These children we are having need a future. They want to study. Life is a bit expensive, so for this we are really asking that we could have something that we can put for the future, that is to say that more or less, that we see, I guess that is it."

Etelvinha: "Since we began with this group, my life has gone badly. I gave birth to three more children ages ten, eight, and six. My husband died just like that, and now my mother died. I am also church-going, so at home we are united and doing well as a family."

Odete: Since that year when you left me with that child named Chissaia, I ended up giving birth to two more children. These children are growing well, except that I was only bearing girls. The last one was a boy, so I saw that God had blessed me. My life is going well, but the year before last I lost my father, and last year I also lost my brother, who died in Zimbabwe. So I am home alone with three children."

Sara: "For me, my life is going reasonably. Since I gave birth to Rosa I have birthed four children. Two lost their lives. My father died, my brother died. Now, living is just such suffering I have. There at home I stay with Mama. Mama is already a very elderly person who needs sustenance, someone to sustain her. Since the brother that I lived with doesn't exist anymore, he already died; now her [mama's] living is just minimal. If we could get going on some projects, I could see how to relieve everyone."

Victoria: "I also give thanks to God. Since I bore Jose when you came to do those consultations, I have borne four children. After that, Jose and then my youngest brother died. For this, I give thanks to God for the protection he is giving us now."

Rosinha: "When we started this thing, I bore Steven. I started with him. Then I had a miscarriage of a boy. I became low in blood, as well. After that I bore another girl. After Steven, I had three and miscarried one time, only I became really weak in my body with problems of bones hurting and my head, problems with my teeth. But when I went to the hospital, they said it wouldn't do to pull them."

Marida: "Since we started with Dona Raquel, it is going well, only that, well, I bore four children. One died. My mother-in-law died, so we were alone. So we left the house where we lived to live where my mother-in-law lived. As such we are living well; there are no misunderstandings and the children God blessed me with are growing well. There is no illness besides my husband's illness. You see the marks on his face. Now, we don't know the causes. When he goes to the hospital, he is prescribed pills, but it doesn't end. Five years have already passed, and so that's how we are. He keeps getting sick, but when we met each other, it wasn't like this." My eyes had left Marida's face for a moment as I play with Victoria's baby boy, but when I look back as her voices wavers, I see she is also unsuccessfully trying to hold back tears.

There are some familiar faces missing from the circle of women, and Javelina reports that Jacinta's husband has died, leaving his five wives and their children to fend for themselves. Joanna's husband has also died. Anita Pedro's husband, then Anita, her mother, and her father-in-law have all died, I learn, of ceremonial tuberculosis or *pitakufa*, an illness caused by the improper treatment of ceremonies involving sexual relations that must occur after a death in the family to ensure the proper passing on of responsibility and property within families, and on other significant occasions. (Since *pitakufa* involves sexual contact between the widow and someone else in the extended family, often the deceased husband's older brother, it has become the focus of debate and concern as HIV infection rates rise.) Tiny Elena was shot by her husband. Four other women in the group I worked with have died over the last five years: Guida Thomas, Saramina, Iris, and Elisa Earnesto. Five children born during the first prenatal study have been orphaned and now live in the care of an older brother, a grandmother, aunts, and godmothers, but in miserable conditions. The women I meet with and find at home as I travel throughout the bairro are all keen to start a small project raising chickens to sell as a way to help support themselves and the orphans from the group. Is it politeness, delicacy, respect, fear? No one has mentioned SIDA (*Síndroma da Imuno-Deficiência Adquirida*, AIDS).

"Nothing is left of Lilia. She left no one behind," Javelina said softly as the two of us settled into the two uncomfortable wooden chairs at her new dining room table after several other women who had come to visit and catch up had left. She has saved this news of her goddaughter, but I doubt it is a secret in the bairro. A year ago, the room we sat in had sky for a roof and a dirt floor. The high walls, bars on the windows, and a padlock on the door had protected piles of bricks and stacks of zinc roofing sheets from robbers in the night. Now this large brick and cement addition to her two-room mud-and-pole house had a shiny waxed cement floor, and the zinc sheets were secured in place overhead. A smooth layer of unpainted cement covered what had been the open brickwork of the walls.

Javelina went on to describe how the parents of Lilia's suitor, Eusébio, had finally agreed to pay the amount of lobolo requested by Lilia's family. The young couple had settled in a small house in Mucessua with Ana, their first child, and then a second child, Solemão. During her third pregnancy, however, Lilia became increasingly sick. She gave birth, but within days the infant died. Weeks afterward, Lilia also died and her two young children both became chronically ill. Unable to cope alone, Eusébio moved back to his parents' compound with the sick children. One after the other, both children developed skin lesions, then other symptoms, and quickly died. Not long after the children's funerals, Eusébio also died.

"*Sentimentos*," I say. On the dirt road outside Javelina's window, I hear a rattling bike zoom by, then a knot of boys kicking a partly inflated soccer ball and an empty soda can, followed by a moment of rare quiet. After a long pause I ask: "What did people blame it on? What did they say?" Even though I choose my words carefully, I am uncomfortably aware that I am gossiping.

"Lilia's death is lamentable," Javelina answered. "That husband of hers went around trading women, and Lilia was the eighth. Between these [women], he had seven children. He got them each pregnant and then was obliged by their parents to pay lobolo. He paid lobolo and then went gathering up his children and sent them to his parents' home in his natal land in Gaza to the south. No one knows the situation of those children, if they are alive or not. And when he married Lilia, that man was already infected, and he was already doing treatment clandestinely in private clinics.

"Since going to stay in her husband's house, [Lilia] went around always sick. Following tradition, her family thought that it was sorcery sent by the other women. Lilia began to get sick after her third pregnancy; she gave birth, but after a few days the baby died. From there on, she did not get better. She became grave and her husband brought her back to her parents' house. He told his parents-in-law that Lilia shouldn't leave their house because she is a spirit's wife (*mukazi we muzimo*), and that this is what made her sick and caused the death of her child.

"The help her parents gave her was the following: fasting, prayers, accompanying her to the hospital. There, she did all the analyses, including the HIV/AIDS test. Results revealed she was HIV-positive. After one or two months passed, she lost her life. You know the rest. In sum, this was the story of our sister Lilia. If antiretroviral treatment had appeared earlier, she would not have died like that, our sister Lilia." Javelina had an amazing way of using just the right language to dignify every situation, and I felt a bit absolved by this short elegy for Lilia.

The Eye of the AIDS Epidemic in Mozambique

When I first arrived in Mozambique in 1991, during the period at the end of the war of destabilization between FRELIMO and RENAMO and the ceasefire, outside of colleagues in the Ministry of Health working in the HIV/AIDS sector, most people were not talking openly about SIDA. Tests were sporadically available as components of isolated research and NGO projects, but few people knew or had even heard of anyone who had AIDS. In the first Manica Province HIV/AIDS Knowledge, Attitude, and Practices (KAP) study conducted as part of my work in the Manica Ministry of Health in 1992, among the minority of people surveyed who had heard of SIDA, many expressed a belief that it was a European disease that could not affect Africans.

But since the mid-1980s, it had been widely recognized that the HIV/AIDS pandemic in sub-Saharan Africa was severe and getting worse (Fleming 1988). Little was known, however, about the gravity of the problem in Mozambique specifically; the first case of AIDS was reported there in 1986. In 1987, the first AIDS prevalence survey was carried out in several urban centers, recording an average prevalence of between 1.2 and 2 percent (UNAIDS 2008a). In 1988, as suspicion turned to panic, the Mozambique National AIDS Control Program (MNACP) was formed. With a lion's share of the international health aid earmarked for HIV/AIDS prevention by outside donors, AIDS prevention quickly became the focus of national health education efforts with an emphasis on community outreach, the production of communication, information, and education materials, and condom distribution.

Out of necessity, other health sectors became handmaidens to this expanding national focus. Program directors from the national to the district levels often had to contort their plans to link underfunded and struggling initiatives to address malaria, infant and maternal health, environmental health, and school and workers' health to the comparatively flush new HIV/AIDS agenda. Although the health system was still reeling from the effects of war, and there was no capacity at the national level for consistent HIV screening; an analysis of AIDS cases reported to the MNACP between 1986 and December 1991 documented the rapid annual increase in clinically diagnosed HIV/AIDS cases, and the rising co-occurrence of tuberculosis as the major opportunistic infection diagnosed among the AIDS cases (Fernandes, Vaz, and Noya 1992).

Of Mozambique's three regions—southern, central, and northern—the central region along the Beira Corridor, where Mucessua is located, continues to be hardest hit by the HIV epidemic (Epstein 2002). Throughout the years I worked in Gondola District, the Beira Corridor breathed life into the sluggish town of Vila Gondola. First, in 1991 it brought Zimbabwean troops in green camouflage personnel carriers like giant metal cockroaches sent by Mugabe to safeguard the Corridor and access for Zimbabwean goods to the Indian Ocean. Local people at times complained that the Zimbabwean soldiers were as exploitive as soldiers on both sides of the civil conflict had been. Blue and white UN peacekeeping patrols later replaced the Zimbabwean troops, their artillery aimed at the silent bush on either side of the road and at the stock-still civilians occasionally caught in the crosshairs of their automatic weapons. The first European UN contingent left in a cloud of scandal that included accusations involving alleged child prostitution. The European troops were soon replaced by Botswanan peacekeepers.

Under the protection of the UN convoys, some speeding freight trucks returned filled with cargo from Tete Province to the north and Malawi and Zimbabwe to the west. Fleets of four-wheel drives burgeoned, bought with foreign aid, their logos blurred in their hurry to help. Even some curious white tourists from Zimbabwe began to come across the Mozambican border at Machipanda, cautiously making their way to the port of Beira to see for themselves the toll that years of war had taken on their formerly idyllic coastal vacation spots. Ever present on the road were the run-down, rickety passenger taxis, trucks and minibuses called *chapa cem* (chapa, sign; cem, one hundred) after the one hundred meticais it once cost to buy a space aboard one of these transports. These assorted vehicles growled by, filled to overflowing with human and animal passengers, their hinges, tailpipes, doors, windshields, door handles, and hoods long gone.

Mucessua and other small bairros and villages huddled up to the sides of the Beira Corridor continue to serve as transit points, market hubs, and rest stops for commercial trucks and buses traveling from Zimbabwe, Zambia, and Malawi to Beira. Sometimes, traveling silently aboard vehicles carrying people who must journey long distances from their homes to work and find solace and company along the way, or people whose work is to provide solace and company for long-distance laborers, is the HIV virus.

During the war, refugees from the central region fled to neighboring countries, especially Malawi and Zimbabwe, where infection rates were already steep by 1990 (UNAIDS/WHO 2004).[1] The Ministry of Health proposed that the virus arrived in the central region at the end of the war in 1992, with the reopening of Mozambique's borders with its neighbors—all of which had higher HIV rates than did Mozambique itself (Agha, Karlyn, and Meekers 2001). Indeed, HIV transmission rates rose rapidly during that period, especially between 1993 and 1994, due to the repatriation of more than two million refugees and the return of some three million internally displaced people to their homes. Though controversial, it was also publicly speculated that elevated HIV rates among Zimbabwean soldiers guarding transport corridors in the central region contributed to high infection rates in the local population (Epstein 2002). Hospital and rural clinic beds began to fill with thin, coughing patients, all wasting, many with diarrhea, thrush, and skin lesions, some of whom came in and lingered, while others came in and quickly died. There was not much that health providers could do besides giving supportive care, antibiotics, antidiarrheals, treating TB and any other opportunistic infections they could.

By the mid-1990s, it was estimated that 8 percent of Mozambicans were HIV-positive, with the highest incidence still in the central region, along other transport corridors in rural communities with large numbers of male migrant laborers returning from South Africa and Zimbabwe (Epstein 2002), and in urban centers. Localities where any of these circumstances overlap continue to bear the greatest HIV-related disease burden. As rates of HIV infection among tuberculosis patients in Mozambique soared as high as 53 percent, depending on the region (Mac-Arthur et al. 2001), the alarmed MNACP predicted that the epidemic would peak by 1997. They further projected that by that time, the country would have 1,650,000 HIV-positive adults fifteen to forty-nine years of age, of whom 500,000 would have developed acquired immunodeficiency syndrome (AIDS), along with 500,000 AIDS orphans. However, the combined pressures of "extreme poverty, the social upheaval and erosion of traditional norms created by years of political conflict and civil war, destruction of the primary health care infrastructure, growth of the commercial sex work trade, and labor migration to and from neighboring countries with high HIV prevalence" continued to accelerate the spread of the HIV virus (AIDS Analysis Africa 1996).

As Mozambique had lagged behind its neighbors in the onset of the HIV epidemic, it has also lagged behind in slowing the spread of the disease. Mozambique was the only country in southern Africa that experienced an increase in prevalence during the surveillance period ending in 2005, according to the Demographic Health Survey in that year (Gouws et al. 2008), and it is still not clear whether the epidemic has reached its peak. With a current national HIV prevalence rate of over 16 percent and rising rapidly, and central and southern provinces registering even higher rates, Mozambique has one of the fastest-growing epidemics in Africa. One thing is certain: the end is not yet in sight.

Although the HIV/AIDS epidemic and national responses to it started later in Mozambique than in its neighbors Uganda, Malawi, and Zimbabwe, the government's response has been concerted. The mid-1990s saw the initiation of HIV/AIDS prevention, education, and community mobilization campaigns throughout the country. Programs included the free distribution as well as social marketing of condoms; peer outreach to sex workers, truckers, and other so-called high-risk groups; prison education (Vaz, Gloyd, and Trindade 1996); theater performances and radio/television programs; and the integration of sex education and STD/AIDS information in primary and secondary schools and university curricula by the Ministry of Education. Some companies distributed condoms to their employees (Mac-Arthur et al. 2001).

In 2001, another level of HIV prevention was initiated in the two central provinces of Manica and Sofala. Voluntary Counseling and Testing was established as a discrete program outside the health sector with freestanding HIV testing sites and a data-gathering system. Prevention of Mother-to-Child Transmission (PMTCT) services began in selected health centers where nurses already working in prenatal care clinics were trained to add testing, data collection, and counseling activities required by HIV screening to their workload. Both programs are prevention-only efforts based on public health research showing that people who get tested for HIV and meet with a trained counselor are more likely to protect themselves and others from spreading the disease. Clients also got referrals to appropriate HIV-related services.

It was not until 2003 that a national plan was rolled out for the national implementation, or "scale-up," of antiretroviral treatment (ART), with major funding and support from the President's Emergency Program for AIDS Relief (PEPFAR); the Global Fund to Fight AIDS, Tuberculosis and Malaria; the Clinton Presidential Foundation; and a range of other donors. In June 2004, Mozambique embarked on an ambitious plan to deliver free HIV care services, including ART, through the public-sector National Health System (NHS). With support for the NHS scale-up plan from international agencies and nongovernmental organizations, the number of people on highly active antiretroviral treatment (HAART) rose from approximately 4,000 in May 2004, to over 20,000 by January 2006, and to 80,000 by September 2007. By early 2009, nearly 130,000 people had started HAART (Pfeiffer et al. 2008).

In the central provinces of Sofala and Manica, the HIV prevalence rates of adults age fifteen to forty-nine are the highest in the country, at 23 percent and 18 percent, respectively (ibid.). Testing and treatment services in the two provinces have been put into place with technical and financial support from Health Alliance International, a US nonprofit affiliated with the University of Washington School of Public Health. HAART has been made available in forty-eight public-sector sites and integrated into primary health care services in these two provinces. By June 2006, 21,000 HIV-positive patients had registered in the treatment clinics and about 3,500 patients had initiated HAART in the two provinces. By September 2007, 10,000 people had been placed on treatment. Adherence has remained very strong (over 90 percent at most sites), and the flow of drugs has been maintained through public-sector systems. By December 2008, ART had been made available in sixty-seven public-sector sites and integrated into primary health care services. Nearly 154,000 HIV-positive patients had registered in the treatment clinics. Almost 30,000 patients have initiated ART across the two provinces, and 22,500 (75 percent) are still on treatment (Health Alliance International 2008).

These numbers are more impressive considering the time-consuming and arduous process that begins after an HIV-positive diagnosis. Following posttest counseling, HIV-positive pregnant women from the antenatal care (ANC) clinics and men and women tested at the Voluntary Counseling and Testing sites are referred to the hospital to undergo a prolonged initial assessment to determine whether they are sick enough to start antiretroviral (ARV) treatment. Clinical assessment involves a physical examination, laboratory tests including CD4 screening to monitor white blood cell levels, and a TB skin test. The first visit also includes a battery of behavioral/psychosocial, adherence, nutritional, and family/household support assessments, all to determine whether the individual has a constellation of living conditions and social support in place to maintain successful follow-through with the complex, as well as time- and resource-draining, drug regimens.

Although ART is ostensibly free for all Mozambicans who need it, the country has been plagued by stock outages and trained personnel shortages, especially pharmacists, laboratory technicians, nurses, and clinicians. When people cannot receive their medications at the state pharmacies, they go without or buy them for higher prices in private pharmacies or in the informal market without prescriptions and usually without prescribed amounts. To add to the challenges faced by Mozambicans living with HIV, even as ARVs have become more accessible and more affordable, securing adequate food raises daily challenges for the more than 50 percent of the population who live on less than a dollar a day (BBC News 2008). It is still more difficult for those who are HIV infected, who must eat well and regularly in order to tolerate the medications and their often toxic and painful side effects.

In September 2007, I sat outside the Beira HIV Voluntary Testing Center with a group of four men living with HIV who had become antiretroviral treatment (TARV) program activists after starting ART themselves. We talked about their work in the hospital assisting people to access HIV testing and to navigate the often-daunting antiretroviral treatment staging process.

Senhor Carvalho described his own experience getting tested for HIV and his struggle to adhere to his treatment regimen:

> When people come in to the hospital for other health problems and get help for that problem, they don't believe if they get tested, they really have HIV. They were not prepared to get tested. They are not ready to understand this *and* resolve the first health problem they came in with. It's too much. They move on until the next time, when they are sicker. People who find out they are HIV-positive when they are sick with something else and then get less sick when they are treated for that first thing are more likely to abandon treatment. People who don't get very sick are more likely to go back to their old ways of life no matter what they have been counseled.
>
> "Eat good foods," one is counseled. "Give up drinking and womanizing." TARV is like a church! You have to give up all your vices. You can't drink, smoke, even do drugs, commit adultery. And, you know, some people do not want to join a church. At least at a church you would get some prayers, someone would pray for you. But the hospital? Nothing but take away your life. Before, you have your vices. A [HIV] positive life is difficult. You start to miss your vices and feel you have been taken out of the world. I think isolation is the most difficult thing keeping people from following up with their treatment. Some people would rather die than have other people know. Once you feel better is when you usually abandon it.

When you consider that for people living with HIV/AIDS, this strict, new AIDS treatment "religion" will continue for the rest of their lives, it is not hard to see why many people here believe that if they learn they are seropositive, they will die faster, and that if they do not know, they will live a longer and healthier life. Yet, the arduous staging process and ongoing monitoring of people living with HIV/AIDS is of critical importance, since people who are put on ARVs too early and those who follow their drug treatment regimens only intermittently run the risk of developing resistance to affordable and available drug courses.

Pregnancy, Prenatal Care, and HIV
Prevention of Mother-to-Child Transmission

Across Africa, the efforts to build systems and implement programs to deliver accessible and affordable HIV/AIDS testing services and antiretroviral treatment since the early 2000s have been impressive. By 2008, the number of people on ART reached 3 million globally, the great majority in Africa, reaching over 30 percent of those in need. The prevention of mother-to-child transmission (PMTCT) of HIV has also been a key goal of these HIV-care program efforts. MTCT is the main source of HIV infection of children throughout sub-Saharan Africa (UNAIDS 2008b). An estimated 1.9 million children under fifteen are living with HIV in sub-Saharan Africa. Some 420,000 children were newly infected with HIV in 2007, and 290,000 died. Without intervention, the risk of an HIV-positive mother transmitting HIV to her infant is 20 to 45 percent—15 to 30 percent transmission risk in utero or at delivery, and 5 to 20 percent risk through breast-feeding (WHO 2004; De Cock et al. 2000).

Current evidence-based practice shows that short courses of ARV drugs started in late pregnancy or during labor can reduce the risk of in utero and peripartum HIV transmission two- to threefold (WHO 2004: 3). MTCT risk can be reduced to below 2 percent by interventions that include antiretroviral prophylaxis given to women during pregnancy and labor and to the infant in the first weeks of life, by obstetrical interventions including elective cesarean delivery (prior to the onset of labor and membrane rupture), and by breast-feeding cessation at six months (Dorenbaum et al. 2002; Cooper et al. 2002; Thorne and Newell 2004).

However, in many resource-poor settings where caesarean delivery is rarely available or safe (Buekens, Curtis, and Alayón 2003), PMTCT efforts have primarily focused on reducing MTCT during labor and delivery (Jackson et al. 2003; Guay et al. 1999; Petra Study Team 2002; Gaillard 2004), followed by the promotion of exclusive breast-feeding for six months, and then complete breast-feeding cessation. PMTCT programs are normally folded into, or linked to, existing antenatal care services. Core aspects of the services include the promotion of antenatal HIV testing and counseling, family-planning counseling, provision of an appropriate antiretroviral regimen for women and newborns, and support for safer infant-feeding options and practices (Lawn and Berber 2006: 113).

Recently, the Ministry of Health in Mozambique launched a national program for universal *opt-out* HIV screening of pregnant women as a core component of newly conceived "integrated" antenatal care services. Integrated antenatal care includes malaria screening, prophylaxis, and treatment for women, as well as screening for HIV/AIDS and other sexually transmitted infections. In opt-out screening, women are offered a number of tests that will be routinely given unless they refuse or opt out of any of them. The Mozambique PMTCT program promotes the delivery of free HIV counseling and testing for pregnant women attending antenatal care, free provision of AZT and nevirapine to prevent transmission during labor and during the postpartum period, and sustained follow-up of HIV-exposed children. By 2008, it was estimated that nearly 85 percent of pregnant women in Mozambique attended prenatal care clinics at some point during pregnancy, and HIV testing rates had risen to nearly 75 percent (>20,000 women). Of the 190 health facilities providing antenatal care services in Sofala and Manica,

168 (89 percent) are now offering PMTCT. HIV-positive pregnant women are also referred from antenatal care services to adult antiretroviral treatment clinics to register for further care and to place eligible mothers (women with CD-4 counts below 350) on antiretroviral treatment.

Lost to Follow-Up?

Alongside this effort, with its infusion of resources and major advances, new challenges have appeared. After nearly seven years of PMTCT expansion throughout Africa, several troubling patterns have emerged. Many pregnant women who test positive for HIV do not return for monitoring and treatment or soon drop out of treatment services, a circumstance labeled loss to follow-up. Major loss to follow-up occurs at each stage of the treatment cascade, from HIV screening and counseling in antenatal care, to institutional birth (where a single dose of nevirapine is given), and through postpartum child follow-up stages. Equally concerning is the significant loss to follow-up among HIV-positive mothers who are referred to antiretroviral treatment services but do not register at ART clinics, and the even greater loss to follow-up among mothers eligible for ART (based on a CD-4 count of <350) who manage to register at clinics but drop out before actually initiating treatment. Despite growing global support for PMTCT programs, less than 10 percent of pregnant women in Africa infected with HIV receive interventions to reduce MTCT, and only one in twenty mother-infant pairs is successfully initiating antiretroviral treatment (UNAIDS 2006a). Few PMTCT programs are able to reach mothers and newborns after discharge to provide support for the infant-feeding choices or to provide ongoing care and treatment (Lawn and Berber 2006: 113).

Loss-to-follow-up rates in PMTCT services vary but are unacceptably high in most sub-Saharan settings. A 2004 study in South Africa showed a loss-to-follow-up rate of 85 percent by the baby's twelve-month visit in health facilities in Johannesburg (Sherman et al. 2004); similarly, 90 percent of babies do not arrive at the health facility for their final HIV diagnosis in the South African province of Gauteng (Jones, Sherman, and Varga 2005). Data from Malawi in 2005 showed cumulative loss-to-follow-up rates of 55 percent as early as at the 36th week of pregnancy, 68 percent at delivery, 70 percent at the first postnatal visit, and 81 percent at the baby's six-month postnatal visit in rural district hospitals (Manzi et al 2005). Recent data from Kenya reveal high dropout rates as well: 31.5 percent are lost before women receive their HIV test results, 53.6 percent did not return to enroll at the HIV clinic, and 80.7 percent did not return for delivery.

When antiretroviral treatment (ART) first became available in Mozambique, HIV-positive pregnant women were referred to free-standing, off-site day hospitals for treatment, but in practice many drop out of the system before getting prophylaxis or treatment for themselves, their infant, or both. Few women came back after testing HIV-positive during a routine prenatal care visit to register at a day hospital for monitoring and treatment. Besides suffering very high loss to follow-up after testing, a very small proportion of mothers who do come back for monitoring and who are found sick enough to be eligible for ART succeed in actually initiating treatment, an even more discouraging development.

As in the rest of Mozambique, the PMTCT efforts in Sofala Province and Manica Province, where Mucessua is located, struggle with high rates of loss to follow-up. In 2009, of the 13 percent of pregnant women who tested HIV-positive during a prenatal care visit, only about 40 percent of those who were referred ended up arriving at the ART clinics to register for monitoring and begin treatment, if needed. Only a handful of that 40 percent who registered managed to start ART while pregnant. And only 25 percent to 29 percent of all HIV-positive mothers—received nevirapine during labor. Women continue to initiate clinical prenatal care late in pregnancy, and the institutional birth rate remains persistently low at about 60 percent in the two provinces. Despite efforts to improve access to pediatric ART, of all those receiving treatment, less than 10 percent are children.

A palpable sense of frustration, urgency, and inadequacy pervades many care providers who are quite aware of the need for ART and the gap in who is getting what they need. In September 2007, on a visit to Ponta Geia Medical Center in the city of Beira, I found Dra. Celia behind a stack of well-worn manila folders bulging with papers, reports, and charts. Dra. Celia was a newly minted twenty-eight-year-old doctor, the new medical director for this health center, the facility with the highest HIV prevalence rates in the country. The stack of charts formed a wall on her desk, blocking her from view of the door. As I entered, she peered over the pile, exhausted, but cheerful as I have always encountered her.

"Ola, Doctora," she greets me, with a beautiful shy grin. "I am doing my own research. I am looking for my babies. These are all my pediatric HIV exposure cases, but we have only a few in treatment." She points, momentarily glum, to the pile of two or three charts she has laid off to one side.

"What is your hypothesis?" I ask.

"Why aren't they getting into treatment? I wish I knew. Even though we have had trainings and gone over this with the SMI (maternal and infant health) nurses, I think they are only registering infants with test results rather than using the clinical protocols, and very few [infants] have those tests. I'm afraid most will die." We leave the piles and walk together through the maternity ward at the health center, the nurses barely hiding their exasperation at having to interrupt what they are doing for a child-doctor many years their junior who has recently become their boss and for another *estrangeira*. The current model for ART in Mozambique has been to build capacity with existing health personnel to take on new tasks related to treating and testing HIV/AIDS rather than developing a whole new cadre of health workers to take on this work. This means more and more work for the already beleaguered care providers. There is no budget for expanding personnel anyway, and even if there were, there are not enough trained personnel.

A Resocialized Framework for HIV/AIDS-Related Stigma

With only a trickle of HIV-positive pregnant women who need ARV treatment receiving it, and even fewer of their HIV-exposed infants, it is imperative to understand why pregnant women hide and stay hidden both before and after delivery. In this moment, it is more crucial than ever that health systems not fail the most vulnerable groups: impoverished women, those who depend on their labor and love, and those who will be born into the world dependent on these women. And yet, once again, this is exactly who is falling through the cracks.

Part of the exigency stems from the dual nature of this moment. On one hand, there is optimism about the real opportunity made possible by the expansion of PMTCT and ART services to the hardest-hit areas of Mozambique, like Mucessua, and elsewhere around the globe. On the other hand, those involved in this work feel trepidation, watching as the need for HIV/AIDS services continues to outstrip by far the capacity of underfunded government systems to provide adequate facilities, drugs, and personnel. With the stakes so high for failing to get HIV prevention and treatment services to women, many people are asking anew the questions I have been seeking to answer for more than ten years. Why are pregnant women disappearing from the system? Where are they going? What has been left out of the treatment picture? From pregnant women's and other community members' perspectives, where does ART fit into women's survival strategies, and what accounts for the lack of integration of AIDS testing and treatment into those strategies? What can be done to improve the situation?

As with the underutilization of prenatal care services by high-risk women, a range of hypotheses has emerged to account for the loss to follow-up of HIV-positive pregnant women in Africa. The problem is often framed as "service operations failure," focusing attention on health system and provider-related barriers at the clinic level. Proposed obstacles range from inadequate counseling, drug stock ruptures, and rude staff to authorized and unauthorized fees for services. There is strong agreement that the cascade of treatment obligatory in most PMTCT programs demands too many clinic visits. Appointments are often uncoordinated, with inconveniently separate appointments for mothers and exposed infants. Appointments for CD4 count measurements are frequently separate from clinical staging where patients get started on treatment. High turnover of health care workers limits patient-provider rapport and interrupts continuity of care (ICAP 2008). Poor pre- and posttest counseling have also been blamed for loss to follow-up, though little research documents the content and influence of different counseling formats and experiences in Africa (Sherman et al. 2004). Poor linkages within programs at the health facility (e.g., ANC, family planning, immunization, etc.) can also create obstacles to program follow-up and adherence. Institutional and structural barriers like the cost of transport and clinics distant from women's homes have been identified as salient barriers to women participating in PMTCT services (Pfeiffer et al. 2008).

Another group of hypotheses fuels ongoing discussions about shame and fear and much speculation about the role of stigma, discrimination, and other social and cultural factors in deterring women from accessing and adhering to ART and PMTCT programs. One study in Kenya found that major causes of loss to follow-up included fear of positive HIV results, chronic illness, stigma and discrimination, an unsupportive spouse, and inability to pay for the services (Moth, Ayayo, and Kaseje 2005). A recent qualitative study in neighboring Malawi came up with a similar list: fear of stigma, discrimination, household conflict, and lack of support from husbands (Jones, Sherman, and Varga 2005). Along the same lines, a recent qualitative study in Sofala Province focusing on maternal care for HIV-exposed children suggests that mothers may stop treatment for themselves and their infants for fear of losing spousal support and of social stigma and because of structural barriers, including lack of basic resources (Blanco 2009). In South Africa, socioeconomic and structural factors such as poverty, geographical relocation, and a lack of paternal support may affect the capacity of families to comply with the PMTCT follow-up program (Manzi et al. 2005). Recent research in Botswana has suggested that the most important consequence of participating in PMTCT was the difficulty associated with breast-feeding cessation. Women participants reported that using formula caused suspicion and prejudice in their local community (Eide et al. 2006).

Fear of discrimination certainly plays a role in how people respond to knowledge or suspicion of HIV infection in themselves and in others. As journalist Kwame Dawes wrote of HIV in his homeland, Jamaica: "[HIV] is one of the few terminal diseases that elicits the question, 'How did you get it?' If you are HIV-positive, everyone knows that you had sex, and it must have been with someone you shouldn't have had sex with or with someone who had sex with someone they shouldn't have had sex with. It suggests a background, values, a lifestyle—history, history, history" (Dawes 2008). Moral judgment and social discrimination have characterized responses to HIV since its early association with groups whose lifestyles were deemed responsible for their choice to expose themselves to HIV, for example, through homosexual partnering or drug use. This moral judgment and prejudice have been extended to whole countries hit hard by the epidemic and especially to the most vulnerable groups in those countries, including poor women. The relationship between AIDS, stigma, and discrimination has thus always been inseparable from narratives of denial and blame (Castro and Farmer 2005: 53).

But what is stigma? Though stigma and discrimination related to HIV/AIDS are frequently articulated within a human rights framework, concepts of stigma invoked in discussions of AIDS vary widely. Some AIDS scholars have claimed that exceptionally high levels of stigma, discrimination, and, at times, collective denial have been as great a challenge to overcome as the disease itself (Parker and Aggleton 2003: 13). Indeed, concern about the role that stigma played in impeding the prevention and now treatment of HIV/AIDS was voiced early in the emergence of the HIV epidemic (ibid.). There is growing intensity in the discussion about AIDS-related stigma, especially as the immensity of the work to scale up antiretroviral treatment lays bare the disappointing incapacity of systems and institutions to deliver treatment to people who need it the most.

The work of sociologist Erving Goffman has shaped much current thinking regarding stigma; Goffman conceptualized stigma as operating through the social enforcement of rules and sanctions that results in the "spoiled identity" of the person or groups concerned and a reduction in their life chances (Goffman 1963). This kind of cognitivist explanation often produces a personalized and individualized narrative of stigma as interpersonal misunderstanding, misinformation, and negative attitudes that lead to "individualistic modes of stigma alleviation" (Castro and Farmer 2005: 54).

Another limitation of this individualizing focus is that it draws attention to stigma as a socially transmitted condition and to the act of stigmatization as modifiable behavior. From this orientation, the aim of responses to AIDS-related stigma, discrimination, and hiding is often to promote stigma reduction, as if stigma, like a virus or other infection, can be stopped from moving through human vectors. Considered in this way, stigma could be treated independently from the continued existence of already stigmatized subject positions. Stigma as bad behavior becomes separated from the consequences of racialized, class, and gendered positions of such deep social and material marginality that people cannot afford personal or public knowledge of their AIDS status. When efforts at stigma alleviation place little emphasis on the larger contexts in which certain categories of people are stigmatized by others, they also become desocialized—that is, "decontextualized from larger social processes that are both historically rooted and linked to persons and processes that are not visible to the survey researcher" (ibid.: 53). Desocialized approaches avoid the economic policies that erode social safety nets, and the ways vulnerable populations pay the price with their bodies and respond in sometimes unexpected ways.

Some anthropologists have begun to critique this framework and propose scrutinizing stigma from a perspective grounded in concepts of power, dominance, hegemony, and oppression. When stigma is redefined not only as a product of uneven relations of power, stigmatization can be seen as a *process* by which hierarchies of social differences are reproduced and challenged, and power dynamics between differently situated social actors are mapped out and contested. In this conceptualization, stigma is less an experience of powerless outcasts than an expression of power "deployed by concrete and identifiable social actors seeking to legitimize their own dominant status within existing structures of social inequality" (Parker and Aggleton 2003: 18). These approaches begin the work of resocializing a framework that would help us understand HIV/AIDS-related stigma and its effects.

Working from this resocialized perspective, what might we make of the fact that in Mozambique, as in Malawi (Manzi et al. 2005), the dropout rate for women in the general antenatal services (with predominantly HIV-negative mothers) is similar to, if not higher than the dropout rate among HIV-positive mothers? This finding might alert us to the possibility that loss to follow-up is unlikely to be a PMTCT-specific problem but instead might reflect a general pattern within the clinic-based antenatal services (Manzi et al. 2005). Further analysis, however, might suggest that the barriers to women accessing hospital-based antenatal service precede the challenges posed by PMTCT services and have not been alleviated by the provision of specialized care for HIV-positive mothers. In most countries in sub-Saharan Africa, between 60 and 90 percent of all deliveries in rural areas do not occur in a hospital, but mostly with traditional birth attendants (Isenalumbe 1990; Walraven and Weeks 1999). Although institutional deliveries in Mozambique have increased on average from 44.2 percent in 1997 to 47.7 percent in 2003, a significant difference remains between urban (71.43 percent) and rural (28.6 percent) areas.

Perhaps we have been asking the wrong questions about loss to follow-up. A question like, "What accounts for the lack of integration of AIDS testing and treatment into women's survival strategies?" might be turned on its head to ask instead, "What kinds of survival do women envision and pursue that does not include accessing clinical services for HIV treatment?" What comes into stark relief is the *structural violence* of daily life—"large-scale social forces that . . . include racism, sexism, political violence, poverty, and other social inequalities that are embedded in historical and economic processes that shape the distribution and outcome of HIV/AIDS" (Castro and Farmer 2005: 54). Uncovering these dynamics means uncovering the dynamics of daily life that I have sought to document to make sense of the patterns in women's hiding and self-protecting, that is, building a structural violence conceptual framework for understanding AIDS-related stigma.

In September 2008, I sat in a meeting of eight women living with HIV in Isarda's sweltering two-room home in Macororo, a peri-urban bairro on the outskirts of Beira. The bare zinc roofing sheets seemed to intensify the white sun that beat down on us throughout the bright afternoon. Isarda, a twenty-five-year-old widow, is an activist working in a church-run program to locate, support, and when needed, assist HIV-positive pregnant women who have not returned after testing to access prevention and treatment services. She brought the group discussion to a halt when she described her struggle to make it as a single mother after losing her husband to HIV, and the torment of decisions she made around transactional sex as an HIV-positive woman: "If you want some help, some currency with a man, when you end up getting into it [sex], everything is secret. You can say a prayer hoping you will live, but it is very secret. We are hiding. Not everyone, but women, like men, conquer [pick up, seduce]. You have got to accept this, end up accepting this, and in this way we pass on the AIDS virus. There are other diseases, too, but you can't speak of it. It is difficult to talk, worse that I am talking . . ."

Her voice trailed off as she looked nervously around the group, and then began again fervently, challenging me, challenging everyone sitting in the circle. "[Women,] the married ones, widows, divorced, I'm telling you, they accept it . . . [long pause] Say what you will, but they end up doing it. [long pause] How are we going to end? We end up contaminating him around this, and it is a secret. A thousand times, it is with the married men. They know how to prevent [HIV infection], but you cannot tell him to or he goes away with his money. He wants it skin against skin. This happens a lot."

Everyone remained silent for what felt like a long time. When the conversation began again, it moved quickly in another direction and did not return to this theme, but no one disagreed. Isarda had made it clear that we cannot look at HIV-positive pregnant women's loss to follow-up without considering the social position of poor women in general, especially poor women with the added weight of living with HIV. Whether measured in secrets, sickness, desperation, loss of dignity, or death, women's vulnerabilities have always told the story of the inabilities of households, communities, and nations to guarantee the basic components of life to its members: food, water, shelter, work, and peace. Women must often bear the burden of these failures and strategize within these constraints (Leclerc-Madlala 2008).

To understand loss to follow-up among pregnant HIV-positive women, then, means paying attention to the vulnerability of all women and the gendered community dynamics of social distrust, competition, and survival. Interpretations of stigma must be informed by the lived experience of those who suffer from it.[2] It means taking into account women's agency as they navigate their own vulnerability by hiding HIV status *and* pregnancy to protect themselves from further vulnerability in the nova vida that has left so many women without economic options and social protection. Women's use of a wide range of non-clinic-based prenatal care options is *transformative labor* that reflects deliberate decisions to protect their pregnancies from social, spiritual, and economic threats that assail them in the nova vida, where HIV risk constitutes yet another level of women's reproductive vulnerability. These strategies have become markedly gendered in more ways than one, for while health care providers wring their hands as they lose track of pregnant women who have tested HIV-positive at enrollment of ART and PMTCT programs and at delivery, this population of women is not lost: they are hiding, and many can be found—in churches.

Transformative Labor: Prophets, Prayers, and the New Politics of Protection

The same impoverished peri-urban communities in Manica and Sofala Provinces where HIV prevalence is highest, and where HAART is now available, have witnessed a rapid ascent and expansion of Pentecostal and African Independent churches (AIC, Zion, Apostolics) over the sixteen years since the end of Mozambique's civil conflict. In some bairros, church membership has grown from an estimated 10 percent in the early 1990s to more than 50 percent. A majority of these new converts are women in the lowest economic stratum. Since the current HIV/AIDS epidemic had not yet made a major impact in the region where church expansion gained its full momentum in the early 1990s, it is unlikely that the church growth is a response specifically to the AIDS crisis (Chapman and Pfeiffer 2008). However, high HIV prevalence and church expansion are certainly entangled, since many of the same social processes fuel both—urbanization, rapid economic change, impoverishment, land alienation, and deepening social inequality. The intersection of church participation and HIV/AIDS is likely to be more direct and complex as the epidemic grows, further underscoring the urgency to understand how churches influence community responses to HIV/AIDS, and why women especially are flocking to churches.

Besides finding lively worship communities, church members find women's groups, tithing, visits and prayer for those who are sick at home, communal gardens, and most importantly, a range of healing techniques for which they are not asked to pay a fee. The most consistent conversion narrative I have heard over the years is of destitute women with reproductive health problems, especially infertility or multiple infants deaths, and women unable to cope with their own or their children's' chronic illness, who had sought treatment from the hospital as well as curandeiros to no avail. Many identify themselves as *mulheres d'espiritos* (wives of spirits). In an attempt to escape the endless cycle of fees and indebtedness acquired while seeking treatment with curandeiros, these women described finally seeking solace and succor in one of the local churches, especially churches that feature the gift of prophecy under the inspiration of the Holy Spirit. This decommodification of healing attracts many members to the independent Zionist churches in Mucessua. While other independent and mission churches offer the material advantages of extended social networks and supposed healing powers of their leaders, there are significant parallels between prophets and traditional Shona spirit mediums. Important ritual similarities exist in both diagnosis and treatment (Chapman and Pfeiffer 2008).

The strongly patriarchal and strict, socially conservative moral codes espoused in church discourses condemn the sex work and transactional sex that are most poor women's primary source of survival (Leclerc-Madlala 2008). Yet a woman's joining a church may help keep people from suspecting, or at least from accusing, her—as an unpartnered woman, an untraditionally partnered woman, or a woman with multiple partners—of being a prostitute or a witch. This is yet another level at which economic austerity amplifies patriarchal repression and control of women (Tsikata and Kerr 2002).

Women are going to churches for social protection, for the "direct face-to-face reciprocities to get things done" that occur among family and neighbors in times of need. Hydén has called this informal and largely invisible political economy the "economy of affection" (Hydén 1980, 2006). This thriving church economy of affection fits Hydén's definition of informal parallel institutions created to provide a buffer from the whims of the market and protection from falling into the wide gap left by the weakened and fettered arms of the state under current neoliberal economic policies (Hydén 2006: 72). The emerging churches in Mucessua institutionalize informal "personal investments in reciprocal relationships with other individuals as a means of achieving goals that are seen as otherwise unlikely to attain" (73). As has been noted in other African settings, in the context of deepening poverty, people's ability to support others diminishes to the point where affective networks break down (MacLean 2003). Through churches, women are able to recollectivize self-help in ways that can change the odds for those at the limit of their social and economic resources. This is no small matter in the nova vida, where social and political relationships have become permeated with a fundamental social logic of *cada um para cada um*, each one for each one, that has eroded both vertical kin and lateral nonkin social interactions.

It is here that sorcery returns as a third strand interwoven in the relationship between church membership and HIV. As I have shown, pregnant women who become chronically sick fear most that they have been the target of sorcery or witchcraft. As people explained, sorcery is born of the hate that comes not so much from destitution as from longing, exclusion, envy, and secrets. The harm attributed to sorcery is animated especially by the hate that leads to murmuring, murmuring, murmuring, the conjuring of ill will into being through verbal repetition, palpable to those vulnerable to it and poisonous to the target and to the source. To be murmured about literally makes people ill at ease. Hate makes people seek ways to poison others—their water, their food, their reputation, their social network, their family ties. People who have something that you do not must have used illicit means, like sorcery or personal witchcraft powers, to get more than you. People who hate you for what you have gained are capable of wanting to harm you. All this hate and longing and the wish to steal—the definition of acquiring things without working, in this case magically—is where witchcraft and sorcery come in. As the women in Victoria's living room explained to me, "sorcery is never-ending," Adelia's answer when I asked whether sorcery continued to be as much of a problem in Mucessua now as it had been in the past.

Ilda: It will always exist, because what causes sorcery is hate.

Adelia: If you say that sorcery exists, it is because sometimes you say to someone, "You, you, wait and see [what will happen to you] or my own daughter will die." Isn't that sorcery? It exists!

Rachel: But why, normally?

Javelina: Hate.

Ilda: Hate.

Rachel: Hate over things? Over life? What, concretely?

Ilda: In life, the case that makes sorcery never ending is hate. To see a person, because people are all different and everyone struggles in his way to better his family. And so, there is someone who also has their own way of struggling just like you, so it doesn't preoccupy you until that other guy over there, for example, builds a house, is eating normally. So I, who don't have this, am going to say, "What's the point? Just look at them! Ah! Hey, these are white people, these are, ah! It's not fair, these have and these [have], but no one else has." And so, from there is when it creates that rancor—that one is passing us by, this one is getting ahead of me, and this is the one who is doing it to me. When actually, no. But, from then on is when this thing gets into your nerves and, pronto, when you want to do these things, it's when you do it.

Rachel: So it is the person who hates that is going to "treat" the other person [with sorcery]?

Ilda: Some person might try to improve the relationship, but another, pronto, it gets on their nerves that you are overtaking me, and at times thinks, "He doesn't want to give me something; now that he already has, he doesn't want to give me some, too." But it becomes difficult when someone, for example, goes with plates of food to give someone without him saying, "Why are you giving this to me? What did you hear?" It becomes difficult, and that is when sorcery is born because he is always going to have [those thoughts] stay with him. He will be murmuring and murmuring, murmuring. And so where a person murmurs [passing on names of whom to harm to a feitiçeiro], we Africans are different, each one has his source, different than others.

Rachel: But can this actually hurt the other person, or doesn't it work these days?

Ilda: It could kill. It works, yes. It can actually kill. You can die from sorcery. In Africa this exists!

Rachel: Well, the last question, I only have one more, I don't know, unless anyone else has another one . . . but at that time [referring to the study that ended in 1998], it was said that when the problem for many women of losing a child, the pregnancy not going well, these were really spiritual things . . . but . . . I don't know . . . if people still have such experiences? . . . So . . . to confront this, people have to also go get a sorcerer? Or what ways are there now?

Ilda: For this [fear of sorcery] there are already many forms. Now people are already inclined more towards the church, that God, as he is more powerful, who made everything on land as in the sky, so let us beg God to see if he will defend us from these types of situations. Plus, in the church there are also other organizations that everyone that belongs to the church tries to do something to not be stopped, just looking at someone who is doing something. Now, we all need to dig in. For example, if there is a sewing project going, a small business and savings, and all the churches in that organization get moving that along, it is to make it understood that to diminish this type of person that only sits and says, "I don't have anything."

And so, no one needs to just sit around. We all must preoccupy ourselves to make sure that [pointing to me] Aunt Rachel has a little, Aunt Sara has a little, everyone has a little. And so, this is to avoid this thing, this endless path of looking at someone and thinking, "This person does not want to give to me." For this reason, many people are now inclined towards the churches. They get support from the Holy Spirit and also this thing of raising a little money to support those people who have nothing. If you don't join a church, you are simply left behind, left out.

Victoria: It [sorcery] is happening. Spirits exist, only no one follows this due to religion. Others really are suffering with spirits at home.

Rachel: How so?

Victoria: In the churches, they pray whether you enter there or not. Then you enter and say, "I want to know how it is, all this I've been hearing about." Then, when you get there you say, "This [seeking help from a curandeiro] in my life, this is not working for me. I tried, but just spent money [on a curandeiro]." At times, a person dies spending money [on traditional healing] and that doesn't work, not like when you go to church. So this is what is helping people. Spirits really exist. That's it.

Javelina: You're finished?

Victoria: I've finished.

Javelina: But what happens when you present yourself at church?

Victoria: The pastors help you, like when they tell you the program. You

might be told that the program is to fast, and so you are given a certain
number of days doing it, and seeing what it is that God will help you in
your life. This is what pastors do to help us, and this is their work. When
you inform the pastors, they inform you that "I have this program that
I am doing in my house," and so they are going to tell you, "Enter this
program and let's see what God will do for you."

Later, in private, Beatrice explained that she had converted and joined
a Pentecostal African Assembly of God Church because she had finally received the results of her HIV test, and she knew her family could not afford her funeral. When Julia's son, Alberto, had become chronically ill with
respiratory infections she suspected were a result of feitiço, she sought out a
prophet who had prescribed a two-month course of weekly enemas for the
boy without charging her. I told Julia I found this course of action deeply
worrisome, but she could not be dissuaded. Before Alberto's treatment was
complete, she had joined the church and was bringing gifts and working in
the communal church fields where produce was being grown to deliver to
church members who were bedridden with chronic illness, including HIV/
AIDS. Working independently or through programs often run by NGOs,
churches have also been the source of the bulk of nonfamily home-based care
for people living with HIV/AIDS in Mozambique. When neither the state
nor, in many instances, households are able to fulfill their role as primary
redistributive mechanisms, and in the absence of the support of a partner
with emotional and material assistance, these are all key elements in drawing
in women to the myriad churches that have mushroomed throughout the
bairro over the last two decades.

In spite of their vitality and reach, these churches have largely been left
out of the national conversation on AIDS, and have not yet been systematically included in any mobilization efforts around AIDS in the country.
The scale-up of HIV/AIDS treatment offers the potential for collaborative
efforts to encourage church members to get tested and treated, and opening up a broader discussion about AIDS within these congregations. There
must certainly be a new or renewed dialogue with churches as autonomous
and lively community institutions that are playing a major if largely unacknowledged role in the survival of the most economically marginalized
communities.

The dialogue that is possible between people in health care and emergent
Pentecostal and African Independent churches in Mozambique has shifted,
now that prevention, and particularly the use of condoms, is not the only
point of entry and inevitable contention. The presence of testing and treatment services could help realign healing discourses from the churches with
the goals and efforts of the health system. However, there is a wide range
of responses from churches to this particular moment—from churches that

prohibit the use of any health services and cast out openly HIV members on one end of the spectrum, to churches whose leadership has come out as HIV-positive and modeled both testing and treatment practices to their followers on the other. Because of this diversity, there is no room for generalizations, complacency, or one-size-fits-all approaches to faith-based outreach and partnerships.

Much more attention, however, must be paid to this growing social force, for as Hydén and others have suggested, "the failure to recognize the prevalence of the economy of affection and its robustness in Africa compared to formal institutions is one of the biggest—if not *the* biggest—challenges to scholars and policy analysts alike; . . . if we wish to understand—and explain—what happens on the scene in Africa, informal institutions must be given the highest priority (Hydén 2006: 73; see also Chabal and Daloz 1999).

It is most important not to mistake these growing institutions as substitutes for an adequate health and social system. While churches may keep those who are sinking "barely floating," they are no substitute for the social security system of the modern welfare state (Hydén 2006: 76).

New Commons: Continuity and Change on the Margins

How can health care providers take into account these issues of secrecy and security? Women in Mozambique need access to confidential reproductive health care in a facility that is not separate from other forms of health services in the clinical setting. Prenatal services based on assumptions that the greatest threats to reproduction are physiological processes, and not social and economic relationships, are inadequate to address women's needs for safe motherhood in an environment of intensifying social inequality and increasing pressure to bear children. What I watched unfold daily in women's lives suggests that the mere provision of prenatal care services may not be enough to reduce reproductive risks for the most socially and economically marginalized, since this vulnerability may prevent women from using available services.

While key modifications in maternal health care programs are essential to improving Safe Motherhood in Mozambique, women's reproductive vulnerability ultimately lies beyond the scope of medical or even public health solutions alone (Turshen 1994). Those who need them most may continue to underuse health services designed to ensure Safe Motherhood for women in Mozambique as long as women remain without economic security, education, and access to services that reduce their social and economic marginality.

These insights will prove even more consequential as rising HIV/AIDS infection rates and the policy of universal HIV/AIDS screening during prenatal care propagate medical diagnoses that are likely to further threaten the fragile claims on safety of marginalized women and their families' already vulnerable social health and economic well-being. Women's social vulnerability is conditioned by their extreme economic insecurity; specifically, women are dependent on others for access to cash and on the life that monetary exchanges both permit and necessitate.

What can we take away from paying attention to the lived details of this moment of opportunity and danger that crystallizes in the reproductive "responses and resistances" of women on the "rough edges" of social and economic life under neoliberal capitalism (Hodgson 1997: 111; Hydén 2006: 72)? What can we learn about what needs to be done? It is not enough to identify this vulnerability, to describe its quality, effects, and textures; not enough to point out that social vulnerability is a core dynamic of modernity. As an unprecedented if inadequate amount of resources flows from the global North to the global South, there is something that we can do now. With these resources and the kind of collective political commitment expressed in the Millennium Development Goal on HIV/AIDS—to halt and reverse the spread of the epidemic by 2015—this is the time to help rebuild the social safety nets that the politics of abandonment have destroyed in much of the world over the last several decades with harrowing results.

Universal Access

Halting and reversing the spread of the HIV/AIDS epidemic by 2015 will require far greater access than is currently available to HIV prevention services and AIDS treatment, care, and support. On December 23, 2005, the UN General Assembly adopted a resolution requesting UNAIDS and its cosponsors to assist in "facilitating inclusive, country-driven processes, including consultations with relevant stakeholders, including non-governmental organizations, civil society and the private sector, within existing national AIDS strategies, for scaling up HIV prevention, treatment, care and support with the aim of coming as close as possible to the goal of universal access to treatment by 2010 for all those who need it" (UNAIDS 2009). "Universal access" is the phrase that has been coined to express the magnitude of the task involved in creating conditions under which all people who need them have access to information and services that are equitable, accessible, affordable, comprehensive, and sustainable.

In June 2006, in signing the Political Declaration on HIV and AIDS, UN member countries worldwide unanimously committed to setting ambitious national targets for scaling up universal access to HIV prevention, treatment, care, and support by 2010. The targets focus on what could be achieved if the following obstacles can be addressed:

predictable and sustainable financing; strengthening human resources and health systems; access to affordable commodities; and stigma, discrimination, gender and human rights. Although the Declaration does not clearly address some of the root causes of HIV transmission—including work targeting injecting drug use, sex work and sex between men—it represented undivided accord on fundamental matters associated with improving planning, financing and implementation of a strategic, long-term global response to AIDS. (UNAIDS 2006b)

A significant part of this work will involve improving PMTCT/ART services for women, reduction of visits through integrated and centralized ART and PMTCT services, and increasingly the provision all PMTCT services as part of quality comprehensive women's health and ART programs. These improvements, however, can occur only within the context of strengthening overall primary health care systems. At this moment in time, the gaps in services to people living with HIV/AIDS are irresolvable without major improvements in health systems, especially the provision of adequately trained and compensated health workers.

Social Protection

Strengthening the health system, while essential, will not address the other problems I have been describing. Major public-sector resources must be channeled to restore and create basic social safety nets that have been eroded over the last decades through policies of economic restructuring and greed. These safety nets could come in the form of social protection models that might provide cash transfers for people living with HIV/AIDS and other chronically vulnerable populations. There have been promising results from Ethiopia (Brandstetter 2004) and elsewhere (Meyer 2007) with the use of cash transfers, cash vouchers, food coupons, or some combination of these. Recently, Mozambique has begun the process of putting in place such a program.

There is no mystery about what is needed to improve women's and infants' health everywhere: large-scale investment in public-sector social programs and safety nets to ensure the economic survivorship of all communities, from subsidized food, clean free water, decent housing, and universal free health care to education, especially for girls and women, adequate access to land, and a toxin-free environment so that people can feed themselves and their children, meaningful work, and protection of workers and workers' rights, including living wages.

This is not work to be done by foreign entities that have as their explicit or default mission the role of substituting for the state. I am proud of the work of organizations like the one I have worked for during these past years, Health Alliance International, or like Partners in Health, which work hard to maintain emancipatory objectives by addressing basic needs and rights to food, water, health care, education, information, and self-determination. However, our most important role may be as valued allies in ongoing advocacy and activism that address the inequity by which African nations pay debts to the very nations that participated in colonization and continue to benefit from neocolonization, the ongoing unequal terms of trade and labor, and the commoditization of natural resources, including labor—a new politics of protection. Through such a new politics of protection we can support "bottom-up activism and critiques from Africans" themselves as to what next steps are required and how we can best partner, following their lead (Bond 2007: 189).

There are signs of this growing bottom-up, grassroots movement and seeds of this "blessed unrest" (Hawken 2007) all across the continent. From a farmer's jury in Mali voting against allowing genetically modified crops into the country, to the youth takeover of oil rigs on the Niger Delta, to the hundreds of university student strikes and demonstrations against Structural Adjustment in cities across Africa, to growing demands by Africans for "reparations for the theft of life, liberty and property during colonialism (which, by the way, is not an ancient phenomenon since most of the countries of Africa were 'decolonized' between 1960 and 1975)," to name just a few examples of an African antineoliberal globalization movement waged since the mid 1980s, long before the Battle for Seattle (Caffentzis 2002).

In Mozambique there are also signs and seeds of this grassroots struggle, from the groups of Mozambican subsistence farmers who traveled in 2001 to Cochabamba, Bolivia, to participate in the People's Global Action meeting as part of a transnational movement to resist privatization of water and other basic resources, to Mozambique's role in contributing to and hosting a screening of the 2009 Non-Competitive Documentary Film Festival and Social Cinema, whose purpose was to promote justice, equality, and social inclusion, the defense of human rights and nondiscrimination, the free exercise of active citizenship, organization, and political participation, the right to free expression, environment defense, and sustainable development.

There is grassroots struggle, from the ongoing solidarity between Canada's Steelworkers Union and Mozambique's National Union of Construction, Wood and Mine Workers, and National Union of Security Guards and the participation of Mozambican activists in Canada's International Labour Research Information Group Globalization School to Mozambique's rejection of Monsanto's genetically modified corn seed in 2002.

The power of grassroots struggle can also be witnessed in the sit-ins staged in 2008 by people living with HIV/AIDS when the provincial Ministry of Health in Manica threatened to shut down free-standing day hospitals delivering HIV/AIDS treatment services. There are churches in Mucessua filling with poor women who cannot and will not pay for health care treatments, leaving the curandeiros and fee-for-services clinics behind. This is blessed unrest.

In September 2008, on my last evening in Mucessua, I stood on the site where I had held my first prenatal care community meeting and where the women had built and rebuilt the preschool after every rainy season, each time a wall or two of sun-baked bricks washed away. Before I left in 1998, I had assisted with purchasing roofing material and kiln-baked bricks for the annual reconstruction. Now we stood, ten years later, in front of the beautiful new primary school. Etelvinha, Rosa, Ilda, Rosinha, Beatriz, Marida, Sara, Adelia, Victoria, Louisa and Javelina were saying goodbye in the fading light as I waited for my ride. Nearby a few women pumped water from the well for the evening chores. A large group of children played and sang in the darkening classrooms of the school.

"So you must be very proud of bringing this school into Mucessua because of your hard work," I said.

"Ahh, nada, Dona Raquel," Ilda shakes her head impatiently. "The school is all well and good, but we women are still suffering here in Mucessua, and we need a clinic for women right here in the bairro. If we women can get the government to build a school, we can get them to build a clinic. When do we start?"

Adelia added, laughing and upbeat: "Women are directing things now. We are no longer oppressed. We unite and stand up, because long ago we were oppressed. Now, we women, when we are three or four of us, we are really going to do this."

Looking straight at me, unsmiling, Ilda asked again, "When do we start?"

Notes

Chapter 1

1. Shortly after Mozambique won independence from Portugal in 1975 through a thirteen-year war, fighting broke out again. FRELIMO, the political party formed to fight for independence from Portugal, had won the support of many Mozambicans by forming agricultural cooperatives and improving access to and quality of education and health care. Interested in Mozambique's natural resources, and alarmed by FRELIMO's compliance with UN sanctions against Rhodesia, the white minority regime of South Rhodesia, later joined by the apartheid regime of South Africa, set out to destabilize the young country, an effort that led to sixteen more years of warfare. In 1982, South Africa increased its involvement to block Mozambique's support for resistance against apartheid in South Africa, targeting and maiming civilians, including children, and the social infrastructure (*c-r.org/our-work/accord/mozambique/historical-context.php*).

2. A *bairro*, Portuguese for "residential neighborhood," in Mozambique refers to an informal peri-urban sprawl, with houses constructed of wood, reeds, mud, tin, or cement.

3. An around-the-corner woman is a girlfriend, mistress, or prostitute who waits for her boyfriend in an out-of-the-way location, thus around the corner.

4. Useful for health workers, clinicians, and others involved in primary health care delivery and health promotion programs, Werner's manual provides practical, easy-to-understand information on how to diagnose, treat, and prevent common diseases. Special attention is focused on nutrition, infection and disease prevention, and diagnostic techniques as primary ways to prevent and treat health problems.

5. During follow-up research in 1998, women in Mucessua made even more accusations that the underpaid nurses at the maternity clinic demanded under-the-table fees to ensure attentive treatment during delivery and postpartum. Women who could not pay were left to give birth alone or mistreated. Informants reported that a particular nurse had been summoned three times before the district tribunal but acquitted of accusations of killing infants of women who could not pay the bribe demanded. Not enough data were gathered to substantiate these rumors; however, their persistence suggested that the commodification of childbirth extended to the formal sector and that women without any access to cash would be trapped between these two potentially predatory systems, leading to the emergence of new birthing practices. Preliminary data collected during the follow-up year suggests that Pentecostal and African Independent churches offering maternity services may attract women who feel unsafe with both home and hospital childbirth. Also see Pfeiffer, Gimbel-Sherr, and Augusto 2007.

6. The names of these nurses are pseudonyms. I refer to all other health personnel by their real names.

7. Abortion is illegal in Mozambique, except in extreme cases when the mother's life is endangered. However, the interpretation of the law has become less restrictive, and

abortions are available on request in a number of hospitals, where doctors have encouraged women to seek medical help rather than use clandestine methods (see Agadjanian 1998; see also Machungo et al. 1997).

8. The SMI strategy adopted in Mozambique encompasses short- and long-term goals of upgrading all levels of care within maternal health services, including: domiciliary deliveries by traditional birth attendants; primary care—family planning, postpartum consultations, maternity deliveries; secondary care—communication and transport, waiting hostels, surgically equipped hospitals; and epidemiologic monitoring (Povey 1990).

9. Although the scope of benefits accrued by routine prenatal care for all women is currently being debated, both researchers and health care providers agree that various components of prenatal care services have been associated with positive pregnancy outcomes for both mother and infant. No prenatal care, as well as late initiation and inadequate number of prenatal care visits, are associated with negative pregnancy outcomes in some cases, including increased maternal and infant mortality.

10. This core element of the Mozambican Safe Motherhood Program is based on WHO's risk approach (WHO 1978a; WHO/UNICEF 1980). Beginning in 1980, a pregnancy control form for health personnel to fill out during initial prenatal examinations was introduced in prenatal clinics throughout the country "to monitor pregnancies and to help direct specialist care to mothers at greatest risk" (Jelley and Madeley 1983: 111).

11. The discussion that follows relies heavily on Crehan's *Fractured Community* (1997); page numbers in parentheses in the text that follows refer to this work unless otherwise noted.

12. I use the term "reproductive loss" to refer to miscarriage, perinatal deaths (stillbirth to seven days postpartum), and infant deaths (one week to one year postpartum). Deaths of infants up to the age of one are included in this category because women believed death of a nursing or weaning-age child to have a negative impact on one's future fertility, a serious threat to conception, pregnancy, and reproduction (Chapman 1998).

Chapter 2

1. A military commander in FRELIMO, Machel (1933–1986) assumed leadership after the assassination of Eduardo Modlane. As a fighter and a leader, he was committed to getting rid of colonial rule and Portuguese settlers, and to transforming society. He died in an airplane crash whose cause is still undetermined. His widow, Graça Machel, later married Nelson Mandela.

2. For in-depth discussion of land use in Mozambique, see Tique 2002 and Hanlon 2004 on the 1997 Land Law and recent land debates.

3. After the failure of the "people's" farms, the government sought other means to increase productivity. In 1980, a *Gabinete de Zonas Verdes* (Green Zones Cabinet) was established to provide administrative and technical support to both cooperative and private farms within the Green Zones. Administratively attached to the Maputo City Council, the Cabinet was also a part of the Ministry of Agriculture (MOA) and worked through the seven MOA agricultural centers located throughout the Maputo area. These centers were designed to offer technical assistance through the services of extension workers and provision of transport, seeds, fertilizer, and the like. The new Green Zone initiative was developed in response to the government's decision to provide greater support to small production units in order to meet the critical need for food in the cities. From the start, however, it was stressed that the project would take a "self-help approach" that would "encourage cooperative workers to regard the results as a fruit of their own work rather than a free gift" (Ayisis 1985).

4. Unless otherwise noted, all translations are to or from Portuguese. I indicate Shona, Tewe, or Ndau terms by "Sh.," "Tewe," or "Ndau."

5. Local justice tribunals were set up throughout Mozambique following Independence in

neighborhoods of the urban areas, in communal villages, and in localities. These tribunals handle problems relating to the family and between families, as well as petty offenses, and are empowered to impose small fines and other limited penalties. In precolonial times this role was played by male chiefs or councils of elders. No official policy stipulated that women be included on these tribunals, but each court in Mucessua had at least one woman member.

6.   With the exception of my research assistant, Javelina Aguiar, all the names of women in Mucessua are pseudonyms.

Chapter 3

1.   See Beach 1980: 88–89 and Bourdillon 1994: 3–6 for discussion and critique of the sources of Shona history. Focusing on Holleman, an influential anthropologist of Rhodesia and Zimbabwe, Donald Moore (2005) has more recently traced and critiqued the role of colonial anthropologists and their analytics and agendas in supporting colonial rule in the region.

Because detailed ethnographic descriptions of Mozambique Shona groups of the Chimoio-Sussundenga peneplain region are rare, the primary sources of Shona ethnography and ethnohistory, including Mozambican groups, are ethnographic and historical accounts of Zimbabwean Shona groups: Beach 1977, 1980, 1994; Bourdillon 1991; Chavanduka 1978; Chigwedere 1980; Gelfand 1968, 1979, 1992; Holleman 1952; and Meekers 1993. The descriptions that follow in the text are based primarily on these works and on my observations and interviews conducted in Manica Province between 1993 and 1995.

2.   Of Portuguese sources of Mozambican ethnography, Antonio Rita-Ferreira is the most widely published (1958, 1959, 1960, 1973). Augusto Cabral, who served as director of indigenous affairs for the Portuguese government, produced a widely cited description of the Chopi and Tonga (1910) and later an account of the indigenous peoples of the colony of Mozambique (1931). J. R. Dos Santos (1933)produced several less useful general descriptions of Mozambican peoples.

3.   During the height of the agricultural season, women in Mucessua are often up at 5 a.m. to build a fire outside the house, heat bathwater for the family, prepare breakfast, sweep the yard, clean up breakfast, walk to the river/neighbor spigot/town fountain to collect water, walk home, clean the house, wash clothes, take care of children, build a fire, prepare lunch, clean up lunch, take care of children, carry water to the farm, hoe the field, plant seeds, water seeds, weed the vegetables, harvest the vegetables, carry vegetables to the market, sell at the market, take care of children, prepare dinner (pound grain or peanuts, grind cassava leaves), build a fire, heat water for men returning home, cook dinner, feed children, eat, clean up dinner, take care of children, go to bed at 11 p.m.

Chapter 4

1.   "Reproductive ethnophysiology" refers to a woman's culturally specific way of understanding and talking about her body and the process of reproduction.

2.   The term "Zionist spirit-type church" is from the typology elaborated in Daneel 1971.

3.   I borrow this use of "unofficial" from Barber 1987: 9–12, 30–40.

Chapter 5

1.   See Modola 2007. This brief article suggests the incentives many families have to marry off their young daughters to pay off debts; see, for example, Mupotsa 2008.

2. National policies may play a part in shaping women's use of government clinics for prenatal care and childbirth, including the continued illegality of abortion except to save maternal life (Machungo, Zanconato, and Bergstrom 1997), and, as in most African countries, the promotion of contraceptives to space out births and protect maternal and child health, rather than as a means to limit births (Bledsoe 1998). Newborns must be presented at the hospital for birth registry, where women who gave birth at home are frequently chastised. Surveillance of pregnant women and pressures on them to use government clinics is also apparent in the practice of requiring all women who arrive to deliver at government clinics to present a prenatal care card documenting that they attended a prenatal clinic. These elements of the national health policy inform the context of women's childbirth choices.

Chapter 6

1. Any woman who has frequent miscarriages or still births or whose children do not survive is suspected of being a spirit wife, as is a woman who has difficulty in delivery, except when she gives birth within the confines of her father's compound. Spirit wives and their offspring are threatened by spirit intervention if their social, especially sexual, behavior knowingly or unknowingly contradicts their status as a *mukadzi we mudzimo* (wife of spirit elder or spirit of a dead relative, Sh.; *mulhere d'espirito*, spirit's wife, Port.).

2. A bill is currently before the Mozambique Assembly of the Republic to legalize abortion on demand, a right promised to women when Mozambique ratified the Maputo Protocol—the Protocol on the Rights of Women in Africa, which came into force on October 26, 2005, having been ratified by the required fifteen member states. The Maputo Protocol covers a broad range of women's rights, including the elimination of discrimination, the right to dignity, the right to life, the integrity and security of the person, the right to education and training, economic and social welfare rights, and health and reproductive rights. Article 14 of the protocol ensures women's rights to health, including sexual and reproductive rights and choice.

3. According to national maternal health norms, when a woman initiates antenatal consultations at a government clinic, a prenatal card is to be filled out. A second card is used to record antitetanus vaccinations given during antenatal clinic visits (*cartão da vaccinação anti-tetano*). The woman is to bring both cards to every follow-up visit to the clinic. These are the only personal records of her maternal clinic visits. The maternity clinic is supposed to keep copies of the prenatal evaluation card for women identified as high-risk obstetric cases (*alto risco obstetrico*). When a woman returns to give birth, information concerning the birth is registered on the prenatal form, which is then filed by month of birth in the maternity records.

Chapter 7

1. Levirate practices sanction the marriage of a widow to her dead husband's brother. Mozambicans acknowledge the "sacred heat" generated by the first intercourse between a man and his brother's wife. Both parties must be cleansed through appropriate ceremonies to avoid harming others with the heat they carry following this taboo act.

2. *Mfuta* (Tewe) is probably the seed from the castor-oil bush (from *pfuta*, Sh.), used for its resin in Shona female initiation practices (see Gelfand 1979: 19).

Chapter 8

1. In Malawi between 1985 and 1993, HIV prevalence among pregnant women (generally quite close to that among male and female adults combined) tested at urban antenatal clinics increased from 2 percent to 30 percent (UNAIDS/WHO 2004). *data.unaids.org/Publications/Fact-Sheets01/malawi_EN.pdf*
2. For anthropologists working in this area, see Alonzo and Reynolds 1995; Farmer 1992; Good and Good 1994; Kleinman and Kleinman 1991; Farmer and Kleinman 1989; Whittaker 1992.

References

Adetunji, Jacob Ayodele. 1992. Church-based obstetric care in a Yoruba community, Nigeria. *Social Science and Medicine* 35(9): 1171–78.

———. 1996. Preserving the pot and water: A traditional concept of reproductive health in a Yoruba community, Nigeria. *Social Science and Medicine* 43 (11): 1561–67.

Agadjanian, Victor. 1998a. Economic security, information resources, and women's reproductive choices in urban Mozambique. *Social Biology* 45(1–2): 60–79.

———. 1998b. Quasi-legal abortion services in a sub-Saharan setting: User profile and motivations. *Family Planning Perspectives* 24(3): 111–16.

Agha, Sohail, Andrew Karlyn, and Dominique Meekers. 2001. The promotion of condom use in non-regular sexual partnerships in urban Mozambique. *Health Policy and Planning* 16(2): 145.

AIDS Analysis Africa. 1996. Risk analysis. HIV/AIDS country profile: Mozambique. *AIDS Analysis Africa* 6(6): 8–11.

Alexander, Jacqui. 1990. Mobilizing against the state and international aid agencies: Third World women define reproductive freedom. In *From Abortion to Reproductive Freedom: Transforming a Movement*, ed. Marlene Gerber Fried, 49–62. Boston: South End Press.

Alexander, Jocelyn. 1994. *Land and Political Authority in Post-War Mozambique: A View from Manica Province*. Oxford: Oxford University Press.

———. 1997. The local state in post-war Mozambique: Political practice and ideas about authority. *Africa* 67(1): 1–26.

Alinsky, Saul. 2001. Rebuilding local capacities in Mozambique: The National Health System and civil society." In *Patronage or Partnership: Local Capacity Building in Humanitarian Crises*, ed. Ian Smillie. Idrc/Kumarian Press. *idrc.ca/en/ev-87954-201-1-DO_TOPIC .html*. Accessed 20 June 2010.

Allen, Denise Roth. 2002. *Managing Motherhood, Managing Risk: Fertility and Danger in West Central Tanzania*. Ann Arbor: University of Michigan Press.

Alonzo, Angelo A., and Nancy R. Reynolds. 1995. Stigma, HIV, and AIDS: An exploration and elaboration of a stigma trajectory. *Social Science and Medicine* 41(3): 303–15.

Alpers, Edward A. 1975. *Ivory and Slaves in East Central Africa: Changing Patterns of International Trade to the Later Nineteenth Century*. London: Heinemann.

Appadurai, Arjun, ed. 1986. *The Social Life of Things: Commodities in Cultural Perspective*. New York: Cambridge University Press.

———. 1996. *Modernity at Large: Cultural Dimensions of Globalization*. Minneapolis: University of Minnesota Press.

Arnfred, Signe. 1988. Women in Mozambique: Gender struggle and gender politics. *Review of African Political Economy* 41:5–16.

Aschwanden, Herbert. 1982. *Symbols of Life: An Analysis of the Consciousness of the Karanga*. Shona Heritage Series, 3. Gweru, Zimbabwe: Mambo Press.

———. 1984. *Symbols of Death: An Analysis of the Consciousness of the Karanga*. Gweru, Zimbabwe: Mambo Press.

————. 1989. *Karanga Mythology: An Analysis of the Consciousness of the Karanga in Zimbabwe*. Shona Heritage Series, 5. Gweru, Zimbabwe: Mambo Press.

Asowa-Omorodion, Francisca Isibhakahome. 1997. Women's perceptions of the complications of pregnancy and childbirth in two Esan communities, Edo State, Nigeria. *Social Science and Medicine* 44(12): 1817–24.

Atkinson, Sarah, and Monica Façanha Farias. 1994. Perceptions of risk during pregnancy amongst urban women in northeast Brazil. *Social Science and Medicine* 41(11): 1577–86.

Avotri, Joyce Yaa, and Vivienne Walters. 1999. You just look at our work and see if you have any freedom on earth: Ghanaian women's accounts of their work and health. *Social Science and Medicine* 48(9): 1123–33.

Ayisis, Ruth Ansah. 1985. Supporting women farmers in the Green Zones of Mozambique. Seeds, no. 17. New York: UNICEF.

Bakker, Isabella, and Stephen Gill. 2003. *Power, Production and Social Reproduction: Human In/security in the Global Political Economy*. Basingstoke, UK: Palgrave/Macmillan.

Bannerman, J. H. 1993. Land tenure in Central Mozambique past and present. Report prepared for Mozambique Agricultural Rural Construction Programme (MAARP), supported by the German Agency for Technical Cooperation. Chimoio, Mozambique: MAARP.

Barnes-Josiah, Debora, Cynthia Myntt, and Antoine Augustin. 1998. The "three delays" as a framework for examining maternal mortality in Haiti. *Social Science and Medicine* 46(8): 981–93.

BBC News. 2008. Country profile: Mozambique. *news.bbc.co.uk/go/pr/fr/-/2/hi/africa/country_profiles/1063120.stm*, 18 June. Accessed 28 June 2010.

Beach, David. 1977. The Shona economy: Branches of production. In *The Roots of Rural Poverty in Central and Southern Africa*, ed. Robin Palmer and Neil Parsons, 37–65. Berkeley: University of California Press.

————. 1980. *The Shona and Zimbabwe, 900–1850*. Gweru, Zimbabwe: Mambo Press.

————. 1984. *Zimbabwe before 1900*. Gweru, Zimbabwe: Mambo Press.

————. 1994. *The Shona and Their Neighbors*. Oxford: Blackwell.

Beckles, Hilary. 1995. Sex and gender in the historiography of Caribbean slavery. In *Engendering History: Caribbean Women in Historical Perspective*, ed. Verene Shepherd, Bridget Brereton, and Barbara Bailey, 125–40. New York: St. Martin's Press.

Berger, Amelie. 1998. *Twice Humanity: Implications for Local and Global Resource Use*. Uppsala, Sweden: Nordic Africa Institute.

Bhila, H.H.K. 1982. *Trade and Politics in a Shona Kingdom: The Manyika and Their African and Portuguese Neighbors, 1575–1902*. United Kingdom and Zimbabwe: Longman Group.

Blanco, Ana Judith. 2009. Maternal characteristics and poor follow-up rates of HIV-exposed infants in Central Mozambique. Master's thesis, University of Washington.

Bledsoe, Caroline. 1990. The politics of children: Fosterage and the social management of fertility among the Mende of Sierra Leone. In *Births and Power: Social Change and the Politics of Reproduction*, ed. W. Penn Handwerker, 81–100. Boulder, CO: Westview Press.

————. 1998. Reproductive mishaps and western contraception: An African challenge to fertility theory. *Population and Development Review* 24(1): 15–57.

Bledsoe, Caroline, with Fatoumatta Banja. 2002. *Contingent Lives: Fertility, Time, and Aging in West Africa*. Chicago: University of Chicago Press.

Bogues, Anthony. 2005. The politics of power and violence: Rethinking the political in the Caribbean. Paper presented at the Conference on Caribbean Studies, Yale University, New Haven, CT.

Bolles, A. Lynn. 2002. The impoverishment of women: A glimpse of the global picture. *Voices* 6(1): 9–13.

Bolton, Pamela, Carl Kendall, Elli Leontsini, and Corinne Whitaker. 1989. Health technologies and women in the third world. *Women and International Development Annual* 1:57–100.

Bond, Patrick. 2007. The dispossession of African wealth at the cost of Africa's health. *International Journal of Health Services* 37(1): 171–92.

Bourdillon, Michael. 1991. *The Shona Peoples: An Ethnography of Contemporary Shona, with Special Reference to Their Religion*. Gweru, Zimbabwe: Mambo Press.

———. 1994. Street children in Harare. *Africa-London-International African Institute* 64(4): 516–32.

Brandström, Per. 1990. Seeds and soil: The quest for life and the domestication of fertility in Sukuma-Nyamwezi thought and reality. In *The Creative Communion: African Folk Models of Fertility and the Regeneration of Life*, ed. A. Jacobson-Widding and W. van Beek. Uppsala Studies in Cultural Anthropology 15. Stockholm: Almqvist and Wiksell International.

Brown, Wendy. 2005. *Edgework: Critical Essays on Knowledge and Politics*. Princeton, NJ: Princeton University Press.

Browner, Carol. 2001. Situating women's reproductive activities. *American Anthropologist* 102(4): 773–88.

Browner, Carol, and Carolyn F. Sargent. 1996. Anthropology and studies of human reproduction. In *Medical Anthropology: A Handbook of Theory and Methods*, ed. Thomas Malcolm Johnson and Carolyn Fishel Sargent, 219–34. New York: Greenwood Press.

Buckley, Thomas, and Alma Gottlieb, eds. 1998. *Blood Magic: The Anthropology of Menstruation*. Berkeley: University of California Press.

Buekens, Pierre, Siân Curtis, and Silva Alayón. 2003. Demographic and health surveys: Caesarean section rates in sub-Saharan Africa. *British Medical Journal* 326(7381): 136.

Bujra, Janet M. 1986. Urging women to redouble their efforts: Class, gender, and capitalist transformation in Africa. In *Women and Class in Africa*, ed. Claire C. Robertson and Iris Berger, 117–41. New York: Africana Publishing.

Bunting, Madeleine. 2008. Pregnancy should be a cause for cheer, not a reason to fear for your life. *Guardian*, 30 June. *guardian.co.uk/commentisfree/2008/jun/30/internationalaidanddevelopment*.

Bush, Barbara. 1990. *Slave Women in Caribbean Society: 1650–1838*. Bloomington: Indiana University Press.

Cabral, Augusto. 1910. *Raças, usos e costumes dos indigenas da districto de Inhambane, acompanhado de um vocabulario em shitsua, guitonga e shishope*. Lourenço Marques, Mozambique: Imprensa Nacional.

———. 1931. *O agonizar da monarchia: erros e crimes, novas revelações*. Lisbon: F. Franco.

Caffentzis, George. 2002. Neoliberalism in Africa: Apocalyptic failures and business as usual practices. *Alternatives: Turkish Journal of International Relations* 1(3). *alternativesjournal.net/volume1/number3/george.pdf*. Accessed 27 June 2010.

Carter, Anthony. 1995. Agency and fertility: For an ethnography of practice. In *Situating Fertility: Anthropology and Demographic Inquiry*, ed. Susan Greenhalgh, 55–85. Cambridge: Cambridge University Press.

Castro, Arachu, and Paul Farmer. 2005. Understanding and addressing AIDS-related stigma: From anthropological theory to clinical practice in Haiti. *American Journal of Public Health* 95(1): 53–59.

Chabal, Patrick, and Jean-Pascal Daloz. 1999. *Africa Works: Disorder as Political Instrument*. London: International African Institute in association with James Currey, Oxford.

Chapman, Rachel R. 1998. Prenatal care and the politics of protection: An ethnography of pregnancy and medical pluralism in Central Mozambique. PhD diss., University of California, Los Angeles.

———. 2003. Endangering safe motherhood in Mozambique: Prenatal care as pregnancy risk. *Social Science and Medicine* 57(2): 355–74.

———. 2004. A nova vida: The commoditization of reproductive health in central Mozambique. *Medical Anthropology* 23(3): 229–61.

Chapman, Rachel, Paulino Davissone, Francisco Machobo, and James Pfeiffer. 1999. Community leadership and health: A rapid ethnographic study of three zones in Manica Province. Report prepared for Mozambique Ministry of Health and Health Alliance International. Chimoio, Mozambique: Health Alliance International.

Chapman, Rachel, and James Pfeiffer. 2008. Mapping a mighty influence: Pentecostal, Zion, and Apostolic Churches and ARV utilization and adherence in central Mozambique. Paper presented at the American Anthropology Association Annual Conference, Washington, DC. December.

Chavanduka, G. L. 1978. *Traditional Healers and the Shona Patient*. Gweru, Zimbabwe: Mambo Press.

Chigwedere, A. S. 1980. *From Mutapa to Rhodes*. London: Macmillan.

Cliff, Julie. 1991. The war on women in Mozambique: Health consequences of South African destabilization, economic crisis, and structural adjustment. In *Women and Health in Africa*, ed. Meredith Turshen, 15–33. Trenton, NJ: Africa World Press.

Comaroff, Jean. 1983. The defectiveness of symbols or the symbols of defectiveness? On the cultural analysis of medical systems. *Culture, Medicine, and Psychiatry* 7: 47–64.

———. 1985. *Body of Power, Spirit of Resistance: The Culture and History of a South African People*. Chicago: University of Chicago Press.

Comaroff, Jean, and John L. Comaroff, eds. 2000. *Millennial Capitalism and the Culture of Neoliberalism*. Durham, NC: Duke University Press.

Cooper, Ellen R., M. Charurat, L. Mofenson, I. C. Hanson, J. Pitt , C. Diaz, K. Hayani, E. Handelsman, V. Smeriglio, R. Hoff, and W. Blattner. 2002. Combination antiretroviral strategies for the treatment of pregnant HIV-1-infected women and prevention of perinatal HIV-1 transmission. *Journal of Acquired Immune Deficiency Syndromes and Human Retrovirology* 29(5): 484–94.

Cooper, Melinda. 2008. *Life as Surplus: Biotechnology and Capitalism in the Neoliberal Era*. Seattle: University of Washington Press.

Coria-Soto, I., M. Zambrana-Castañeda, H. Reyes-Zapata, and A. M. Salinas-Martinez. 1997. Comparison of two methods for the discrimination of avoidable perinatal deaths. *Journal of Perinatal Medicine* 25:205–12.

Cornwall, Andrea. 2002. Spending power: Love, money, and the reconfiguration of gender relations in Ado-Odo, southwestern Nigeria. *American Ethnologist* 29:963–80.

———. 2005. *Readings in Gender in Africa*. London: International African Institute.

Crandon-Malamud, Libbet. 1991. *From the Fat of Our Souls: Social Change, Political Process, and Medical Pluralism in Bolivia*. Comparative Studies of Health Systems and Medical Care Series. Berkeley: University of California Press.

Crehan, Kate. 1997. *The Fractured Community: Landscapes of Power and Gender in Rural Zambia*. Berkeley: University of California Press.

Daneel, M. L. 1971. *Old and New in Southern Shona Independent Churches I: Background and Rise of the Major Movements*. The Hague: Mouton.

Das, Veena. 1996. Rumours as performative: A contribution to the theory of perculutionary speech. Sudhir Kumar Bose Memorial Lecture, St. Stephens College, University of Delhi, India.

Davis, Mike. 2004. Planet of slums. *New Left Review* 26 (March–April): 5–34.

———. 2006. *Planet of Slums: Urban Involution and the Informal Working Class*. London: Verso.

Davis-Floyd, Robbie. 2003. Home-birth emergencies in the US and Mexico: The trouble with transport. *Social Science and Medicine* 56(9): 1911–31.

———. 2004. *Birth as an American Rite of Passage*. Berkeley: University of California Press.

Davis-Floyd, Robbie, and Carolyn F. Sargent, eds. 2004. *Childbirth and Authoritative Knowledge: Cross-Cultural Perspectives*. Berkeley: University of California Press.

Dawes, Kwame. 2008. Learning to speak: The new age of HIV/AIDS in the other Jamaica. *Virginia Quarterly Review* 84(2): 100–123. *vqronline.org/articles/2008/spring/dawes-aids-jamaica/*. Accessed 27 June 2010.

De Cock, Kevin M., Mary Glenn Fowler, Eric Mercier, Isabelle de Vincenzi, Joseph Saba, Elizabeth Hoff, David J. Alnwick, Martha Rogers, and Nathan Shaffer. 2000. Prevention of mother-to-child transmission in resource poor countries: Translating research into policy and practice. *Journal of the American Medical Association* 283(9): 1175–82.

Delaney, Carol. 1991. *The Seed and the Soil: Gender and Cosmology in a Turkish Village Society.* Berkeley: University of California Press.

Demble, D. M. 2002. Trade liberalization and poverty in sub-Saharan Africa. In *Black Women, Globalization, and Economic Justice*, ed. Filomina Chioma Steady, 72–91. Rochester, VT: Schenkman Books.

Desjeaux, Dominique. 1987. *Strategies Paysannes en Afrique: Le Congo—Essai sur la Gestion de l'Encertitude.* Paris: L'Harmattan.

di Leonardo, Micaela. 1991. Gender, culture, and political economy: Feminist anthropology in historical perspective. In *Gender at the Crossroads of Knowledge: Feminist Anthropology in the Postmodern Era*, ed. Micaela di Leonardo, 1–30. Berkeley: University of California Press.

Dorenbaum, Alejandro, Coleen K. Cunningham, Richard D. Gelber, Mary Culnane, Lynne Mofenson, Paula Britto, Claire Rekacewicz, Marie-Louise Newell, Jean Francois Delfraissy, Bethann Cunningham-Schrader, Mark Mirochnick, and John L. Sullivan. 2002. Two-dose intrapartum/newborn nevirapine and standard antiretroviral therapy to reduce perinatal HIV transmission: A randomized trial. *Journal of the American Medical Association* 288(2): 189–98.

do Rosário, Domingos Artur. 1999. *Cidade de Chimoio: Ensaio histórico-sociológico.* Colecção Embondeiro, 14. Chimoio, Mozambique: ARPAC.

Dos Santos, J. R. 1933. *As Pinturas Pre-Historicas do Cachao da Rapa.* Porto, Portugal: Instituto de Antropologia da Univ. do Porto.

Dujardin B., G. Clarysse, B. Criel, V. De Brouwere, and N. Wangata. 1995. The strategy of risk approach in antenatal care: Evaluation of the referral compliance. *Social Science and Medicine* 40(4): 529–35.

Ebron, Paulla A. 2002. *Performing Africa.* Princeton, NJ: Princeton University Press.

Eggleston, Elizabeth. 2000. Unintended pregnancy and women's use of prenatal care in Ecuador. *Social Science and Medicine* 51(7): 1011–18.

Eide, Magnhild, Marte Myhre, Morten Lindbæk, Johanne Sundby, Peter Arimi, and Ibou Thior. 2006. Social consequences of HIV-positive women's participation in prevention of mother-to-child transmission programmes. *Patient Education and Counseling* 60:146–51.

Ekejiuba, Felicia I. 1995. Down to fundamentals: Women-centered hearth-holds in rural West Africa. In *Women Wielding the Hoe: Lessons from Rural Africa for Feminist Theory and Development Practice*, ed. Deborah F. Bryceson, 47–61. Oxford and Washington, DC: Berg.

El-Mouelhy, Mawaheb, Hind Khattab, Nabil Younis, and Huda Zurayk. 1989. Measurements and determinants of reproductive morbidity with special reference to Middle Eastern society. Typescript.

Epstein, Helen. 2002. The hidden cause of AIDS. *New York Review of Books. nybooks.com /articles/archives/2002/may/09/the-hidden-cause-of-aids/.* Accessed 27 June 2010.

Etuk, S. J., H. Itam, and E.E.J. Asuquo. 1999. Role of the spiritual churches in antenatal clinic default in Calabar, Nigeria. *East African Medical Journal* 76(11): 639–43.

Farmer, Paul. 1992. *AIDS and Accusation: Haiti and the Geography of Blame.* Berkeley: University of California Press.

Farmer, Paul, and Arthur Kleinman. 1989. AIDS as human suffering. *Dædalus* 118(2): 135–60.

Fayorsey, Clara Korkor. 1992. Commoditization of childbirth: Female strategies towards autonomy among the Ga of southern Ghana. *Cambridge Anthropology* 163:19–45.

———. 1993. Economy, kinship, and fertility among the Ga of southern Ghana. PhD diss., Cambridge University, U.K.

Federici, Silvia. 2004. *Caliban and the Witch: Women, the Body, and Primitive Accumulation.* New York: Autonomedia.

———. 2006a. Capital and the body: A rejoinder to Salvatore Engel-Di Mauro. *Capitalism, Nature, Socialism* 17(4): 74–77.

———. 2006b. Women, gender oppression, and science. *Science and Society* 70(4): 550–55.

Feldman-Savelsberg, Pamela. 1994. Plundered kitchens and empty wombs: Fear of fertility in the Cameroonian Grassfields. *Social Science and Medicine* 39(4): 463–74.

Ferguson, James. 2006. *Global Shadows: Africa in the Neoliberal World Order*. Durham, NC: Duke University Press.

Fernandes, A., R. G. Vaz, and A. Noya. 1992. AIDS in Mozambique. International Conference on AIDS. 1992 Jul 19–24; 8: B215 (abstract no. PoB 3747). National AIDS Control Programme, Maputo, Mozambique.

Firmino, Gregório Domingos. 2002. *A questão linguística na Africa pós-colonial: O caso do Português e das línguas autóctones em Moçambique*. Colecção Identidades, 13. Maputo, Mozambique: Promédia.

Fleming, A. F. 1988. AIDS in Africa—an update. *AIDS Forschung* 3:116–38.

Fortunati, Leopoldina. 1995. *The Arcane of Reproduction: Housework, Prostitution, Labor, and Capital*. New York: Autonomedia.

Foster, George. 1998. Disease etiologies in non-Western medical systems. In *Understanding and Applying Medical Anthropology*, ed. Peter Brown, 110–17. Mountainview, CA: Mayfield Publishing.

Foucault, Michel. 1991. *Discipline and Punish: The Birth of the Prison*. Harmondsworth, UK: Penguin Books.

Gaillard, Philippe, Mary-Glenn Fowler, Francois Dabis, Hoosen Coovadia, Charles van der Horst, Koen van Rompay, Andrea Ruff, Taha Taha, Tim Thomas, Isabelle de Vincenzi, and Marie-Louise Newell. 2004. Use of antiretroviral drugs to prevent HIV-1 transmission through breast-feeding: From animal studies to randomized clinical trials. *Journal of Acquired Immune Deficiency Syndromes and Human Retrovirology* 35(2): 178–87.

Galli, Rosemary Elizabeth. 2003. *Peoples' Spaces and State Spaces: Land and Governance in Mozambique*. Lanham, MD: Lexington Books.

Geertz, Clifford. 1973. *The Interpretation of Cultures: Selected Essays*. New York: Basic Books.

Gelfand, Michael. 1968. *African Crucible*. Cape Town: Juta.

———. 1979. *Growing Up in Shona Society*. Gweru, Zimbabwe: Mambo Press.

———. 1992 [1973]. *The Genuine Shona*. Gweru, Zimbabwe: Mambo Press.

Gengenbach, Heidi. 1998. "I'll bury you in the border!": Women's land struggles in post-war Facazisse (Magude District), Mozambique. *Journal of Southern African Studies* 24(1): 7–36.

Geronimus, Arlene. 2000. To mitigate, resist, or undo: Addressing structural influences on the health of urban populations. *American Journal of Public Health* 90(6): 867–72.

Geschiere, Peter. 1997. *The Modernity of Witchcraft*. Charlottesville: University Press of Virginia.

Giddens, Anthony. 1979. *Central Problems in Social Theory: Action, Structure, and Contradiction in Social Analysis*. Berkeley: University of California Press.

Gilman, Sander L. 1985. *Difference and Pathology: Stereotypes of Sexuality, Race and Madness*. Ithaca: Cornell University Press.

Ginsburg, Faye D., and Rayna Rapp, eds. 1995. *Conceiving the New World Order: The Global Politics of Reproduction*. Los Angeles and Berkeley: University of California Press.

Goffman, Erving. 1963. *Stigma: Notes on the Management of a Spoiled Identity*. New York: Simon and Schuster.

Goldin, Carol S. 1994. Stigmatization and AIDS: Critical issues in public health. *Social Science and Medicine* 39(9): 1359–66.

Good, Byron J., and Mary-Jo Del Vecchio Good. 1994. In the subjunctive mode: Epilepsy narratives in Turkey. *Social Science and Medicine* 38(6): 835–42.

Goodburn, Elizabeth, and Oona Campbell. 2001. Reducing maternal mortality in the developing world: Sector-wide approaches may be the key. *British Medical Journal* 322(7291): 917–20.

Gouws, Eleanor, Karen Stanecki, Rob Lyerla, and Peter D. Ghys. 2008. The epidemiology of HIV infection among young people aged 15–24 years in southern Africa. *AIDS* 22 (Suppl 4): S5–S16.

Granja, Ana Carla. 1996. O Aborto É o Direito de Controlar o Seu Corpo. *Noticias de Moçambique*, no. 76:5–7. 7 April. *mol.co.mz/notmoc/1996/76e.html*. Accessed 28 June 2010.

Granja, Ana Carla, F. Machungo, A. Gomes, and S. Bergstrom. 2001. Adolescent maternal mortality. *Mozambique Journal of Adolescent Health* 28(4): 303–6.

Green, Edward C. 1999. *Indigenous Theories of Contagious Disease*. Walnut Creek, CA: Rowman Altamira.

Green, Edward C., Annamarie Jurg, and Armando Djedje. 1994. The snake in the stomach: Child diarrhea in Central Mozambique. *Medical Anthropology Quarterly* 8(1): 4–24.

———. 1997. Purity, pollution, and the invisible snake in southern Africa. *Medical Anthropology* 17(1): 83–100.

Greenhalgh, Susan. 1994. Controlling births and bodies in village China. *American Ethnologist* 21(1): 3–30.

———. ed. 1995. *Situating Fertility: Anthropology and Demographic Inquiry*. Cambridge: Cambridge University Press.

Guay, Laura A., Philippa Musoke, Thomas Fleming, Danstan Bagenda, Melissa Allen, Clemensia Nakabiito, Joseph Sherman, et. al. 1999. Intrapartum and neonatal single-dose nevirapine compared with zidovudine for prevention of mother-to-child transmission of HIV-1 in Kampala, Uganda: HIVNET 012 randomised trial. *Lancet* 354(9181): 795–802.

Guldin, Gregory Eliyu. 1997. *Farewell to Peasant China: Rural Urbanization and Social Change in the Late Twentieth Century*. Armonk, NY: M. E. Sharpe.

Gunewardena, Nandini. 2002. Attention to women's poverty in International Development strategies. *Voices* 6(1): 14–22.

Gurolla-Bonilla, Silvia. 1995. *Avaliaçãao dos Conselhos de Lideres Comunitarios*. Chimoio, Mozambique: Mozambican Health Committee.

Gwaltney, John Langston. 1980. *Drylongso: A Self-Portrait of Black America*. New York: Random House.

Hammonds, Evelynn M. 1997. Toward a genealogy of black female sexuality: The problematic of silence. In *Feminist Theory and the Body: A Reader*, ed. Janet Price and Margaret Shildrick, 249–59. New York: Routledge.

Hanlon, Joseph. 1984. *The Revolution under Fire*. London: Zed Press.

———. 1996. *Peace without Profit: How the IMF Blocks Rebuilding in Mozambique*. Portsmouth, NH: Heinemann.

———. 1997. Strangling Mozambique: International Monetary Fund "stabilization" in the world's poorest country. *Multinational Monitor*, July–August, 17–21.

———. 2004. Renewed land debate and the "cargo cult" in Mozambique. *Journal of Southern African Studies* 30(3): 603–25.

———. 2006. The tobacco debate: Priority for factories or peasants? *O País*, 19 May. *open.ac.uk/technology/mozambique/pics/d60678.doc*. Accessed 28 June 2010.

Hannan, Michael. 1984. *Standard Shona Dictionary*. Harare/ Bulawayo: College Press.

Hannerz, Ulf. 1996. *Transnational Connections: Culture, People, Places*. London: Routledge.

Hansson, Gurli. 1996. Mwana ndi mai: Toward an understanding of preparation for motherhood and child care in the transitional Mberengwa District, Zimbabwe. Studia missionalia Upsaliensia, 65. Uppsala, Sweden: Swedish Institute of Missionary Research.

———. 1998. Motherhood as fulfillment. In *Twice Humanity: Implications for Local and Global Resource Use*, ed. Amelie Berger, 45–56. Uppsala, Sweden: Nordic Africa Institute.

Hart, Gillian. 2002. *Disabling Globalization: Places of Power in Post-Apartheid South Africa.* Berkeley: University of California Press.

Hartmann, Betsy. 1987. *Reproductive Rights and Wrongs: The Global Politics of Population Control and Contraceptive Choice.* New York: Harper and Row.

Harvey, David. 1985a. *Consciousness and the Urban Experience.* Baltimore: Johns Hopkins University Press.

———. 1985b. *The Urbanization of Capital.* Baltimore: Johns Hopkins University Press.

———. 1989a. *The Condition of Postmodernity: An Enquiry into the Origins of Cultural Change.* Cambridge, MA: Blackwell.

———. 1989b. *The Urban Experience.* Baltimore: Johns Hopkins University Press.

———. 2006. [1982]. *The Limits to Capital.* London: Verso.

Hawken, David. 2007. *Blessed Unrest.* New York and London: Viking Penguin.

Health Alliance International. 2008.*Quarterly Report.* Maputo, Mozambique. Health Alliance International and Department of Global Health, University of Washington, Seattle.

Hodgson, Dorothy. 1997. Embodying the contradictions of modernity: Gender and spirit possession among Maasai in Tanzania. In *Gendered Encounters: Challenging Cultural Boundaries and Social Hierarchies in Africa*, ed. Maria Grosz-Ngate and Omari Kokole, 111–29. New York and London: Routledge.

Hodgson, Dorothy, and Sheryl McCurdy, eds. 2001. *"Wicked" Women and the Reconfiguration of Gender in Africa.* Portsmouth, NH: Heinemann.

Holleman, J. F. 1952. *Shona Customary Law.* Cape Town, London, New York: Oxford University Press.

Hughes, David McDermott. 1999. Refugees and squatters: Immigration and the politics of territory on the Zimbabwe-Mozambique border. *Journal of Southern African Studies* 25(4): 533–52.

Hydén, Goran. 1980. *Beyond Ujamaa in Tanzania: Underdevelopment and an Uncaptured Peasantry.* Berkeley: University of California Press.

———. 2006. *African Politics in Comparative Perspective.* Cambridge: Cambridge University Press.

ICAP [International Center for AIDS Care and Treatment Programs]. 2008. Collaborative PMTCT and Pediatric HIV Strategic Planning. Workshop in Partnership with Tygerberg Children's Hospital, South Africa and S2S. Cape Town, South Africa.

INE [Instituto Naçional de Estatística]. 1999. Ii reçenseamento geral da população e habitação, 1997: Província de Manica [Second General Census 1997: Manica Province]. Maputo, Mozambique: Government of Moçambique.

Inhorn, Marcia C. 2003a. *Local Babies, Global Science: Gender, Religion, and In Vitro Fertilization in Egypt.* New York: Routledge.

———. 2003b. The risks of test-tube baby making in Egypt. In *Risk, Culture, and Health Inequality: Shifting Perceptions of Danger and Blame*, ed. Barbara Herr Harthorn and Laury Oaks, 57–78. Westport, CT: Praeger.

Isaacman, Allen. 1996. *Cotton Is the Mother of Poverty: Peasants, Work, and Rural Struggle in Colonial Mozambique, 1938–1961.* Portsmouth, NH: Heinemann.

Isaacman, Allen, and Barbara Isaacman. 1983. *Mozambique: From Colonialism to Revolution, 1900–1982.* Boulder, CO: Westview Press.

———. 1984. The role of women in the liberation struggle of Mozambique. *Ufahamu* 13 (2–3): 128–85.

Isenalumbe, A. E. 1990. Integration of traditional birth attendants into primary health care. *World Health Forum* 11:192–98.

Jackson, J. Brooks, Philippa Musoke, Thomas Fleming, Laura A Guay, Danstan Bagenda, Melissa Allen, Clemensia Nakabiito, et al. 2003. Intrapartum and neonatal single-dose nevirapine compared with zidovudine for prevention of mother-to-child transmission of HIV-1 in Kampala, Uganda: 18-month follow-up of the HIVNET 012 randomised trial. *Lancet* 362(9387): 859–68.

Jelley, Diana, and Richard Madeley. 1983a. Antenatal care in Maputo, Mozambique. *Journal of Epidemiology and Community Health* 37:111–16.

———. 1983b. Preventive health care for mothers and children in Maputo, Mozambique. *Journal of Tropical Medicine and Hygiene* 86:229–36.

Jenkins, Gwynne L., and Marcia Inhorn. 2003. Editorial: Reproduction gone awry: Medical anthropological perspectives. *Social Science and Medicine* 56:1831–36.

Jessop, B. 1982. *The Capitalist State.* Oxford: Martin Robertson.

Jirojwong, Sansnee. 1996. Health beliefs and the use of antenatal care among pregnant women in Southern Thailand. In *Maternity and Reproductive Health in Asian Societies*, ed. Pranee Liamputtong Rice and Lenore Manderson, 61–82. Amsterdam: Harwood Academic Press.

Jok, Madut Jok. 1998. *Militarization, Gender, and Reproductive Health in South Sudan.* New York: Edwin Mellen Press.

Jolly, Margaret. 2002. From darkness to light? Epidemiologies and ethnographies of motherhood in Vanuatu. In *Birthing in the Pacific: Beyond Tradition and Modernity?* ed. Vicki Lukere and Margaret Jolly, 148–77. Honolulu: University of Hawai'i Press.

Jones, S. A., G. G. Sherman, and C. A. Varga. 2005. Exploring socio-economic conditions and poor follow-up rates of HIV-exposed infants in Johannesburg, South Africa. *AIDS Care* 17: 466–70.

Jordan, Brigitte. 1997. Authoritative knowledge and its construction. In *Childbirth and Authoritative Knowledge: Cross-Cultural Perspectives*, ed. Robbie Davis-Floyd and Carolyn F. Sargent, 55–79. Berkeley: University of California Press.

Jules-Rosette, Bennetta. 1980. Changing aspects of women's initiation in southern Africa: An exploratory study. *Journal of African Studies / Revue Canadienne des Études Africaines* 13(3): 389–405.

Jurg, Annemarie, Taju Tomas, and J. De Jong. 1991. Fornecedores e utentes de cuidados modernos ou tradicionais de saude em Maputo, Moçambique: opinões e preferencias mutuas em Moçambique. Maputo: Instituto Nacional de Saude, GEMT.

Kaler, Amy. 2000. Who has told you to do this thing? Toward a feminist interpretation of contraceptive diffusion in Rhodesia, 1970–1980. *Signs: Journal of Women in Culture and Society* 25(3): 677–708.

———. 2003. *Running after Pills: Politics, Gender, and Contraception in Colonial Zimbabwe.* Portsmouth, NH: Heinemann.

Kleinman, Arthur, and Joan Kleinman. 1980. *Patients and Healers in the Context of Culture.* Berkeley: University of California Press.

———. 1986. Somatization: The interconnections among culture, depressive experience, and meanings of pain. In *Culture and Depression: Studies in the Anthropology and Cross-Cultural Psychiatry of Affect and Disorder*, ed. Arthur Kleinman and Byron Good, 429–90. Berkeley: University of California Press.

———. 1991. Suffering and its professional transformation: Toward an ethnography of interpersonal experience. *Culture, Medicine, and Psychiatry* 15(3): 275–301.

Kruks, Sonia, and Benjamin Wisner. 1984. The state, the party and the female in Mozambique. *Journal of Southern African Studies* 11 (October): 106–28.

———. 1989. Ambiguous transformations: Women, politics, and production in Mozambique. In *Promissory Notes: Women in the Transition to Socialism*, ed. Sonia Kruks, Rayna Rapp, and Marilyn Blatt Young, 148–71. New York: Monthly Review Press.

Lafort, Yves. 1994. *Final Report: Prenatal Care Consultations.* Chimoio, Mozambique: Mozambique Health Committee.

Lamphere, Louise. 1974. Strategies, cooperation, and conflict among women in domestic groups. In *Woman, Culture, and Society*, ed. Michelle Z. Rosaldo and Louise Lamphere, 97–112. Stanford, CA: Stanford University Press.

———. 1975. Political and economic strategies in domestic groups. In *Being Female: Reproduction, Power, and Change*, ed. Dana Raphael, 117–30. The Hague: Mouton.

————. 1987. Feminism and anthropology: The struggle to reshape our thinking about gender. In *The Impact of Feminist Research in the Academy*, ed. Christie Farnham, 11–33. Bloomington: Indiana University Press.

Lancaster, Roger N., and Micaela Di Leonardo, eds. 1997. *The Gender/Sexuality Reader: Culture, History, Political Economy*. New York: Routledge.

Lave, Jean. 1988. *Arithmetic Practices and Cognitive Theory: An Ethnographic Inquiry*. Cambridge: Cambridge University Press.

Lawn, Joy, and Lisa Berber, eds. 2006. *Opportunities for Africa's Newborns: Practical Data, Policy, and Programmatic Support for Newborn Care in Africa*. Geneva: WHO / Partnership for Maternal, Newborn and Child Health.

Leclerc-Madlala, Suzanne. 2008. Age-disparate and intergenerational sex in southern Africa: The dynamics of hypervulnerability. *AIDS* 22(Suppl 4): S17–S25.

Lilley, P. J., and Jeff Shantz. 2004. The world's largest workplace: Social reproduction and wages for housework. *Northeastern Anarchist* 9 (Summer/Fall). *nefac.net/node/1247*. Accessed 16 June 2010.

Livingston, David. 1857. *Missionary Travels and Research in South Africa*. London: John Murray.

Lubkemann, Stephen C. 2001. Rebuilding local capacities in Mozambique: The national health system and civil society. In *Patronage or Partnership: Local Capacity Building in Humanitarian Crises*, ed. Ian Smillie, 77–106. Ottowa: IRDC/Kumarian Press.

Lupton, Deborah. 1999. *Risk*. New York: Routledge.

Lyons, Tanya. 2003. *Guns and Guerilla Girls: Women in the Zimbabwean National Liberation Struggle*. Trenton, NJ: Africa World Press.

MAARP [Mozambique Agricultural Rural Reconstruction Programme]. 1995a. *Integrated Rural Development Strategy Plan for Manica Province (IRDSP): Agriculture Final Report*. Chimoio, Mozambique: GTZ.

————. 1995b. *Land Use Issues in Nhambonda Locality of Gondola District*. Chimoio, Mozambique: GTZ.

Mabala, Richard. 2006. Programming with and for adolescents and young people in Africa: Lessons learned (and not learned, yet). Presentation at Africa Regional Youth Forum on Reproductive Health, June, Dar es Salaam.

Mac-Arthur Jr., A., S. Gloyd, P. Perdigão, A. Noya, J. Sacarlal, and J. Kreiss. 2001. Characteristics of drug resistance and HIV among tuberculosis patients in Mozambique. *International Journal of Tuberculosis and Lung Disease* 5(10): 894–902.

Machungo, Fernanda, Giovanni Zanconato, and Staffan Bergstrom. 1997. Reproductive characteristics and post-abortion health consequences in women undergoing illegal and legal abortion in Maputo. *Social Science and Medicine* 45(11): 1607–13.

MacLean, Lauren Morris. 2003. State social policies and social support networks: The unintended consequences of state policymaking on informal networks in Ghana and Cote d'Ivoire. *International Journal of Public Administration* 26(6): 665–91.

Madhavan, S. and C. Bledsoe. 2001. The compound as the locus of fertility decision-making: The case of the Gambia. *Journal of Culture, Health and Sexuality* 3(4): 451–68.

Magadi, Monica Akinyi, Nyovani Janet Madise, and Roberto Nascimento Rodrigues. 2000. Frequency and timing of antenatal care in Kenya: Explaining the variations between women of different communities. *Social Science and Medicine* 51(4): 551–61.

Magode, José, ed. 1996. *Moçambique: Etnicidades, Nacionalismo e o Estado: Transição Inacabada*. Maputo, Mozambique: CEEI.

Magode, José, and A. Khan. 1996. O Estado unitário e a questão nacional. Uma reflexão sobre o caso moçambicano. In *Moçambique: Etnicidades, Nacionalismo e o Estado: Transição inacabada*, ed. José Magode, 40–106. Maputo, Mozambique: CEEL.

Mamdani, Mahmood. 1973. *The Myth of Population Control: Family, Caste, and Class in an Indian Village*. New York: Monthly Review Press.

Manning, Carrie L. 2002. *The Politics of Peace in Mozambique: Post-conflict Democratization, 1992–2000*. Westport, CT: Praeger.

Manzi, M., R. Zachariah, R. Teck, L. Buhendw, J. Kazima, E. Bakali, P. Firmenich, and P. Humblet. 2005. High acceptability of voluntary counselling and HIV-testing but unacceptable loss-to-follow-up in a prevention of mother-to-child HIV transmission programme in rural Malawi: Scaling-up requires a different way of acting. *Tropical Medicine and International Health* 10(12): 1242–50.

Marcus, George E., and Michael M. J. Fischer. 1999. *Anthropology as Cultural Critique: An Experimental Moment in the Human Sciences.* Chicago: University of Chicago Press.

Marlene, Rosa, Rachel Chapman, and Julie Cliff. 2000. Lovers, hookers, and wives: Unbraiding the social contradictions of urban Mozambican women's sexual and economic lives. In *African Women's Health*, 2d ed., ed. Meredith Turshen, 49–68. Trenton, NJ: Africa World Press.

Marlins, Robert. 2000. Legacies of violence: Spirit possession and constructions of gender and illness in central Mozambique. PhD diss., Rutgers University.

Marshall, Judith. 1988. *Structural Adjustment in Mozambique: The Human Face.* Ottawa: Canadian International Development Agency.

———. 1989. Training for Empowerment: A Kit of Materials for Popular Literacy Workers Based on an Exchange among Educators from Mozambique, Nicaragua and Brazil. Toronto: Doris Marshall Institute.

Martin, Emily. 1990. The ideology of reproduction: The reproduction of ideology. In *Uncertain Terms: Negotiating Gender in American Culture*, ed. Faye Ginsburg and Ana Lowenhaupt-Tsing, 300–314. Boston: Beacon Press.

Marx, K. 1973. *Grundrisse: Foundations of the Critique of Political Economy.* Trans. Martin Nicolaus. London: Penguin Books.

———. 1976. *Capital: A Critique of Political Economy.* Vol. 1. Harmondsworth: Penguin Books.

———. 1978. *The Marx-Engels Reader.* Ed. Robert C. Tucker. New York: W. W. Norton.

Mass, Bonnie. 1976. *Population Target: The Political Economy of Population Control in Latin America.* Toronto: Women's Press.

Massey, Doreen. 1993. Power-geometry and a progressive sense of place. In *Mapping the Futures: Local Cultures, Global Change*, ed. Jon Bird, Barry Curtis, Tim Putnam, George Robertson, and Lisa Tickner, 59–69. London: Routledge.

Mate, Rekopantswe. 2002. Wombs as God's laboratories: Pentecostal discourse of femininity in Zimbabwe. *Africa: Journal of the International African Institute* 72(4): 549–68.

Matenga, Edward. 1997. Images of a fertility complex: Iron Age figurine from Zimbabwe. In *Legacies of Stone: Zimbabwe Past and Present*, vol. 1, ed. William Joseph Dewey, 57–75. Tervuren, Belg.: Royal Museum for Central Africa.

Maternowska, M. Catherine. 2006. *Reproducing Inequities: Poverty and the Politics of Population in Haiti.* New Brunswick, NJ: Rutgers University Press.

Maxwell, David J. 1993. Local politics and the war of liberation in northeast Zimbabwe. *Journal of Southern African Studies* 19(3): 361–86.

———. 2005. The Durawall of faith: Pentecostal spirituality in neo-liberal Zimbabwe. *Journal of Religion in Africa* 35(1): 4–32.

Mazarire, Gerald Chikozho. 2003. "The politics of the womb": Women, politics, and the environment in pre-colonial Chivi, southern Zimbabwe, c. 1840 to 1900. *Zambezia* 30(1): 35–50.

McDaniel, Susan. 1996. Towards a synthesis of feminist and demographic perspectives on fertility. *Sociological Quarterly* 37(1): 83–104.

Meekers, Dominique. 1993. The noble custom of roora: The marriage practices of the Shona of Zimbabwe. *Ethnology* 32(1): 93–105.

Merchant, Carolyn. 1980. *The Death of Nature: Women, Ecology, and the Scientific Revolution.* San Francisco: Harper and Row.

Metraud, Claire. 1993. *Baseline Assessment of Traditional Birth Attendants and Birth Practices in Manica Province.* Chimoio, Mozambique: Mozambique Health Committee.

Meyer, John. 2007. *The Use of Cash/Vouchers in Response to Vulnerability and Food Insecurity: Case Study Review and Analysis.* TANGO International, Special Initiative for Cash and Voucher Programming. WFP South Africa.

Mies, Maria. 1986. *Patriarchy and Accumulation on a World Scale: Women in the International Division of Labour.* London: Zed Books.

Mikell, Gwendolyn, and Elliot Percival Skinner. 1989. *Women and the Early State in West Africa.* East Lansing: Michigan State University.

Modola, S. 2007. Zimbabwe: Daughters fetch high prices as brides. *IRIN*, 27 July. irinnews.org /Report.aspx?ReportId=73272. Accessed 27 June 2010.

MOH [Government of Mozambique, Ministry of Health]. 1993. *Boletim de Nutricao.* No. 26. Department of Nutrition. Maputo, Mozambique: Government of Mozambique.

Moore, Donald S. 2005. *Suffering for Territory: Race, Place, and Power in Zimbabwe.* Durham, NC: Duke University Press.

Moore, Donald S., and Terence Ranger. 2006. Review of books—Suffering for Territory: Race, Place, and Power in Zimbabwe. *Africa: Journal of the International African Institute* 76(3): 440.

MOPF [Government of Mozambique, Ministry of Planning and Finance]. 1998. *Understanding Poverty and Well-Being in Mozambique: The First National Assessment (1996–1997).* Maputo, Mozambique: MOPF.

Morsy, Soheir A. 1995a. Deadly reproduction among Egyptian women: Maternal mortality and the medicalization of population control. In *Conceiving the New World Order: The Global Politics of Reproduction,* ed. Faye Ginsburg and Rayna Rapp, 162–76. Berkeley: University of California Press.

———. 1995b. Political economy in medical anthropology. In *Medical Anthropology: Contemporary Theory and Method,* ed. Carolyn F. Sargent and Thomas M. Johnson, 26–46. New York: Praeger.

Moth, I. A., A.B.C.O. Ayayo, and D. O. Kaseje. 2005. Assessment of utilisation of PMTCT services at Nyanza Provincial Hospital, Kenya. *Journal of Social Aspects of HIV/AIDS* 2(2): 244–50.

Mudenge, S. I. G. 1988. *A Political History of Munhumutapa c. 1400–1902.* Harare: Zimbabwe Publishing House.

Mukonyora, Isabel. 1999. Women and ecology in Shona religion. *Word and World* 19(3): 276–84.

Mullings, Leith. 1995. Households headed by women: The politics of race, class, and gender. In *Conceiving the New World Order: The Global Politics of Reproduction,* ed. Faye Ginsburg and Rayna Rapp, 122–39. Berkeley: University of California Press.

Mupotsa, Danai S. 2008. Sex, money, and power: Considerations for African women's empowerment. *Economic Empowerment of African Women* 7 (January–April), africafiles.org/article.asp?ID=17172. Accessed 27 June 2010.

Murata, P., E. McGlynn, M. Leff, A. Siu, and R. Brook. 1992. *Prenatal Care: A Literature Review and Quality Assessment Criteria.* Santa Monica, CA: Rand Publications.

Mutambirwa, Jane Makuto. 1984. Shona pathology, religio-medical practices, obstetrics, paediatrics and concepts of growth and development in relation to scientific medicine. PhD diss. University of Zimbabwe.

Myer, Landon, and Abigail Harrison. 2003. Why do women seek antenatal care late? Perspectives from rural South Africa. *Journal of Midwifery and Women's Health* 48(4): 268–72.

Navarro, Vicente. 1986. *Crisis, Health, and Medicine: A Social Critique.* New York: Tavistock.

Ndyomugyenyi, R., S. Neema, and P. Magnussen. 1998. The use of formal and informal services for antenatal care and malaria treatment in rural Uganda. *Health Policy and Planning* 13:94–102.

Nelkin, Dorothy. 2003. Foreword: The social meaning of risk. In *Risk, Culture, and Health*

Inequality: Shifting Perceptions of Danger and Blame, ed. Barbara Herr Harthorn and Laury Oaks, vii–xiii. Westport, CT: Praeger.

Newitt, Malyn. 1995. *A History of Mozambique.* London: Hurst.

Nichter, Mark. 1990–91. *African Health Care Systems and the War in Mozambique, a Six-Part Study.* Maputo, Mozambique: Mozambican Ministry of Health.

———. 2002. Social relations of therapy management. *New Horizons in Medical Anthropology*, ed. Mark Nichter and Margaret Lock, 81–110. New York: Routledge.

———. 2003. Harm reduction: A core concern for medical anthropology. In *Risk, Culture, and Health Inequality: Shifting Perceptions of Danger and Blame*, ed. Barbara Herr Harthorn and Laury Oaks, 13–33. Westport, CT: Praeger.

Oaks, Laury, and Barbara Herr Harthorn. 2003. Introduction: Health and social and cultural construction of risk. In *Risk, Culture, and Health Inequality: Shifting Perceptions of Danger and Blame*, ed. Barbara Herr Harthorn and Laury Oaks, 3–12. Westport, CT: Praeger.

Oboler, Regina Smith. 1986. Nandi widows. In *Widows in African Society*, ed. Betty Potash, 66–84. Stanford, CA: Stanford University Press.

Omorodion, Francisca Isi. 1993. Sexual networking of market women in Benin City, Edo State, Nigeria. *Health Care for Women International* 14(6): 561–71.

Parker, Richard, and Peter Aggleton. 2003. HIV and AIDS-related stigma and discrimination: A conceptual framework and implications for action. *Social Science and Medicine* 57(1): 13–24.

Parson, J. 1985. The "labour reserve" in historical perspective: Toward a political economy of the Bechuanaland Protectorate. In *The Evolution of Modern Botswana*, ed. Louis Picard. London: Rex Collins.

Pearce, Tola Olu. 1995. Women's reproductive practices and biomedicine: Cultural conflicts and transformation in Nigeria. In *Conceiving the New World Order: The Global Politics of Reproduction*, ed. Faye Ginsburg and Rayna Rapp, 195–208. Berkeley: University of California Press.

Petra Study Team. 2002. Efficacy of three short-course regimens of zidovudine and lamivudine in preventing early and late transmission of HIV-1 from mother to child in Tanzania, South Africa, and Uganda (Petra study): A randomised, double-blind, placebo-controlled trial. *Lancet* 359(9313): 1178–86.

Pfeiffer, James. 1997. Desentendimento em casa: Income, intrahousehold resource allocation, labor migration and child growth in Central Mozambique. PhD diss., University of California, Los Angeles.

———. 2002. African independent churches in Mozambique: Healing the afflictions of inequality. *Medical Anthropology Quarterly* 16(2): 176–99.

———. 2003. International NGOs and primary healthcare in Mozambique: The need for a new model of collaboration. *Social Science and Medicine* 56(4): 731–43.

———. 2005. Commodity fetichismo, the holy spirit, and the turn to Pentecostal and African independent churches in central Mozambique. *Culture, Medicine, and Psychiatry* 29(3): 255–83.

Pfeiffer, James, Kenneth Gimbel-Sherr, and Orvalho Joaquim Augusto. 2007. The Holy Spirit in the household: Pentecostalism, gender, and neoliberalism in Mozambique. *American Anthropologist* 109(4): 688–700.

Pfeiffer, James, Pablo Montoya, Mark Micek, Wendy Johnson, Kenny Sherr, Baptista Marina, Shelagh Barrot, and Steve Gloyd. 2008. *Integration of HIV/AIDS Services into African Primary Health Care: A Health System Strengthening Approach in Mozambique.* Seattle: Health Alliance International.

Phiri, Isabel Apawo. 1997. *Women, Presbyterianism, and Patriarchy: Religious Experience of Chewa Women in Central Malawi.* Kachere Monograph no. 4. Blantyre, Malawi: CLAM.

Pitcher, Anne. 2000. Celebration and confrontation, resolution and restructuring: Mozambique from Independence to the Millennium. In *The Uncertain Promise of Southern Africa*, ed. York Bradshaw and Stephen Ndegwa, 188–213. Bloomington: Indiana University Press.

———. 2008. *Transforming Mozambique: The Politics of Privatization, 1975–2000*. Cambridge: Cambridge University Press.

Povey, George. 1990. Safe Motherhood in Mozambique. Ministry of Health Proposal at the National Seminar, 4–8 November. Maputo, Mozambique.

Raikes, Alanagh. 1989. Women's health in East Africa. *Social Science and Medicine* 28(5): 447–59.

Rakodi, Carole. 1997. Global forces, urban change, and urban management in Africa. In *The Urban Challenge in Africa: Growth and Management of Its Large Cities*, ed. Carol Rakodi, 17–73. Tokyo: United Nations University Press.

Randall, Sarah. 1998. The consequences of drought for populations in the Malian Gourma. In *Population and Environment in Arid Regions*, ed. J. Clarke and D. Noin, 149–76. Paris: UNESCO and Parthenon.

Ranger, Terence. 1974. The meaning of Mwari. *Rhodesian History* 5: 5–17.

———. 2001. Priestesses and environment in Zimbabwe. In *Sacred Custodians of the Earth? Women, Spirituality, and the Environment*, ed. Alaine Low and Soraya Tremayne, 95–106. Oxford: Berghahn Books.

———. 2002. The invention of tradition revisited: The case of colonial Africa. In *Development: A Cultural Studies Reader*, ed. Susanne Schech and Jane Haggis, 283–91. Hoboken, NJ: Blackwell.

Rita-Ferreira, António. 1958. *Agrupamento e Caracterizacao Etnica dos Indigenas de Mocambique*. Lisbon: Junta de Investigacaoes do Ultramar.

———. 1959. Documentação etnológica de Moçambique. *Boletim da Sociedade de Estudos da Provincia de Moçambique* 117 (July and August): 117–32.

———. 1960. Labor migration among the Moçambique Thonga: Comments on a study by Marvin Harris. *Africa: Journal of the International African Institute* 30(2): 141–52.

———. 1973. *Povos de Mocambique: Historia e Cultura*. Porto, Portugal: Edicoes Afrontamento.

Roesch, Otto. 1984. Peasants and collective agriculture. In *Mozambique: The Politics of Agriculture in Tropical Africa*, ed. J. Barker, 291–316. Beverly Hills: Sage Publications.

———. 1986. Socialism and rural development in Mozambique: The case of Aldeia Comunal 24 de Julho. Ph.D. diss., University of Toronto.

Rohde, J. E. 1995. Removing risk from safe motherhood. *International Journal of Gynecology and Obstetrics* 5(2): S3–S10.

Root, Robin, and Carole Browner. 2001. Practices of the pregnant self: Compliance with and resistance to prenatal norms. *Culture, Medicine, and Psychiatry* 25(2): 195–223.

Roseberry, William. 1990. *Anthropologies and Histories*. New Brunswick, NJ: Rutgers University Press.

Ross, Edward Alsworth. 1925. *Report on Employment of Native Labor in Portuguese Africa*. New York: Abbott.

Saad, Shirley. 2002. Book of the week: Birthing a nation. *UPI Perspectives*, 19 November.

Salmon, Enrique. 2000. Kincentric ecology: Indigenous perceptions of the human-nature relationship. *Ecological Applications* 10(5): 1327–32.

Sargent, Carolyn F. 1982. *The Cultural Context of Therapeutic Choice: Obstetrical Care Decisions among the Bariba of Benin*. Dordrecht, Holland: D. Reidel.

———. 1989. *Maternity, Medicine, and Power: Reproductive Decisions in Urban Benin*. Berkeley: University of California Press.

Sargent, Carolyn, and Dennis Cordell. 2003. Polygamy, disrupted reproduction, and the state: Malian migrants in Paris, France. *Social Science and Medicine* 56:1961–72.

Sargent, Carolyn, and Joan Rawlins. 1991. Factors influencing prenatal care among low-income Jamaican women. *Human Organization* 50(2): 179–87.

Sassen, Saskia. 2003. The repositioning of citizenship: Emergent subjects and spaces for politics. *New Centennial Review* 3(2): 41–66.

Saude, Artur. 1999. Homenagem de Eduardo Mondlane nada tem que ver com Eleições. *Domingo*, 21 February.

Scheper-Hughes, Nancy. 1982. Virgin mothers: The impact of Irish Jansenism on childbearing and infant tending in Western Ireland. In *Anthropology of Human Birth*, ed. Margarita Artschwage Kay, 267–87. Philadelphia: F. A. Davis.

———. 1992. *Death without Weeping: The Violence of Everyday Life in Brazil*. Berkeley and Los Angeles: University of California Press.

Schmid, Thomas, Omari Kanenda, Indu Ahluwalia, and Michelle Kouletio. 2001. Transportation for maternal emergencies in Tanzania: Empowering communities through participatory problem solving. *American Journal of Public Health* 91(10): 1589–90.

Schmidt, Elizabeth. 1992. *Peasants, Traders, and Wives: Shona Women in the History of Zimbabwe, 1870–1939*. Social History of Africa Series. Portsmouth, NH: Heinemann.

Scott, James. 1985. *Weapons of the Weak: Everyday Forms of Peasant Resistance*. New Haven, CT: Yale University Press.

———. 1990. *Domination and the Arts of Resistance: Hidden Transcripts*. New Haven, CT: Yale University Press.

Senanayake, P. 1995. The Impact of Unregulated Fertility on Maternal and Child Survival. *International Journal of Gynecology and Obstetrics* 50(Suppl 2): S11–S17.

Sesia, Paola M. 1997. Women come here on their own when they need to: Prenatal care, authoritative knowledge, and maternal health in Oaxaca. In *Childbirth and Authoritative Knowledge: Cross Cultural Perspectives*, ed. Robbie Davis-Floyd and Carolyn F. Sargent, 397–420. Berkeley: University of California Press.

Shefer, Tamara, and Don Foster. 2001. Discourses on women's heterosexuality and desire in a South African local context. *Culture, Health, and Sexuality* 3(4): 375–90.

Sheldon, Kathleen. 1994. Women and revolution in Mozambique: *A Luta Continua*. In *Women and Revolution in Africa, Asia, and the New World*, ed. Mary Ann Trétreault, 33–61. Columbia: University of South Carolina Press.

———. 2002. *Pounders of Grain: A History of Women, Work, and Politics in Mozambique*. Portsmouth, NH: Heinemann.

Sherman, G. G., S. A. Jones, A. H. Coovadia, M. F. Urban, and K. D. Bolton. 2004. PMTCT from research to reality—results from a routine service. *South African Medical Journal* 94:289–92.

Shumba, R. 1995. UNDP Representative. Interview in Chimoio, Mozambique, 12 March.

Siegel, James. 2006. *Naming the Witch*. Stanford, CA: Stanford University Press.

Silverblatt, Irene Marsha. 1987. *Moon, Sun, and Witches: Gender Ideologies and Class in Inca and Colonial Peru*. Princeton, NJ: Princeton University Press.

Steady, Filomina Chioma. 2001. Global perspectives on the black woman: Race, gender, and economic justice in the age of globalization. In *Black Women, Globalization, and Economic Justice*, ed. Filomina Chioma Steady, 37–60. Rochester, VT: Schenkman Books.

Stewart, Julie, Welshman Ncube, Mary Maboreke, and Alice Armstrong. 1990. The legal situation of women in Zimbabwe. In *The Legal Situation of Women in Southern Africa*, ed. Julie Stewart and Alice Armstrong, 165–222. Harare: University of Zimbabwe Press.

Stewart, Pamela, and Andrew Strathern. 2003. *Witchcraft, Sorcery, Rumors, and Gossip*. Cambridge: Cambridge University Press.

Stoner, Bradley P. 1986. Understanding medical systems: Traditional, modern, and syncretic health care alternatives in medically pluralistic societies. *Medical Anthropology Quarterly* 17(2): 44–48.

Susser, Ida. 2004. Globalization. Review of Globalization, by Arjun Appadurai, ed. *American Anthropologist* 106(3): 612–13.

Swantz, Marja Liisa. 1979. Community and healing among the Zaramo in Tanzania. *Social Science and Medicine* 13B(3): 169–73.

Taringa, Nisbert Taisekwa. 2004. African metaphors for God: Male or female? *Scriptura: Tydskrif Vir Bybelkunde* 86:174–79.

Tatira, Liveson. 2004. Beyond the dog's name: A silent dialogue among the Shona people. *Journal of Folklore Research* 41(1): 85–98.

Taussig, Michael T. 1980. *The Devil and Commodity Fetishism in South America*. Chapel Hill: University of North Carolina Press.

Taylor, Janelle. 2004. A fetish is born: Sonographers and the making of the public fetus. In *Consuming Motherhood*, ed. Janelle S. Taylor, Linda L. Layne, and Danielle F. Wozniak, 187–210. New Brunswick, NJ: Rutgers University Press.

Tesh, Sylvia Noble. 1988. *Hidden Arguments: Political Ideology and Disease Prevention Policy*. New Brunswick, NJ: Rutgers University Press.

Thompson, Guy. 2000. Cultivating conflict: Modernism and improved agriculture in colonial Zimbabwe, 1920–1965. PhD diss., University of Minnesota.

Thorne, Claire, and Marie-Louise Newell. 2004. Are girls more at risk of intrauterine-acquired HIV infection than boys? *AIDS* 18(2): 344–47.

Tique, César A. 2002. Rural land markets in Mozambique, its impact on land conflicts. Paper presented at SARPN Workshop on Land Markets and Poverty in Moçambique, Maputo, 5 April. *sarpn.org/EventPapers/mozambique_april2002/tique/rural_land_markets.pdf*. Accessed 27 June 2010.

Tsikata, Dzodzi, and Joanna Kerr. 2002. *Demanding Dignity: Women Confronting Economic Reforms in Africa*. Ottawa: North-South Institute; Accra: Third World Network-Africa.

Turshen, Meredeth. 1994. *Trends in the Health Sector: With Special Reference to Zimbabwe*. Madison: Global Studies Research Program, University of Wisconsin.

Udvardy, Monica L. 1995. The lifecourse of property and personhood: Provisional women and enduring men among the Giriama of Kenya. *Research in Economic Anthropology* 16:325–48.

UNAIDS. 2006a. *Report on the Global AIDS Epidemic*. Geneva: Joint United Nations Program on HIV/AIDS (UNAIDS).

———. 2006b. Statement: 2006 High Level Meeting on HIV—Political Declaration on HIV/AIDS. *data.unaids.org/pub/PressStatement/2006/20060620_PS_HLM_en.pdf*.

———. 2008a. *Country Profile: Mozambique*. UNAIDS 2008 Report on Global AIDS Epidemic. Geneva: UNAIDS.

———. 2008b. *Report on the Global AIDS Epidemic*. Geneva: UNAIDS. *unaids.org*. Accessed October 2008.

———. 2009. *Towards Universal Access*. *unaids.org/en/PolicyAndPractice/TowardsUniversalAccess/default.asp*. Accessed 28 June 2010.

UNAIDS/WHO. 2004. *UN Epidemiological Fact Sheets on HIV/AIDS and Sexually Transmitted Infections*. Malawi: UNAIDS/WHO.

UNDP [United Nations Development Program] Mozambique. 1998. *Mozambique United Nations Development Program Report*. Geneva: UNDP.

UNDP [United Nations Development Program]. 2005. *Mozambique National Human Development Report 2005*. *undp.org.mz/en/publications/global_reports/national_human_development_report_2005*. Accessed 28 June 2010.

———. 2008. *Human Development Reports 2007/2008: Mozambique*. *hdrstats.undp.org/countries/data_sheets/cty_ds_MOZ.html*.

UNICEF. 1991. *The Situation of Women and Children in Mozambique*. Maputo, Mozambique: United Nations.

UN Mozambique. 2008. *Key Development Indicators*. *unmozambique.org/eng*. Accessed 28 June 2010.

Urdang, Stephanie. 1983. Women, oppression, and liberation. *Review of African Political Economy* 27/28(Winter): 8–32.

———. 1989. *And Still They Dance: Women, War, and the Struggle for Change in Mozambique*. New York: Monthly Review Press.

———. 2006. The care economy: Gender and the silent AIDS crisis in southern Africa. *Journal of Southern African Studies* 32(1): 165–77.

Van Hollen, Cecilia. 2003. *Birth on the Threshold: Childbirth and Modernity in South India.* Berkeley: University of California Press.

Vaz, Rui Gama, Stephen Gloyd, and Ricardo Trindade. 1996. The effects of peer education on STD and AIDS knowledge among prisoners in Mozambique. *International Journal of STD and AIDS* 7(1): 51–54.

Virtanen, Pekka. 2005. Tradition, custom, and otherness: The politics of identity in Mozambique. *Identities: Global Studies in Culture and Power* 12(2): 223–48.

Walraven, Gijs, and Andrew Weeks. 1999. The role of traditional birth attendants with midwifery skills in the reduction of maternal mortality. *Tropical Medicine and International Health* 4(8): 527–29.

Walt, Gillian, and Angela Melamed. 1983. *Mozambique: Towards a People's Health Service.* Third World Studies. London: Zed Books.

Walt, Gillian, and P. A. Smith. 1980. From the classroom to the community: Teaching primary health workers. *Journal of Tropical Medicine and Hygiene* 83(4): 161–64.

Weiss, Brad. 1996. *The Making and Unmaking of the Haya Lived World: Consumption, Commoditization, and Everyday Practice.* Durham, NC: Duke University Press.

Wekker, Gloria. 2006. *The Politics of Passion: Women's Sexual Culture in the Afro-Surinamese Diaspora.* New York: Columbia University Press.

Werbner, Richard P., and Terence O. Ranger. 1996. *Postcolonial Identities in Africa: Postcolonial Encounters.* Atlantic Highlands, NJ: Zed Books.

West, Harry. 2001. Sorcery of construction and socialist modernization: ways of understanding power in postcolonial Mozambique. *American Ethnologist* 28(1): 119–50.

———. 2005. *Kupilikula: Governance and the Invisible Realm in Mozambique.* Chicago: University of Chicago Press.

White, Luise. 1997. The traffic in heads: Bodies, borders, and the articulation of regional histories. *Journal of Southern African Studies* 23(2): 325–38.

———. 2007. Review of Witchcraft, Violence, and Democracy in South Africa, by Adam Ashforth. *Journal of Modern African Studies* 45(1): 171–72.

Whittaker, A. M. 1992. Living with HIV: Resistance by positive people. *Medical Anthropology Quarterly* 6(4): 385–90.

Wiesner, Merry E. 1986. *Working Women in Renaissance Germany.* New Brunswick, NJ: Rutgers University Press.

WHO [World Health Organization]. 1978a. *The Risk Approach on Maternal and Child Health.* Offset 39. Geneva: WHO.

———. 1978b. Social and Biological Differences in Peri-Natal Mortality. Vol. 1. Geneva: WHO.

———. 1985a. Report of the First Inter-Regional Meeting on Prevention of Maternal Mortality. Geneva: WHO.

———. 1985b. Safe Motherhood Initiative (SMI). Geneva: WHO.

———. 1994. Mother-Baby Package: Implementing Safe Motherhood in Developing Countries (WHO/FHE/MSM/94.11.). Geneva: WHO.

———. 1997. *Integrated Management of Childhood Illness Information Packet.* Division of Child Health and Development. September. Geneva: WHO.

———. 2004. Antiretroviral Drugs for Treating Pregnant Women and Preventing HIV Infection in Infants. Department of HIV/AIDS. Geneva: WHO.

———. 2007. Maternal mortality in 2005: Estimates developed by WHO, UNICEF, UNFPA, and the World Bank. Geneva: WHO.

WHO/UNICEF. 1980. Country Decision Making for the Achievement of the Objective of Primary Health Care. (Report from the People's Republic of Mozambique). Geneva: WHO.

———. 1997. *State of the World's Children Report.* Geneva: UNICEF/WHO.

WHO/UNICEF/UNFPA [UN Populations Fund]. 2004. *Maternal Mortality in 2000.* Geneva: World Health Organization, UNICEF, UNFPA.

Wolf, M. 1972. *Women and the Family in Rural Taiwan*. Stanford, CA: Stanford University Press.

World Bank. 1993. *World Development Report: Investing in Health*. Washington, DC: World Bank.

Young, Sherilynn. 1977. Fertility and Famine: Women's Agricultural History in Southern Mozambique. In *The Roots of Rural Poverty in Central and Southern Africa*, ed. Robin Palmer and Neil Parsons, 66–81. Berkeley: University of California Press.

Zahr, C. A., and E. Royston. 1991. *Maternal Mortality: A Global Sourcebook*. Geneva: WHO.

Index

The letter *t* following a page number denotes a table.